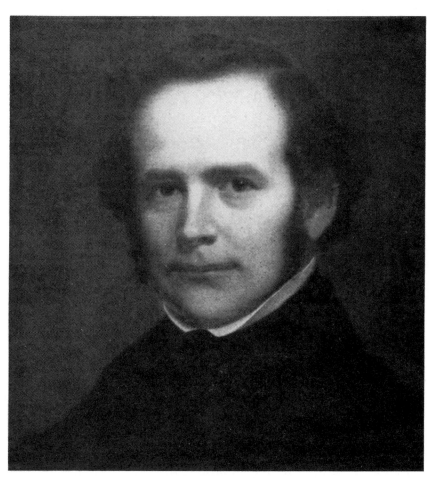

Horace Wells

With contributions by:

HAROLD DINER, D.D.S., M.A.

Associate Professor of Dentistry (Pedodontics),
Albert Einstein College of Medicine;
Director of Dentistry, Rose F. Kennedy
Center for Research in Mental Retardation
and Human Development

Adaptations from:

ARTHUR C. GUYTON, M.D.

Professor and Chairman of the
Department of Physiology and Biophysics,
University of Mississippi School of Medicine

BRIAN CURTIS, Ph.D.

Associate Professor of Physiology and
Assistant Dean for Undergraduate Medical Education,
Peoria School of Medicine,
College of Medicine,
University of Illinois

STANLEY JACOBSON, Ph.D.

Professor of Anatomy,
Tufts University Schools of
Medicine and Dental Medicine

SECOND EDITION

RELATIVE ANALGESIA IN DENTAL PRACTICE

Inhalation Analgesia and Sedation with Nitrous Oxide

HARRY LANGA, B.S., D.D.S., F.A.C.D., F.I.C.D.

Past President, American Analgesia Society;
Fellow of the New York Academy of Dentistry;

Guest Lecturer in Analgesia at the Schools of
Dentistry of Temple University, Case Western
Reserve University, University of Detroit,
University of the Pacific, New York University,
University of Indiana, University of California,
University of Southern California, University of
Kentucky, Marquette University, State University of
New York, Fairleigh Dickinson University,
Emory University, Washington University,
University of Louisiana

W. B. SAUNDERS COMPANY
Philadelphia, London, Toronto

W. B. Saunders Company: West Washington Square
Philadelphia, PA 19105

1 St. Anne's Road
Eastbourne, East Sussex BN21 3UN, England

1 Goldthorne Avenue
Toronto, Ontario M8Z 5T9, Canada

Library of Congress Cataloging in Publication Data

Langa, Harry.

Relative analgesia in dental practice.

Includes bibliographies and index.

1. Nitrous oxide.   2. Anesthesia in dentistry.   I. Diner,
Harold.   II. Title. [DNLM: 1. Analgesia.
2. Anesthesia, Dental.   3. Nitrous oxide—
Pharmacodynamics. WO460 L271r]

RK512.N55L36 1976   617'.967'6   76–1223

ISBN 0–7216–5621–8

Relative Analgesia in Dental Practice   ISBN 0-7216-5621-8

Last digit is the print number: 9   8   7   6   5   4   3   2

To Sara
and to Bob, Roz, and Steve

Foreword

Dr. Harry Langa, in preparing this text, *Relative Analgesia in Dental Practice,* has performed an outstanding service to dentists and to their patients. He has taken a giant step forward in removing the misunderstanding and doubt that have surrounded the use of this method of fear, anxiety and pain control in the practice of dentistry. It seems almost unreal that so many untruths and half-truths could have persisted for so long a period of time. The author, by his teachings and demonstrations, and now by this first full length scientific book on the subject, places within reach of all interested practitioners an authentic and proven source of information. Based on my forty years of teaching pain control in dental practice, I can recall no single work in this field which makes a greater contribution to the literature regarding nitrous oxide analgesia in dentistry.

LEONARD M. MONHEIM, M.S., D.D.S.

The late Professor and Head, Department of Anesthesia,
University of Pittsburgh School of Dentistry;
Associate Professor, Department of Anesthesia,
University of Pittsburgh School of Medicine.

Preface

Ample clinical experience has clearly demonstrated these facts:

1. When nitrous oxide and oxygen are administered from a continuous flow machine with an open air valve and no rebreathing, patients *can* be maintained easily for hours in the lighter planes of the analgesic stage without passing into the excitement stage. When an intermittent flow machine is employed, the same objective may be attained without the use of an open air valve because of the high proportions of oxygen and the low pressures employed.

2. The practitioner and the patient are in complete control of the level of analgesia. Since the dental practitioner works on the oral cavity and since closure of the mouth (when no mouth props are employed) is a sign of increasing analgesic depth, he has an excellent guide to the patient's status. When a physician is treating other parts of the body not requiring an open mouth, the patient is taught to decrease depth of analgesia by oral inhalation. Moreover, because the action of nitrous oxide is so readily reversible, analgesic depth can be lightened quickly by either the operator or the patient long before the excitement stage is reached.

3. Fear of the dental experience can be eliminated *on a continuing basis* only by maintaining the patient in the lighter planes of the analgesic stage.

4. This modality is one of extreme safety and great value in the hands of the average practitioner, whether he is a generalist or a specialist. He treats a patient whose protective reflexes are functioning fully at all times.

5. The use of relative analgesia permits the practitioner to treat more patients (or perform more work) in a given period of time, without hurrying, without diminishing the excellence of the work performed, and without having created fear, anxiety, or pain in the patient.

6. To be socially acceptable, treatment must be humanely given. In these days of rapid social change, of modifications in the relationship between society and members of the healing arts, of expanded duties of auxiliary personnel, and of more efficient means of health care delivery, all safe, practical and effective means of attaining these objectives should be employed. Use of nitrous oxide and oxygen for relative analgesia is one very valuable approach to this end, not only for the dental practitioner, but for *all* practitioners of the healing arts.

7. The term "relative analgesia" was introduced by the author many years ago. Some prefer to call it "nitrous oxide sedation." Neither term is all-encompassing, since both sedation and analgesia can be attained. At this writing, many who use the term "nitrous oxide sedation" state that no analgesia can result from the use of this instrument — and that local anesthesia must *always* be employed with it for pain relief. This is an incorrect assumption, which obviously is based on a paucity of clinical experience with this modality in the general practice of dentistry.

With a greater understanding of the behavioral sciences and their intimate relationship to the physical sciences, and with the development of an approach to the patient based on this knowledge, the practitioner soon learns and recognizes the close interrelationship of fear and pain. The term "relative analgesia" defines an instrument which functions within three well-defined parameters: (a) at least 20 per cent of the mixture of gases administered must be oxygen; (b) the patient must be capable of maintaining an open mouth without the use of a mouth-prop, and must be capable of following directions; (c) the depth of analgesia does not create fear or anxiety.

Within these parameters, sedation is *always* attained; analgesia attained varies from partial to *complete — and very frequently it is complete in the patient's estimation*. In this respect, we can assuredly believe the patient over measurements of machines, for it is not necessary to eliminate all pain stimuli to gain a painless experience!

HARRY LANGA

Acknowledgments

No book can ever be the product of one individual. I am grateful to all those whose pertinent thoughts and words of wisdom I have been privileged to include herein.

Much gratitude to the late Dr. Leonard M. Monheim for his graciousness in writing the Foreword for this book, and for his encouragement along the way.

I shall ever be grateful to Dr. Harry M. Fisk for having started me on a career of teaching the use of analgesia and for his continuing advice over many years. This teaching led inevitably to the writing of this text.

My thanks to Dr. Philip E. Shipper for his invaluable assistance in the teaching of analgesia and for his many valuable and constructive suggestions during the writing of the manuscript.

I am thankful to Dr. Norman Menken for his valuable, constructive criticism and for having permitted me to use his photographs, a great number of which are included in this text.

To Dr. Harold Diner go my thanks for having given us all the benefit of his extensive experience in the use of analgesia with handicapped patients.

My thanks also to Dr. Mortimer J. Shulman, who began to administer relative analgesia at about the same time as I did. Our sharing of experiences over a period of many years proved extremely helpful and encouraging.

I extend thanks to Dr. Alfred C. Waldrep, Jr., for his contribution on precautions for patients on drug therapy, alerting all practitioners to the possibility of iatrogenesis.

I thank all those friends who were kind enough to send me photographs for use in this text.

I am grateful to my wife, Sara, not only for her forbearance during the long writing period, but also for her active and extremely valuable assistance in the many typings of the manuscript.

Perforce, the task of writing has kept me from paying full attention to all details of my daily work. My thanks to my secretary, Virginia Rickman, and my assistant, Ruth Fowls, for having kept the wheels of progress in action.

I cannot conceive of having accomplished my purpose in the writing of this text without the very able assistance and cooperation of Mr. Carroll Cann (Dental Editor) and Ms. Catherine Fix (Manuscript Editor) of the W. B. Saunders Company.

HARRY LANGA

Contents

HISTORICAL BACKGROUND OF ANESTHESIA AND INHALATION ANALGESIA

1

ANESTHESIA*

Despite the fact that this book deals with one particular facet of anesthetic treatment, I think it both fruitful and pertinent to discuss the origins of anesthesia as a concept and as a viable modality. Then, too, many of the early attempts to produce anesthesia resulted in analgesia.

Pain is a universal scourge which man has tried to avoid instinctively. In the early history of the human race attempts to control pain were crude and ineffectual. However, the concept of anesthesia must have arisen at a very early time in history, for the classic picture of a patient under anesthesia appears in the story of the Creation. The Creator "caused a deep sleep to fall upon Adam" ere He plucked the rib from his side to form Eve. It seems to have been ordained at that time, too, that the concept of anesthesia and the wherewithal to produce it should be dangled before the eyes of man for countless centuries before he was permitted to see, to understand, and to make use of what existed.

Ancient man discovered that pain from sprains or bruises was relieved by the cold water of a river or a lake. At other times the sun's heat, and later heat from fires or stoves, gave him surcease from pain. Primitive peoples attempted to eradicate pain by treating it as a demon, and to frighten this demon away by tattooing the skin, wearing rings in the ears and nose, or wearing talismans or amulets such as a tiger's claw.

Anthropologists tell us that primitive man lived in a matriarchal society. It is conceivable, then, that the first anesthetist was a woman. She was the priestess and the sorceress, the mistress of the healing arts who was called upon to relieve the pain of primitive man. Spells, magic, and conjurations were used. Even at this early time human beings realized the powerful influence of the mind on the degree of pain experienced. Later, under the patriarchal state, the priestess and the sorceress were replaced by the medicine man, the conjurer and the shaman. Their incantations and battles with the invisible demon who was causing pain afforded relief.

---

*Adapted from Thomas E. Keys: History of Surgical Anesthesia. New York, Abelard-Schuman, 1945.

The birth of Christianity gave rise to the concept of the relief of pain through divine healing by touch and prayer. This power was passed down through the ages from Christ to his Disciples, to the Church Fathers, and finally to all those with ministerial duties. So it came about that the Church of the early Middle Ages functioned as a healing institution and that all priests, monks, and nuns were thought to be able to relieve pain. As early as 1513 monks used alcoholic fumes to control pain prior to and during surgical procedures. The early Christian kings created the theory of the "divine right of kings" for their own protection. Thus, they were thought to have the power to cure disease and relieve suffering by the laying on of hands.

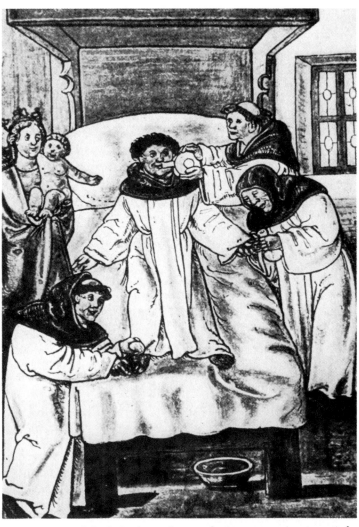

Figure 1-1   Early use of alcoholic fumes for anesthetic purposes in monastic hospital. From Diebold Schilling's *Swiss Chronicle*, 1513.

The Early Use of Drugs

The use of drugs to cause unconsciousness brought us to another stage in the development of anesthesia. Drugs were initially compounded from various roots, barks, herbs, berries, seeds, and the blossoms of flowers. It is of more than passing interest to note how the literature abounds in the mention of the more commonly used medicaments, such as henbane, poppy, Mandragora, and hemp. A Babylonian clay tablet of about 2250 B.C. describes a remedy for the pain of dental caries. Cement consisting of henbane seeds in powdered form was mixed with gum mastic and applied to the cavity.

The Odyssey of Homer states that Helen, the daughter of Zeus, prepared a drug, possibly opium, dissolved in wine to sleep off grief and anger and to forget pain. The Greeks also used anodyne poultices to deaden pain. Aesculapius, the god of medicine, was supposed to have used a potion, nepenthe, to produce insensibility in his patients prior to surgical intervention. The Greeks and later the Romans also utilized a type of local anesthesia. They applied the "Stone of Memphis" treated with vinegar. It is thought that the anesthetic effect was obtained by the action of the vinegar on the carbonates of the stone, releasing carbon dioxide.

The Semites used compression of the veins before a circumcision. Egyptians and Assyrian physicians created artificial sleep in their patients by quickly compressing the carotid vessels of the neck, thus probably causing temporary cerebral anemia.

Dioscorides, a famous Greek physician of the first century A.D., administered the root of the Mandragora plant boiled in wine before operating. Galen used this plant experimentally to paralyze sensation and movement. The ancient Scythians inhaled fumes produced by a certain form of hemp. This caused an initial state of mental excitation followed by sleep. The Egyptians and the Arabians also inhaled the fumes of this same hemp, which they called hashish. In the third century, Hua T'O, a Chinese physician, utilized Indian hemp to render his patients unconscious.

Anesthesia During the Renaissance

In the thirteenth century, use was made of a soporific agent with opium as a base. This medicament also included hemlock, henbane, and the leaves of Mandragora and wild ivy. Administered on a sponge, it was apparently successful in producing anesthesia for some surgical procedures. In order to revive the patient, sponges filled with vinegar were held under his nose. Of course, the results produced by the medicated sponge could not be foretold or controlled, and it soon fell into disuse. There was no attempt at standardization of the drugs used. This was no doubt one of the reasons why the development of anesthesia took so long a time. Many physicians were afraid to use these drugs, which sometimes caused death. Additionally, pain was considered in a holy light, as ordained by God. The elimination of pain was therefore considered by many to be sacrilegious.

In this same century, Raymundus Lullius, a prominent Spanish alchemist, noticed a white fluid which he called "sweet vitriol." Two centuries later, Paracelsus, the great physician, experimentally mixed sulfuric acid with alcohol. He distilled this mixture and rediscovered sweet vitriol, which was not called ether until 1730 by Frobenius of Germany. As early as 1540 Valerius Cordus described the synthesis of what came to be called ether. He correctly noted that ether promotes the flow of mucus secretion from the respiratory tract and that it afforded relief from whooping cough. He also commented on its high volatility.

Paracelsus seems to have a strong claim to being the founder of anesthesia. In writing of his experiments with fowl, he says:

> However, the following should be noted here with regard to this sulphur, that of all things extracted from vitriol it is most remarkable because it is stable. And besides, it has associated with it such a sweetness that it is taken even by chickens, and they fall asleep from it for a while but awaken later without harm. On this sulphur no other judgment should be passed than that in diseases which need to be treated with anodynes it quiets all suffering without any harm, and relieves all pain, and quenches all fevers and prevents complications in all illnesses.

William Bullein's work entitled *Bulwarke of Defence Against All Sickness* was printed in 1562. The first mention of an anesthetic agent in a medical book printed in English is found here. Therein is described the preparation and properties of Mandragora. In that same year, Arthur Brooke's *The Tragicall Historye of Romeus and Juliet* was published. In this poem, reference is made to a sleeping potion that a friar gives to Juliet. In Shakespeare's version there is a remarkable description of the signs of profound anesthesia. In the works of Shakespeare there are quite a few references to poppy, Mandragora, and "drowsy" syrups.

At the beginning of the seventeenth century, Valverdi used a type of regional anesthesia. He compressed nerves and blood vessels near the region to be operated on. This was similar to the procedures followed by the ancient Semites and Assyrians. Others followed this procedure even into the eighteenth century.

During the Renaissance much emphasis was placed on the development of chemistry and physics. A genuine search was made in these fields for pain-relieving agents. This period also saw the rise of many pseudoscientific thinkers who began to expound their views on the cause and cure of disease. One of these was Franz A. Mesmer, who introduced the doctrine of vitalism. Vitalism was based on the assumption that some men possess the ability to transmit the "harnessed powers of the cosmic energies," these latter having the power to relieve pain and suffering. Mesmer and his ideas were opposed by the physicians and scientists of his time. They considered him a quack. One of Mesmer's pupils later accidentally stumbled upon an offshoot of mesmerism called somnambulism. Some physicians in the British Isles found that somnambulism (or hypnotism) was very successful, but the leading surgeons were highly skeptical after having failed to relieve operative pain with its use.

Up to this point the search for relief from pain was desultory, erratic, and very unscientific from the modern point of view. Many factors served to hold back the discovery of anesthesia as a practical modality. Fear of the unknown is always a factor in human thinking. Superstitions, religious opposition, bondage to the traditional, and intellectual inertia all served their usual ends. As knowledge increased, many European surgeons dared to use various concoctions of Mandragora and opium. The development of modern chemistry was the golden key that opened the door, because it made possible the study of the effects of pure chemical agents.

The Development of Modern Anesthesia

THE DISCOVERY OF NITROUS OXIDE AND OXYGEN

This volume discusses the use of nitrous oxide and oxygen as an analgesic agent, and it can be stated with full justification that the man who made possible the ultimate development of this instrument was Joseph Priestley. This dedicated man discovered oxygen (1771) and nitrous oxide (1772) as well as carbonic acid gas (date unknown). His fundamental research on gases became the foundation of experiments which led to modern surgical anesthesia. Because Priestley suggested that the inhalation of oxygen could possibly be of benefit in certain pulmonary diseases, some members of the medical profession developed "pneumatic medicine." Soon not only oxygen but hydrogen and nitrogen as well were being used for the treatment of such diverse conditions as asthma, catarrh, consumption, paralysis, scurvy, hysteria, and cancer. For a while it was a fad that was employed by quacks as well as by reputable physicians.

THE EXPERIMENTS OF HUMPHRY DAVY

Although Priestley discovered nitrous oxide, it remained for a young, curious apprentice physician to discover some of its anesthetic properties. In 1798, Humphry Davy prepared to risk his life for the cause of science by inhaling "dephlogisticated nitrous air." He must have been an unusually brave soul, for shortly before this, Dr. Samuel Latham Mitchell of New York City, then an unquestioned authority, had declared that this "oxide of septon" was deadly, that it caused fever, cancer, scurvy, leprosy, and plague, and that it might possibly be the contagium for the spread of epidemics. Dr. Mitchell's opinions, being then accepted without reservation, prevented most physicians from attempting to make use of nitrous oxide for many years. In spite of this, young Davy proceeded to inhale the gas. His attitude was that the whole question was open to discussion until verified by experimentation.

When Davy inhaled nitrous oxide for the first time, instead of dying he experienced many pleasurable sensations. He felt giddy and experienced a relaxation of the muscles. He noticed that his hearing became more acute and that he felt like laughing. In short, he felt euphoric. After Davy completed his apprenticeship to a surgeon-apothecary, he accepted a position as assistant to

Dr. Thomas Beddoes, who had recently established his "Pneumatic Institute" for the treatment of diseases by inhalation. Here he could more easily continue his study of nitrous oxide, for the institute had facilities for making large quantities of gas in a relatively pure state. In April, 1799 Davy inhaled nitrous oxide in the presence of Dr. Beddoes and described the effects as analogous to gentle pressure on all the muscles and a pleasurable thrilling sensation in the chest and extremities:

> The objects around me became dazzling and my hearing more acute. Towards the last inspirations, the thrilling increased, the sense of muscular power became greater, and at first an irresistible propensity to action was indulged in. I later recalled but indistinctly what followed; I know that my motions were varied and violent.

Later Davy tried the gas on volunteers. One of these, Samuel Taylor Coleridge, after his first experience with inhaling nitrous oxide, wrote, "I experienced the most voluptuous sensations. The outer world grew dim and I had the most entrancing visions. For three and a half minutes I lived in a world of new sensations."

Up to this point only the pleasurable and unusual sensations afforded by the inhalation of nitrous oxide had been noted. This was so until an occasion when Davy was suffering from a severe toothache and gingival inflammation. He writes of his experience as follows:

> On the day when the inflammation was the most troublesome, I breathed three large doses of nitrous oxide. The pain always diminished after the first four or five inspirations; the thrilling came on as usual, and uneasiness was for a few minutes swallowed up in pleasure. As the former state of mind returned, the state of organ returned with it; and I once imagined that the pain was more severe after the experiment than before.

Here was the first mention of the possible value of nitrous oxide as an anesthetic. In 1800 Humphry Davy published the results of his studies on nitrous oxide in *Researches, Chemical and Philosophical; Chiefly Concerning Nitrous Oxide.* This most important treatise not only outlined his basic researches but also suggested the possible anesthetic properties of nitrous oxide by stating: "As nitrous oxide in its extensive operation appears capable of destroying physical pain, it may probably be used with advantage during surgical operations in which no great effusion of blood takes place." Unfortunately, no surgeon took the hint. Organized medicine looked upon the science of chemistry with considerable contempt at that time, and Davy never went further with his experiments on anesthesia.

ETHER INHALATION

Michael Faraday, who was a student of Humphry Davy, was the next investigator to make an important contribution to the modern application of anesthesia. He did a great deal of original experimentation on the isomerism of butylene with ethylene and on the chlorides of carbon. He also liquefied many gases. During his experiments he observed the soporific properties of ether vapor. In 1818 he wrote about the effects of inhaling the vapor of sulfuric ether in the quarterly *Journal of Science and the Arts*, noticing the similarity of the effects of ether and nitrous oxide:

> In trying the effects of the ethereal vapour on persons who are peculiarly affected by nitrous oxide, the similarity of sensation produced was very unexpectedly found to have taken place. One person who always feels a depression of spirits on inhaling the gas [nitrous oxide], had sensation of a similar kind produced by inhaling the vapour [ether].

In the United States great interest developed in the use of ether and nitrous oxide. Stockman of New York demonstrated the exhilarating effects of nitrous oxide in 1819. Many American physicians followed Beddoes' advice, using ether in the treatment of pulmonary diseases.

CARBON DIOXIDE INHALATION

Henry Hill Hickman, a scholarly Englishman, made a further contribution to the development of surgical anesthesia. In 1824 he experimented with the use of carbon dioxide as a general anesthetic during surgical intervention in animals. Even though he succeeded in operating without causing pain, the many prejudices of the time still prevented surgeons from trying this approach with their patients. Hickman's contribution was extremely valuable, however. He was the first modern investigator to prove (on animals) that the pain of surgical operation could be abolished by the inhalation of a gas. He further recognized the importance of the maintenance of a constant flow of blood and of the necessity for being prepared to deal with circulatory collapse.

From "Laughing Gas" to Surgical Anesthesia

Looking back on this period, it is sometimes difficult to understand why it took so many more years for anesthesia to become a practical medium. Here was a world that was waiting for pain elimination during surgical intervention, a world in which surgical patients died from shock as well as from postoperative infection. It remained for two of our dental colleagues, Horace Wells and William Morton, to make this world aware of the value of the application of the long-known drugs to surgical anesthesia. It is ironic that, while the medical world searched for an anesthetic aid to surgery, nitrous oxide and ether gained great popularity as sources of amusement. However, it must be admitted that it was the employment of nitrous oxide (and ether) for pleasurable purposes that eventually contributed to the use of these gases as anesthetic agents.

It became fashionable at dinner parties to inhale "laughing gas," and this diversion became the vogue among university students in the United States. Sensing a good chance for profit, showmen, "lyceum lecturers," and itinerant "professors" traveled through the towns and villages lecturing on the properties of nitrous oxide and demonstrating its exhilarating effects. Very often these demonstrations involved the inhalation of ether vapor or nitrous oxide by members of the audience. Very soon, many of these people were amusing themselves without the lectures. "Laughing gas" parties and ether "frolics" became the vogue.

The Application of Nitrous Oxide Inhalation to Surgery

In 1842, William E. Clarke, a medical student who had held some of these "ether entertainments," administered ether from a towel to a young woman while one of her teeth was extracted painlessly by a dentist, Dr. Elijah Pope. This appears to be the first recorded use of ether anesthesia.

Dr. Crawford W. Long of Jefferson, Georgia, was sufficiently stimulated by one of these public demonstrations to remove a small tumor from the neck of one of his patients while the latter was under the influence of ether. The operation was successfully and painlessly performed. Long was the first to use ether for a nondental operation.

It was at an exhibition of the exhilarating effects of nitrous oxide gas that the next important development in the history of anesthesia took place. On the evening of December 10, 1844, Dr. Gardner Q. Colton was demonstrating the effects of "laughing gas" before an enthusiastic audience at Union Hall in Hartford, Connecticut. According to Colton's own story, one of the young men who volunteered to try the gas was Samuel A. Cooley, a druggist's clerk. He immediately came under the influence of the gas and while jumping about, struck his leg on a wooden settee. He bruised it badly. After taking his seat he was astonished to find his leg bloody. He felt no pain until the effects of the gas had worn off. Dr. Horace Wells, one of the town's leading dentists, who had sat next to Cooley and had himself sniffed the gas at Colton's urging, noticed this circumstance. When the audience was retiring, Dr. Wells asked Dr. Colton why a man could not have a tooth extracted without pain while he was under the influence of this gas. Dr. Colton replied that he did not know, because the idea had not occurred to him. Dr. Wells believed it could be done and persuaded Colton to bring a bag of gas to his office the next morning, December 11, 1844. Dr. John M. Riggs, a colleague (for whom Riggs' disease, or alveolar pyorrhea, is named), was called in to extract one of Wells' own teeth. Dr. Colton administered the nitrous oxide and Riggs extracted a molar. Dr. Wells, on recovery, was said to have exclaimed, "It is the greatest discovery ever made! I didn't feel it so much as the prick of a pin!"

At Dr. Wells' request, Dr. Colton taught him how to prepare the gas and then left Wells and continued his lectures on the exhilarating powers of nitrous oxide. Dr. Wells made and tested the effects of the gas and then journeyed to Boston to make known the discovery. He called on Dr. William Thomas Green Morton, a former student and partner, as well as other dentists and physicians, stating his discovery. According to Colton, they treated him as a visionary enthusiast.

Wells obtained permission from Dr. John C. Warren to address the class in surgery at Harvard Medical School. At the close of his remarks, Wells administered the gas to a boy and extracted a tooth. Most unfortunately, the boy screamed out, for anesthesia had not been complete. Later, the patient admitted he had suffered no pain and did not know when the tooth had been drawn. At the time, however, the students hissed and pronounced the so-called discovery a hoax. Had Dr. Wells' demonstration proved successful to all parties concerned, nitrous oxide probably would have been adopted for surgical anesthesia. But even though Wells returned to Hartford and used nitrous oxide successfully in his dental practice in 1845, as the deposition of some 40 respected citizens of Hartford indicates, the use of this gas was abandoned until June, 1863, when Dr. Colton revived it in New Haven, Connecticut. He administered it for Dr. J. H. Smith, a distinguished dentist of that city. Although Wells had failed to convince the world of the value of nitrous oxide as an anesthetic agent, he is credited with conceiving the idea of anesthesia and publicizing the possibility of its use.

The Application of Ether Anesthesia to Surgery

William Morton had witnessed the unsatisfactory demonstration of his former partner and teacher, Horace Wells, under whom he studied dentistry. At that time Morton had been a student at the Harvard Medical School, where he had for his preceptor Dr. Charles A. Jackson. Dr. Jackson was not only a qualified physician but also a chemist of note and among other accomplishments was well known for his researches in geology.

In the practice of dentistry, Morton, according to Miller, had invented an improved process for making artificial teeth. This required that his patients submit to the painful process of having the roots of their teeth extracted before Morton's artificial teeth could be fitted. The pain of extraction of such roots was tremendous, and the procedure was unsatisfactory. Morton was constantly thinking of a means of alleviating this pain.

THE LOCAL APPLICATION OF ETHER

One day in July, 1844, a patient, Miss Parrot, asked to have a tooth filled, a process which ordinarily caused excessive pain. Many times Jackson had mentioned that ether sprinkled on the skin could relieve pain. Morton's patient could not endure the pain caused by the necessary preparation for filling. To deaden the pain locally, Dr. Morton applied sulfuric ether to the adjacent tissue as recommended by Jackson. He was able to continue his work without hurting the patient. Because the action of ether as he administered it was slow, it was necessary for the patient to return on several subsequent days. One day, in using the ether a bit freely, Morton noticed its numbing effects on the surrounding parts of the face. The idea occurred to Morton that if the whole system could be brought under the influence of this drug, a valuable means of relief might be afforded for more difficult dental surgery.

THE GREAT BREAKTHROUGH IN SURGICAL ANESTHESIA

Morton thought of the inhalation of ether. But he thought it would endanger life. He had learned on reading Pereira's *Materia Medica* that a small amount of ether inhaled was not dangerous, but that inhalation of large amounts was dangerous. He began to experiment. First he submitted a puppy to the inhalation of ether. This was successful. Next he tried to anesthetize goldfish. He also experimented on insects, caterpillars, and worms. One day the puppy sprang against a glass jar containing ether and broke it. The contents fell to the floor and Morton soaked his handkerchief in the portion that

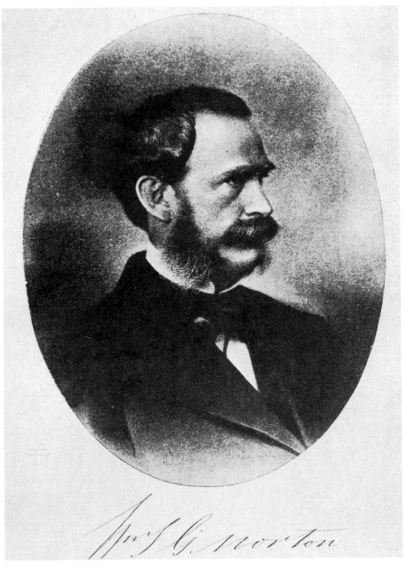

Figure 1–2   William T. G. Morton

remained and applied it to his own mouth and nostrils. He felt the effects of the vapor and thought he might have had a tooth pulled without feeling pain.

Morton next tried to experiment on his two dental assistants, Thomas Spear and William Leavitt. But when they inhaled ether both students became greatly excited, not subdued. Something was wrong. He consulted Dr. Jackson. Jackson recommended that he try pure sulfuric ether. Morton professed ignorance of the use of sulfuric ether, and Jackson later based his claim to the discovery on his suggestion to Morton that ether would anesthetize the patient. Morton did find out from Jackson, however, that pure sulfuric ether would serve his purpose better than the commercial product. After experimenting on himself he was ready for the proper patient.

On September 30, 1846, an opportunity presented itself for Morton to test his theoretic discovery. On the evening of that day a patient, Eben H. Frost, came to Morton's office. An ulcerated tooth was causing him considerable pain and he wished to have it extracted. Dreading the operation, Frost asked to be mesmerized. Morton said he had something better and induced his patient to inhale sulfuric either. The success of his first dental operation under anesthesia produced by ether is best told by the *Boston Journal*, which printed an account of the operation the following day:

> Last evening, as we were informed by a gentleman who witnessed the operation, an ulcerated tooth was extracted from the mouth of an individual, without giving him the slightest pain. He was put into a kind of sleep, by inhaling a preparation, the effects of which lasted about three-quarters of a minute, just long enough to extract the tooth.

Shortly after the painless extraction of Eben Frost's tooth, Morton called on Dr. John C. Warren, explained his discovery, and asked permission to try it at some operation. In reply to his visit he received the following historic note from Dr. C. F. Heywood, house surgeon to the Massachusetts General Hospital:

> Dear Sir: I write at the request of Dr. J. C. Warren, to invite you to be present on Friday morning at 10 o'clock, at the hospital to administer to a patient who is then to be operated upon the preparation which you have invented to diminish the sensibility to pain.
>
> Yours respectfully,
> C. F. HEYWOOD,
> House Surgeon to the General Hospital
> Dr. Morton, Tremont Row, October 14, 1846.

On that famous Friday morning, October 16, 1846, members of the staff of the hospital filled the operating room. Because Morton had to wait for the completion of his inhaling apparatus, which was being constructed for him by an instrument maker, he arrived a few minutes late at the hospital. Meanwhile, Dr. Warren, believing that Morton did not intend to fulfill his mission, prepared to proceed with the operation in the usual manner. Then Morton appeared on the scene and, after apologizing for his slowness, induced the patient, a young man named Gilbert Abbot, to inhale the vapor from his new apparatus.

As to the actual operation, the removal of a tumor of the jaw, the report of the surgeon, John C. Warren, may be consulted:

> On October 17th (i.e., the 16th), the patient being prepared for the operation, the apparatus was applied to his mouth by Dr. Morton for about three minutes, at the end of which time he sank into a state of insensibility. I immediately made an incision about 3 inches long through the skin of the neck, and began a dissection among important nerves and blood vessels without any expression of pain on the part of the patient. Soon after he began to speak incoherently, and appeared to be in an agitated state during the remainder of the operation. Being asked immediately afterward whether he had suffered much, he said that he had felt as if his neck had been scratched; but subsequently, when inquired of by me, his statement was, that he did not experience pain at the time, although aware that the operation was proceeding.

On the next day, Dr. Hayward performed an operation on a patient anesthetized with ether. He removed a large fatty tumor of the arm. Morton was the anesthetist. The operation was a success and there was no evidence of pain, excepting some occasional groans during the last stage.

NITROUS OXIDE AND OXYGEN

Pursuing another approach to anesthesia, Edmund W. Andrews, a Chicago surgeon, in 1868 found some difficulty in using pure nitrous oxide as an anesthetic agent. He reasoned that the oxygen contained in nitrous oxide was not available for the proper oxidation of the blood. When any attempt was

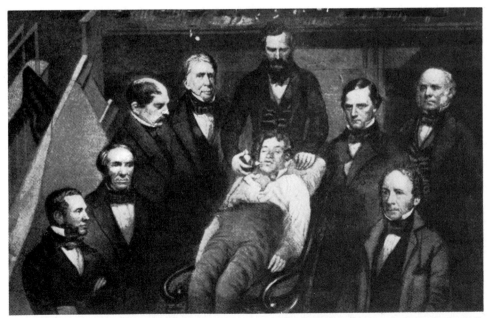

Figure 1–3   The first public demonstration of anesthesia with ether. Engraving by H. B. Hall. Reproduced from Rice, N. P.: *Trials of a public benefactor.* New York, Pudney & Russell, 1858.

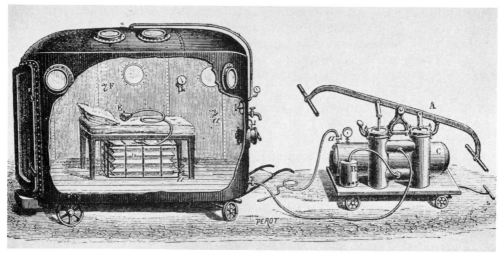

Figure 1-4   Paul Bert's anesthetic apparatus.

made to continue its anesthetic action, the patient began to show the signs of asphyxia. Nitrous oxide alone, therefore, was not a satisfactory anesthetic for operations of long duration. To overcome this difficulty, Andrews experimented to see if the addition of oxygen to nitrous oxide would make for a safe anesthetic. He found that in rats a mixture of one-fourth oxygen and three-fourths nitrous oxide was satisfactory. Andrews used a mixture of one-third oxygen and two-thirds nitrous oxide (the mixture having been already compressed into cylinders) successfully for operations of short duration upon a few of his own patients. He felt, however, that the best proportion of oxygen would be one-fifth by volume, which he had computed would equal the proportion in atmospheric air.

Paul Bert was one of the outstanding pupils of Claude Bernard. Like his teacher he was keenly aware of the shortcomings of anesthesia and searched for an anesthetic agent that would be without any danger to the patient and still have the desirable qualities. The use of nitrous oxide for operations of short duration had by this time become popular, especially for the extraction of teeth. Bert, without previous knowledge of the work of Andrews, found that the administration of pure nitrous oxide could not be prolonged for more than two minutes without bringing on symptoms of asphyxia of dangerous appearance.

Bert, profiting by his profound knowledge of the pressures of gases, was able to remove this difficulty. He used a mixture of three-quarters nitrous oxide and one-quarter oxygen, with the mixture being breathed under a slightly increased barometric pressure. He thus introduced into the blood of an experimental animal the quantity of oxygen necessary to maintain respiration and the quantity of nitrous oxide sufficient to maintain anesthesia. He was able in this manner to overcome the dangers of asphyxia.

Because of his success with animals, Bert recommended the use of nitrous oxide–oxygen anesthesia under increased atmospheric pressure for operations upon human beings. Its use proved successful, but unfortunately, Bert's method, while brilliantly conceived, lacked practicability, since it necessitated cumbersome and expensive apparatus.

Bert carried out his researches on other anesthetic agents, especially chloroform, but felt that nitrous oxide was the superior agent for the following reasons: (1) the absence of the usual period of excitation with nitrous oxide; (2) the tranquility it gives to the surgeon, who has the assurance that the dosage of the anesthetic agent cannot change during the operation and consequently that the patient has nothing to fear; (3) the almost instantaneous return to complete sensibility even after 25 minutes of anesthesia; (4) the almost general absence of discomfort, nausea, and vomiting, and (5) its remarkable harmlessness.

THE DEVELOPMENT OF ANESTHESIA EQUIPMENT

Now a proper anesthesia apparatus had to be developed. Perhaps the first modern gas inhaler was that constructed by James Watts, an engineer, for Thomas Beddoes. Humphry Davy's "gas machine," too, was constructed for Davy by Watts in 1799.

In the United States ether inhalers, such as the one perfected by Morton, were soon discarded and replaced by the ether sponge. The sea sponge, probably similar to the sponge of Thedoric of the thirteenth century, was hollowed

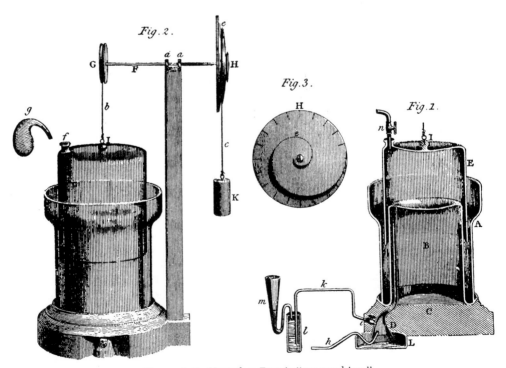

Figure 1–5   Humphry Davy's "gas machine."

to fit the face. It was then saturated with ether. It provided, by its extensive surface, sufficient ether vapor for the purpose of anesthesia.

Dr. Edmund W. Andrews, as has already been mentioned, introduced the use of a mixture of oxygen with nitrous oxide into the practice of anesthesia in 1868. The feasibility of this method, however, was not demonstrated until Sir Frederic Hewitt many years later adapted it. Hewitt was the first to develop an apparatus that was practicable. By using semielastic bags, he overcame the terrific pressures of nitrous oxide and oxygen. The bags were kept almost full from the high pressure tanks by means of an intermittent flow of the gases. The gases were controlled directly by hand valves and the tanks, which acted against the high pressures.

Joseph Clover in 1874 reported a supplemental bag which provided for rebreathing a portion of the anesthetic agent, and in 1876 introduced the gas-ether sequence. To do this he added to the bag of the inhaler a tap through which nitrous oxide could be admitted for the production of anesthesia.

S. J. Hayes, a Pittsburgh dentist, in 1882 patented an apparatus for generating and applying anesthetic agents. Ether and chloroform were mixed and heated by means of a water bath. In 1885, Frederic Hewitt described a face piece used for rebreathing nitrous oxide. The S. S. White Dental Manufacturing Company in 1899 brought out a machine which measured the relative quantities of the gases. This was their nitrous oxide–oxygen apparatus. It was constructed similarly to a machine that Hewitt had perfected in England.

Charles K. Teter, a Cleveland dentist, while practicing his profession in Upper Sandusky, Ohio, became interested in developing an apparatus for administering nitrous oxide and oxygen as well as other anesthetic agents. His first machine was manufactured in 1903 by the Cleveland Dental Manufacturing Company. It was very well received, and it is due somewhat to Teter's influence that the use of nitrous oxide–oxygen anethesia became widespread.

About 1909, according to Heidbrink, the A. C. Clark machine was developed. By means of this machine the maintenance of constant pressure in the bags was attempted. A central valve with a slot for each gas was designed to proportion the gases, but this arrangement did not afford fine enough control to give good results in gas anesthesia.

From 1906 to 1910, E. I. McKesson, of Toledo, and J. A. Heidbrink worked independently in an attempt to build a machine which would provide better control of the gases. McKesson invented a machine which produced pressure on the bags individually. This was similar to the Clark machine, but it had a better proportioning valve. In 1910 McKesson perfected the first "intermittent flow" nitrous oxide and oxygen anesthesia machine. It contained an accurate percentage control for the two gases. In 1910 McKesson introduced the principle of fractional rebreathing. He found it possible to save the first part of each expiration for rebreathing. The expiratory valve made provision for the escape of the last part of each expiration.

Meanwhile, Heidbrink was developing his machines. He perfected a machine called the "OO." Later, after a few minor changes, this machine was called the "model T." Heidbrink made use of the reducing valve on his machine as a flowmeter. He was an early exponent of "timed anesthesia."

Willis D. Gatch in 1910 published his important article on nitrous oxide–

oxygen anesthesia produced by his rebreathing method. His apparatus is described therein. Gatch also provided for a sight-feed dropper, and in some cases ether was administered after the gas. Karl Connell also invented a gas machine about this time. In 1918, a government order for gas machines was divided among McKesson, Connell, von Foregger, and Heidbrink.

In 1911 J. T. Gwathmey and William C. Woolsey began experimenting with gas machines. A nitrous oxide–oxygen apparatus was built for them by Langsdorf in 1912. That same year the Ohio monovalve anesthesia machine was put on the market by the Ohio Chemical and Manufacturing Company of Cleveland. That year, too, marked the appearance of the Boothby-Cotton sight-feed apparatus. To ensure an even flow of gas, this machine provided for the use of automatic reducing valves. In 1914, Boothby furnished accurate calibration for the sight-feed valves.

Richard von Foregger in 1914 built a nitrous oxide–oxygen machine without a reducing valve. The first Gwathmey apparatus built by von Foregger, without reducing valves but with control valves for oxygen and nitrous oxide, appeared in 1915. H. E. G. Boyle modified the early Gwathmey machine.

Many others during the period from 1910 to 1923 developed gas machines. These included Coburn, Cunningham, Flagg, Guedel, Peariro, Miller, Morgan, and Lundy. In 1923, John S. Lundy specified the first Seattle model gas machine. This was a four-valve apparatus for the utilization of oxygen, nitrous oxide, carbon dioxide and ethylene. It was the first apparatus to employ all four gases. Dr. Lundy in 1925 worked with Dr. Heidbrink on the first Lundy-Heidbrink model. One of the first machines was delivered to the Mayo Clinic on August 20, 1925.

From these beginnings has evolved the equipment used in anesthesia and analgesia in medical and dental practice today.

THE STATUS OF ANESTHESIOLOGY TODAY

After many years of trials and tribulations, of successes and failures, the stage was finally set for the more rapid development of anesthesiology as a highly important specialty of medicine and dentistry. Beecher has said that the introduction of anesthesia into the clinic probably altered the practice of medicine more than any other single advance up to that time. With the improvement of the equipment, with the discovery of a diversity of anesthetic agents, anesthesiology has come into its own as an important and highly specialized facet of medical and dental treatment.

It is more than one and one-quarter centuries since the discovery of anesthesia. We have learned how to make use of it, but how it is effectuated is still not definitely known. There are over 25 theories relating to the cellular changes that take place in the central nervous system under anesthesia. Those most commonly accepted pertain to anoxia, lipoids, surface tension, adsorption, cell permeability, dehydration, and coagulation. We theorize, but we still do not know how to explain anesthesia. Nevertheless, this theorizing and experimentation have led us a long way from the empirical use of Mandragora, hemp, and the "Memphis Stone." We have learned a great deal about various types of chemicals which block either the conduction of or the reaction to pain. We have been able to modify chemical agents to produce a greater or lesser degree of central nervous system depression and to control undesirable side-effects. We will keep striving to discover the secret of anesthesia and to find the ideal anesthetic agent.

INHALATION ANALGESIA

Nitrous oxide was first used as an analgesic during labor by S. Klikovitsch of St. Petersburg in 1881. It is thought that its use for the same purpose was introduced in the United States by a French obstetrician in the early part of the twentieth century. The use of nitrous oxide analgesia for cavity preparation dates back to 1889 in Liverpool, England.[8] By this time gas machines had been somewhat improved and oxygen had been added to the nitrous oxide administered. Of course, by current standards the machines were still relatively crude and the gases were far from pure. Many dentists used to make their own nitrous oxide.

After Horace Wells' demonstration at the Massachusetts General Hospital and the introduction of ether by Morton, interest in nitrous oxide as an anesthetic agent waned in the medical profession. However, some dentists thought that it might have value for removing teeth painlessly. Various names for nitrous oxide, such as "sweet air" and "nap a minute" began to appear. At some point between the introduction of ether and the invention of the hollow needle and local anesthesia, members of the dental profession who were using gas machines for oral surgery began to think of inhalation analgesia with nitrous oxide and oxygen. Its use in obtunding pain during labor no doubt served as a stimulus. Then, too, cavity preparation with hand instruments and foot drills was so painful that many patients would rather submit to the painless loss of the tooth than endure the agonies involved in the efforts to save it.

The pioneers in the dental profession who reasoned that cavity preparation might be done painlessly with milder doses of nitrous oxide had great obstacles to overcome. As has been mentioned, the gas machines were not finely calibrated, and the gases were impure. This led to a great deal of nausea, vomiting, and excitement-stage symptoms. Many men drew away from a situation which seemed to be uncontrollable.

During the first half of the twentieth century there were two periods of renewed interest in nitrous oxide as an analgesic for dental operative procedures. These periods (1913–1918 and 1932–1938) were inevitably followed by an almost complete loss of interest. The loss of interest was engendered by a high incidence of failure in the administration of nitrous oxide, for despite improved machines and pure gases success came to relatively few. Indeed, given these circumstances, it is astounding that the concept of inhalation analgesia survived. If these two flurries of interest produced no real, general progress in introducing analgesia as a normal instrument of the dentist, or in introducing analgesia into the dental school curriculum, either on an undergraduate or a postgraduate level, they did serve to make known the valuable potential of this modality to a select few of the dentists who tried it. It is to these few men that the dental profession owes the survival of this very valuable instrument. It seems that they were the ones to discover its marvelous ability to eliminate fear of the dental experience.

In general, the use of analgesia was condemned in the 1930's because of the lack of training of men who attempted its use and because of the generally poor results. Of course, there was no place to turn to in order to obtain that training. At one time, dentists permitted the manufacturers of gas machines to come into the dental office to teach the use of the machine. With no background or training in the chemistry, physics, physiology, or the art of anesthesia, and with no supervised clinical experience, failure and condemnation followed. It has been unfortunate that the dental profession, which gave anesthesia to the world, has until lately been remiss in the teaching of this subject. The undergraduate student completes his training with little or no instruction in anesthesia administration, but with a vivid remembrance of the possible untoward results of its administration. Thus, he leaves dental school adversely conditioned to the use of general anesthesia and inhalation analgesia, because in his mind they are but one instrument.

As the 1930's gave way to the 1940's more and more dentists attempted the use of inhalation analgesia. Success still came to relatively few, but now it was not due to improper equipment or impure gases. Failure in administration ensued because of misconceptions on the part of the operator relating to his main objective in using analgesia, to the stage of analgesia in which he was keeping his patient, and to proper dosage. In the 1880's a French anesthetist wrote a paper on the use of nitrous oxide analgesia for obstetric patients. He described his technique with the use of 80 per cent nitrous oxide and 20 per cent oxygen. It seems that this proportion became inviolate, to the extent that most leading writers and lecturers on inhalation analgesia for dentistry recommended this rigid proportion. They failed to mention total minute volume, in addition to percentages, or to draw any guidelines for evaluating the patient's reactions. It has been unfortunate that for many years much of the guidance for the use of nitrous oxide in analgesia has been forthcoming from men who have indicated no personal experience with the use of analgesia, although expert in the administration of general anesthesia.

Searching the dental literature back to the beginning of the twentieth century, one finds a goodly number of published articles on the subject of nitrous oxide analgesia. Elimination of pain was stressed as its main objective. Where control of fear was mentioned as a possible result, it was not stressed as being overly important, but rather described as an additional dividend of secondary importance. It was only when the greater importance of its fear-eliminating properties was realized that analgesia began to assume the importance that it has today. The changed objective led to a change in technique, in dosage, and in approach to the patient, and these modifications have led to the successful adaptation of the instrument to the practice of dentistry.

In the United States the writings and teachings of several men showed a true insight into the value of inhalation analgesia with nitrous oxide. Outstanding among them are Harry M. Seldin and James F. Henegan. Seldin's textbook, *Practical Anesthesia for Dentistry and Oral Surgery*, contains an excellent chapter on the signs, symptoms, and introduction of analgesia.[9] Henegan was probably one of the first to use a continuous flow apparatus for the administration of analgesia.[4] I owe a great debt to these men, for they inspired me to look further into the subject.

Inhalation analgesia with nitrous oxide also developed in Europe, but with more difficulty because legal restrictions were put on the administration of inhalation anesthetics by dentists. (In the United States there have been no such restrictions.) In Switzerland there have been such strong and enthusiastic advocates as Maurice de Trey, H. P. Lugeon, T. Gordonoff, A. S. Held, and Paul Vonow. Vonow has written an excellent treatise on the application of nitrous oxide analgesia to dental practice.[11] In Germany since 1951 Soehring, Schuchardt, Schön, Fuchs, and Krüger-Janson have written on the use of nitrous oxide in dentistry. J. J. Holst, Professor of Operative Dentistry at the Royal Dental College in Copenhagen, wrote to me in 1962, as follows:

> I took over a seat in a governmental commission in 1930, which was appointed to find out whether dentists in this country should be allowed to use nitrous oxide—oxygen analgesia. We tried our best then, but failed. It was not until 1955 that dentists were given permission to use this very valuable procedure.
>
> Since 1955 we have held many postgraduate courses for practicing dentists. In addition, a regular course in the administration of inhalation analgesia with nitrous oxide—oxygen is included in the undergraduate curriculum of both Danish Dental Schools. We feel that with the use of this instrument we have a method that permits us to treat many cases in a far better way than would be possible with local anesthesia. Our students are taught to use the analgesia machine as routinely as the dental handpiece.

The continued success in the use of nitrous oxide in Denmark is illustrated by the following article by Henning Ruben, which appeared in the *British Dental Journal* on March 7, 1972[12]:

Nitrous Oxide Analgesia in Dentistry: Its Use During 15 Years in Denmark[12]

Fifteen years have passed since dentists in Denmark were authorized to administer general analgesia with nitrous oxide, oxygen, and air, provided that they had attended an undergraduate or postgraduate course. The present investigation aimed at assessing the usefulness of the method as expressed by the frequency of its application, taking into consideration also any complications involved.

METHOD OF ANALGESIA ADMINISTRATION

Using a continuous flow anesthesia apparatus, the patient inhales a mixture of nitrous oxide, oxygen, and air through a nasal mask, no premedication being used. For conservative dental treatment, flows per minute of about 3 liters of nitrous oxide and 2 to 5 liters of oxygen (the minimum flow rate of oxygen used) are usually suitable. This corresponds to about 30 to 35 per cent nitrous oxide in the inhaled mixture. When necessary, the flow of nitrous oxide may be slightly increased or decreased, usually by 0.5 to 1 liter. Extractions and other painful operations demand an essentially higher flow of nitrous oxide, usually at least 6 to 8 liters/minute, the oxygen flow being as above. The administration of nitrous oxide analgesia, however, remains reserved mainly for conservative dental treatment and superficial gingival operations. As regards the more painful operations, it will be possible and useful to supplement the procedure with injection analgesia.

According to regulations, the apparatus used by the dentists must fulfill certain requirements for safety, first and foremost that the delivered gas mixture never contain less than 20 per cent oxygen.

With this end in view, the apparatus has been constructed so that no less than a set minimum flow of oxygen and no more than a set maximum flow of nitrous oxide can be turned on. Furthermore, its construction ensures that nitrous oxide can flow only when oxygen is flowing.

Owing to the relative resistance to flow of gases through the tubing to the nasal mask and the resistance to gas flow through an opening to the atmosphere in the nasal mask, the possibility of rebreathing is extremely limited, even if the flow of gases should be interrupted.

Either full analgesia or hypalgesia is obtained. In the latter case, the patient does not feel uncomfortable since the most essential part of the inhalation apparently is its pronounced sedative effect. During general analgesia, the patient will still be able to react properly to commands by the dentist and there will be no amnesia.

Induction of, as well as recovery from, the analgesia takes 1 to 2 minutes. Since the anesthetic state thus obtained is very superficial, the protective reflexes of the airways will not be depressed and the circulation is not impaired. These are the main reasons why the following procedure which, no doubt, may appear controversial, has been the routine in Denmark:

After treatment, the patient leaves unaccompanied. As a matter of fact, he is even allowed to drive a car on his own, provided he feels fit to do so, as he generally does within 5 to 10 minutes.

No restrictions concerning intake of food have been found necessary; in other words, the general analgesia can be used at any time and even on the spur of the moment.

The nitrous oxide analgesia is administered by the person who is in charge of the treatment—namely, the dentist himself. If necessary, treatment may be carried out while the patient is sitting upright in the chair, because fainting during this analgesia will be easily detected.

CONCLUSIONS:

Since the use of nitrous oxide was adopted by Danish dentists 15 years ago, at least 3 million general analgesias, on an estimate, have been administered. This high number, together with the steady rise in its use, suggests that it is a useful aid in dental treatment.

Taking into consideration this substantial number of administrations, the absence of complications is remarkable, bearing in mind that the analgesia, without any restriction whatsoever, has been administered by the dentist in his capacity of operator/anesthetist to outpatients. Thus, the degree of safety of this method is remarkably high.

A Postgraduate Course in Relative Analgesia

I had the good fortune to be one of the men exposed to use of nitrous oxide analgesia during its second period of resurgence (1936). After extensive use of this modality for 13 years, we began postgraduate teaching of the subject, this teaching continuing to the present day. The invaluable experience gained from teaching over 6000 dental practitioners has graphically and emphatically demonstrated that the dental profession has at its command an instrument of extreme safety, of great value to both patient and dentist, a modality that can be easily learned and applied by *every* dental practitioner.

Postgraduate instruction has taught us that initially the dentist's fear of the gas machine has to be eliminated. The average dental school graduate starts practice with little or no knowledge of anesthesia administration; however, he seems to remember vividly all the untoward results that may ensue from such administration. This fear is transferred to his thoughts about analgesia. The solution for this proved to be detailed instruction in the manipulation of the machines and clear differentiation between (1) total analgesia and relative analgesia and (2) relative analgesia and general anesthesia. After practice on several different types of machines and with the realization that the patient is at all times conscious and cooperative, with all protective reflexes functioning fully, fear of the procedure is rapidly eliminated. Only then can the dentist realize the importance of first eliminating the patient's fear of the machine and the procedure by a simple, planned psychological approach.

Six thousand dental practitioners were taught the use of nitrous oxide and oxygen analgesia in groups of 20 to 60. Instruction consisted of lectures, demonstrations, and student participation. Each group had 15 to 20 hours of instruction. It was stressed that the main objective for the use of this instrument was elimination of fear of the dental experience and that the elimination of pain itself, even though highly important, was a secondary objective. A clear differentiation was made between the planes of total analgesia and relative analgesia and between relative analgesia and general anesthesia. The necessity and importance of the introductory administration of analgesia was stressed.

Members of the class were given detailed instructions in proper psychological conditioning of the patient, proper range of dosage, and interpretation of patient reactions. Five or six different types of gas machines were used. The application of this method to all phases of dental treatment was shown in great detail, and the advantages offered to both the patient and the dentist were stressed. The relationship between inhalation analgesia with nitrous oxide and other modalities used for fear and pain control were also covered.

These included general anesthesia, intravenous sedation, and local analgesia, as well as drugs given by mouth or by injection.

From questionnaires sent to all practitioners about one year after they had completed the course in nitrous oxide–oxygen analgesia, additional valuable information has been gained:

1. *As a result of taking the course, are you using analgesia in your practice?*

Yes – 88 per cent
No – 12 per cent

Although these results are now being bettered, they are still excellent when one considers that those who took instruction many years ago were pioneers in their individual areas of practice.

2. *Has the use of analgesia proved to be a practice builder?*

Yes – 88 per cent
No – 12 per cent

The ability of analgesia to expand a practice in such a short time stresses the great need for eliminating fear of the dental experience.

3. *Have you found that you can accomplish more work per unit of time with the use of analgesia?*

Yes – 72.3 per cent
No – 27.7 per cent

It should be stressed that these figures reflect increased production without increased speed of operation. Also, allowing for the use of analgesia over a period greater than one year, more experience would change a great many "no's" to "yes's."

4. *Does the use of analgesia control the patient's fear?*

Yes – 99.8 per cent
No – 0.2 per cent

These figures speak for themselves. A result so universally encountered by diverse personalities must be considered a truth.

5. *Has the use of analgesia enabled you to treat children more easily?*

Yes – 88 per cent
No – 12 per cent

An appreciable number of practitioners answering "No" mentioned that they had few or no children in their practice. It has been shown that the use of analgesia has encouraged dental practitioners to treat the younger generation.

6. *Have you found that you are less tired and more relaxed in your daily work when using analgesia?*

Yes—78 per cent
No—22 per cent

7. *Do you encounter much nausea and vomiting?*

Yes—0.2 per cent
No—99.8 per cent

8. *Have you ever administered general anesthesia?*

Yes—10 per cent
No—90 per cent

It is significant here that success was obtained in the use of analgesia by men who had little or no experience with a gas machine.

9. *Will you make greater use of analgesia in the future?*

Yes—86 per cent
No—14 per cent

About one-third of those answering "No" to this question stipulated that they were using analgesia to the maximum at present.

10. *In your opinion, is the use of nitrous oxide–oxygen analgesia important enough to warrant its inclusion in a dental school curriculum?*

Yes—99.8 per cent
No—0.2 per cent

It is now being taught in a number of schools of dentistry at the undergraduate level.

11. *After one year, how extensive is the use of analgesia in your practice?*

Very little—13 per cent
Moderate—51 per cent
A great deal—36 per cent

It was found that the dentists using analgesia very little after one year deliberately chose the patients to whom they offered it. This is a very difficult choice to make and presupposes an omniscience that few individuals possess. Even the so-called good dental patient will be happier in the dental chair when he is cushioned by a state of euphoria, distracted and less annoyed by noises, sights, instrumentation, and the spraying of water. Those practitioners who were using it extensively after one year chose the proper approach by attempting to introduce analgesia to almost every patient. The purpose of this final question was to ascertain the time factor involved in introducing analgesia into a dental practice.

The answers to this questionnaire have helped us to evaluate the efficacy of the teaching and the *value* and *safety* of nitrous oxide–oxygen analgesia in the hands of the *average dental practitioner*. It was found that nitrous oxide–oxygen analgesia when used primarily to eliminate fear of the dental experience is a safe and valuable instrument. Its use is advantageous to both the patient and the dentist.

The greatly expanded application of inhalation analgesia with nitrous oxide by the general dental practitioner has resulted in bringing under the canopy of dental treatment many people who formerly remained untreated because of physical, mental, or emotional reasons. It has served to make the dentist's daily task easier and, by dissociating dental treatment from fear and pain, it serves to create an atmosphere in which the public places a higher valuation on the dental profession.

REFERENCES

1. Archer, W. H.: Life and letters of Horace Wells, the discoverer of anesthesia. J. Amer. Coll. Dent., 11:83, 1944; 12:85, 1945.
2. Breitman, F.: Psychology does half the work in nitrous oxide analgesia. Dent. Survey, 27:1081, 1951.
3. Fechtner, J. L.: Pain control in dentistry for children. J. Dent. Child., 24:163, 1957.
4. Henegan, J. F.: Nitrous oxide and oxygen analgesia. New York J. Dent., 11:207, 1941.
5. Holst, J. J.: Use of nitrous oxide–oxygen analgesia in dentistry. Inter. Dent. J., 12:47, 1962.
6. Holst, J. J.: Personal communication, 1962.
7. Keys, T. E.: History of Surgical Anesthesia. New York, Abelard-Schuman, 1945.
8. Lippe, H. T.: Nitrous oxide analgesia in cavity preparation. Temple Dent. Rev., 14:7, Feb., 1944.
9. Seldin, H. M.: Practical Anesthesia for Dentistry and Oral Surgery. Philadelphia, Lea & Febiger, 1947.
10. Thorwald, J.: The Century of the Surgeon. New York, Pantheon Books, Inc., 1956.
11. Vonow, P.: Die Lachgas-Analgesie in der Zahnärztlichen Praxis. Bern and Stuttgart, Medizinisher Verlag Hans Huber, 1956.
12. Ruben, H.: Nitrous oxide analgesia in dentistry. Its use during 15 years in Denmark. Brit. Dent. J., 132:195–196, 1972.

THE NERVOUS SYSTEM

2

Brian Curtis and Stanley Jacobson*

Anesthetic drugs can act as such because they influence the functioning of the nervous system. It is germane, therefore, to discuss some of the basic modern concepts of the anatomy and physiology of the nervous system.

Man has always wondered and speculated about the function of the brain. The ancients understood that the brain was the seat of thought and behavior. Scientific inquiry over a period of several hundreds of years has revealed a great deal about the functions of the human nervous system and the localization of those functions within the various structures of the nervous system. Systematic and careful investigation has revealed the rich interconnections between these structures. This knowledge is of great importance to the practitioner, since correct and more effective use of a drug must be based on knowledge of the structures it affects and the mechanisms involved.

The basic units of the nervous system are called *nerve cells*. Each has a *cell body* and one long process, the *axon*, and many short processes, the *dendrites*. These cells are capable of propagating an electrical disturbance received by the dendrites through the cell body and down the axon. The axon forms many connections or *synapses* with dendrites of other cells.

There are two basic divisions of the nervous system: The *peripheral nervous system* and the *central nervous system*. The peripheral nervous system connects the central nervous system to the rest of the body. It lies primarily outside the bony structures of the skull and vertebral column. The central nervous system, on the other hand, is completely encased in these bony structures. It forms the integrative and thinking portions of the nervous system.

THE CENTRAL NERVOUS SYSTEM

The central nervous system consists of the *spinal cord*, lying within the vertebral column, and the *brain*, lying within the skull.

The *spinal cord* serves both as a connecting link between the brain and the body and as a lower level center for the integration of motor activity.

*Adapted from Curtis, B. A., Jacobson, S., and Marcus, E. M.: An Introduction to the Neurosciences. Philadelphia, W. B. Saunders Co., 1972.

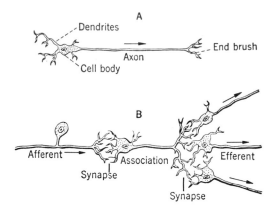

Figure 2–1 *A*, A typical motor or efferent neuron, which transmits impulses to muscles or glands. *B*, All three types of neurons are shown as they appear in the reflex arc. (From N. L. Munn: Psychology. 3rd ed. Boston, Houghton Mifflin Co., 1956.)

The Brain

The *brain* consists of three major parts, the cerebrum, the brain stem, and the cerebellum. One great difference between the human brain and the brain of lower animals is the extensive development of the *"new brain"* or *cerebral cortex* of man. Phylogenetically, the cerebral cortex is considered to be of recent origin. The cerebrum is by far the largest part of the brain, and occupies the upper portion of the skull. Through histological studies of its cells, the cortex has been subdivided into areas of specific structure in the belief that structural differences denote differences in function. From these studies it has been deduced that all parts of the cerebral cortex can both receive and give off impulses and that there are provisions for the spread of impulses horizontally,

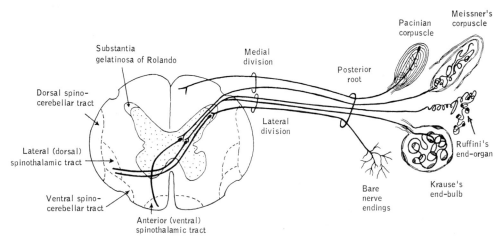

Figure 2–2 The various receptor organs and their course into the spinal cord. Note that the pacinian corpuscle and Meissner's corpuscle, which are both tactile, or touch, end organs, pass into the cord through the medial division of the dorsal root. Ruffini's end organ (warmth), Krause's end bulb (cold), and bare nerve endings (pain) pass through the lateral division of the dorsal root. (From B. E. Finneson: Diagnosis and Management of Pain Syndromes. Philadelphia, W. B. Saunders Co., 1962.)

Central Nervous System

Brain

Spinal cord

Peripheral nerve

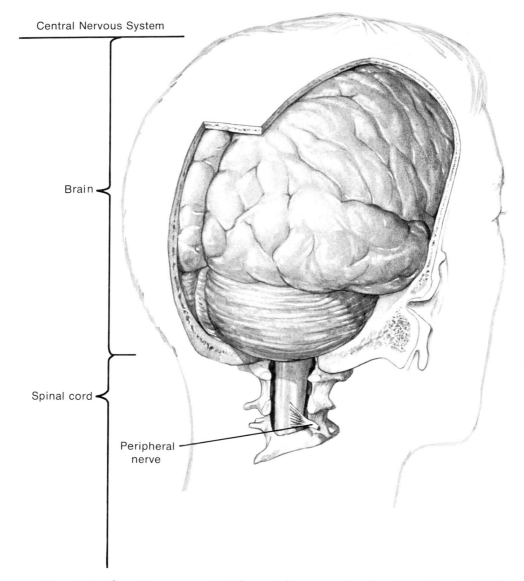

Figure 2–3 The major components of the central nervous system in relationship to the head and neck. (From B. A. Curtis, S. Jacobson, and E. M. Marcus: An Introduction to the Neurosciences. Philadelphia, W. B. Saunders Co., 1972.)

so that efferent discharges can be generated in one part of the cortex as a result of impulses it receives from other cortical areas. Practitioners of the healing arts are particularly interested in the cerebrum, for it is here that pain is interpreted as such by the patient.

THE CEREBRUM

Most of those functions of the nervous system with which we are familiar are conscious functions which are located in the cerebrum; that is, the final

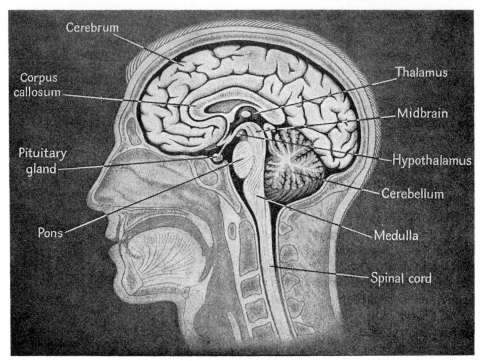

Figure 2–4   This side view of the brain shows the major anatomical and functional parts. The two cerebral hemispheres are connected through the corpus callosum, while the lobes of the cerebellum are connected through the pons. (From N. L. Munn: Psychology, 3rd ed. Boston, Houghton Mifflin Co., 1956.)

integrative or "conscious" action occurs in the cerebrum. The *cerebrum* is a paired structure, with right and left cerebral hemispheres, each governing the opposite side of the body. Voluntary movements of the right hand are "willed" in the left cerebral hemisphere. The surface of the hemisphere called

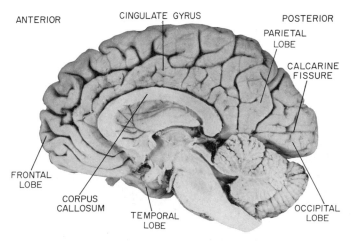

Figure 2–5   The four lobes of the cerebrum shown on a photograph of the medial surface of a hemisection of the same atrophied brain shown in Figure 2–6. (From Curtis, Jacobson, and Marcus, 1972.)

the cortex receives sensory information from skin, eyes, ears, and other sensory receptors on the opposite side of the body. This information is compared to previous experience and produces movements in response to these stimuli.

Each hemisphere consists of several layers. The outer layer consists of a dense collection of nerve cells which look gray when examined in a fresh state and are thus called *gray matter*. This outer layer, about 3 mm. in thickness, is called the *cerebral cortex* and is molded into *gyri* (ridges) and *sulci* (valleys), the deepest sulci being termed *fissures*. The deeper layers of the hemisphere consist of axons, or *white matter*, and collections of cell bodies (nuclei).

Some of the integrative functions of the cerebrum can be localized within specific regions of the cortex, whereas others are more diffusely distributed.

THE LATERAL SURFACE OF THE CEREBRUM

The major dividing landmark of the cerebral cortex is the *lateral fissure*, which runs on the lateral surface of the brain from the open end in front, posteriorly and dorsally (backwards and up). The lateral fissure defines a tongue of cortex ventral to it, the *temporal lobe*. This lobe contains the *primary auditory cortex*, which is that part of the cortex receiving auditory impulses via pathways leading from the auditory receptors in the inner ear.

The *primary auditory cortex* is localized on the *transverse temporal gyrus*

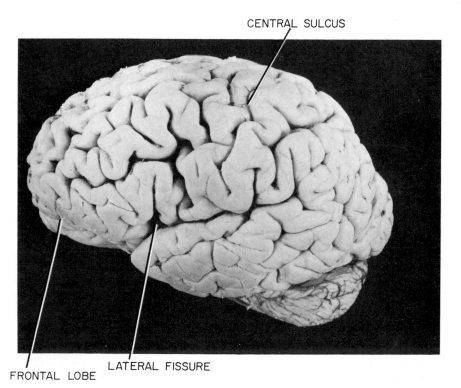

Figure 2-6 The frontal lobe shown on a photograph of a markedly atrophied human brain. The sulci are much wider than normal. (From Curtis, Jacobson, and Marcus, 1972.)

which is located at the posterior and dorsal margin of the temporal lobe, buried on the inner slope of the lateral fissure. To see it, we must pull the temporal lobe out and down. When a recording electrode is placed on this gyrus at the time of neurosurgery, a large and characteristic electrical response follows when noise is played into the patient's ear. If a weak current is passed into a stimulating electrode in this same location, the conscious patient will report "hearing" tones or noise. The primary auditory cortex is an excellent example of a function which can be precisely located on the cortex.

In right-handed individuals, the left temporal lobe surrounding the transverse temporal gyrus is involved in the more complex interpretation of auditory signals. If the cells of this area die, the patient will not be able to interpret sounds as words. The function of the cells on the homologous surface of the right hemisphere is unknown. They can be removed without causing any overt clinical problems. Consequently, the neurosurgeon will not hesitate to cut through the right temporal lobe of a right-handed person to reach a tumor, but he will try some other approach on the left side. The functions of the rest of the temporal lobe, particularly the anterior tip, are more difficult to specify, but storage of long-term memory is one of them.

Another major landmark of the cerebral cortex is the *central sulcus*. It delimits the posterior border of the *frontal lobe*. The gyrus immediately anterior to the central sulcus is the *precentral gyrus*, which functions as the *primary motor cortex*. From this gyrus signals run down through the brain stem to the spinal cord and out via the peripheral nervous system to control the skeletal muscles. Lesions of part of the precentral gyrus will cause partial paralysis on the opposite side of the body.

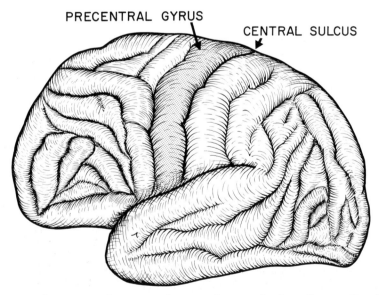

PRECENTRAL GYRUS

CENTRAL SULCUS

Figure 2–7 The precentral gyrus in relation to the central sulcus. Can you identify the precentral gyrus on the brain in Figure 2–6? (From Curtis, Jacobson, and Marcus, 1972.)

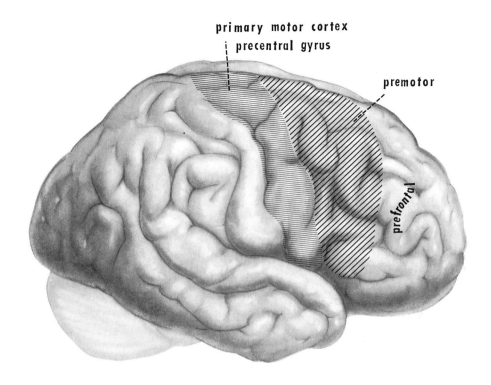

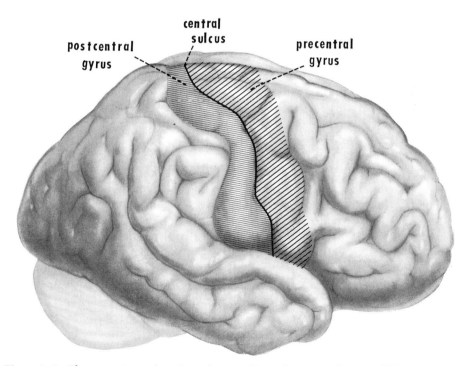

Figure 2–8 The premotor and prefrontal areas. (From Curtis, Jacobson, and Marcus, 1972.)

Further anterior in the frontal lobe is an area of *premotor cortex*. Here more complex motor movements, such as speech, are organized. The anterior and inferior portions of the frontal lobe are involved in *control of emotional behavior*. These areas, referred to as *prefrontal,* appear to have an inhibitory function predicated on the future consequences of present actions. Patients who have had prefrontal lobectomies (removal of the lobe) seem to have little awareness of the social consequences of their actions.

Immediately behind the central sulcus lies the *parietal lobe*. Several component areas of the parietal lobe may be distinguished. Immediately posterior to the central sulcus is the postcentral gyrus. This is the *primary sensory cortex* which receives impulses from all the sensory receptors of the skin. Each little area along the gyrus is related to a particular part of the body; for example, the legs on the medial end, the hand in the center, and the face on the end next to the lateral fissure. We can "feel" pain, touch, and pressure at lower levels of the nervous system, particularly the brain stem, but we cannot determine where the stimulus was applied. The following example is helpful. A patient loses a small portion of the hand-area in the left postcentral gyrus. When a pin is stuck into his right hand, he will know that a pin has been stuck into him, but he cannot tell the examiner where the pin was placed.

If a recording electrode is appropriately placed during a neurosurgical procedure, cortical response can be elicited by tactile stimuli to the hand of the opposite side of the body. Likewise, if a stimulus is applied through the same electrode, the patient will report a tingling sensation in this hand. Higher order sensory discrimination, such as recognizing a number drawn on the palm of the hand, is organized solely in the parietal lobe. Destruction of the parietal lobe leads to a loss of this ability. The patient will still know he is being touched but cannot tell where or what is being drawn. The awareness of body is also organized in the parietal lobe.

The *occipital lobe* is the last and most posterior lobe. Only a small portion is present on the lateral surface of the cerebrum.

THE MEDIAL SURFACE OF THE CEREBRUM

If the cerebral hemisphere were cut apart at the midline and separated, the medial surface would be seen. All four lobes extend onto the medial surface. The tissue on either side of the *calcerine fissure in the occipital lobe* is the *primary visual cortex*. Light flashed into the eyes evokes large electrical potentials from electrodes placed over this area of the cortex. The remainder of the occipital lobe is involved in *interpreting and categorizing visual sensations*.

The *corpus callosum* is a prominent structure on the medial surface. This wide band of nerve fibers interconnects the two cerebral hemispheres and serves to transfer information between them.

Immediately surrounding the corpus callosum is the *cingulate gyrus*. This area is involved in *emotional responses*. It functions in conjunction with other areas of the brain, such as the phylogenetically newer frontal lobe and other, phylogenetically older areas of the brain stem.

THE BRAIN STEM

The brain stem is composed of four regions: *medulla oblongata, pons, midbrain, and diencephalon.* These regions have discrete functions, and each of them contains groupings of cell bodies (nuclei) and bundles of axons (tracts). The *medulla oblongata* is a direct continuation of the spinal cord. It contains the same fiber tracts as the spinal cord. It also contains groups of motor and sensory nuclei for the segments it controls, mainly the throat, neck, and mouth. Of interest to the practitioner administering relative analgesia are those functions of the medulla oblongata concerned with respiration and the cardiovascular system. The medullary centers exhibit integrative functions as regards reflex activities involved in the control of respiration. They are sensitive to changes in the partial pressures of carbon dioxide and oxygen in the blood. Stimulation of one side of the medulla (and the pons) affects equally the respiratory muscles on both sides of the body.

The nerves connecting directly to the brain are called *cranial nerves.* There are 12 pairs of cranial nerves, 11 of which enter the brain stem; the olfactory nerve enters the cerebrum directly. The cell bodies of each cranial nerve, both sensory and motor, are grouped together and are very distinct within the brain stem, in contrast to the continuous nature of the gray matter of the spinal cord.

The *pons* contains cranial nerve nuclei associated with sensory input and

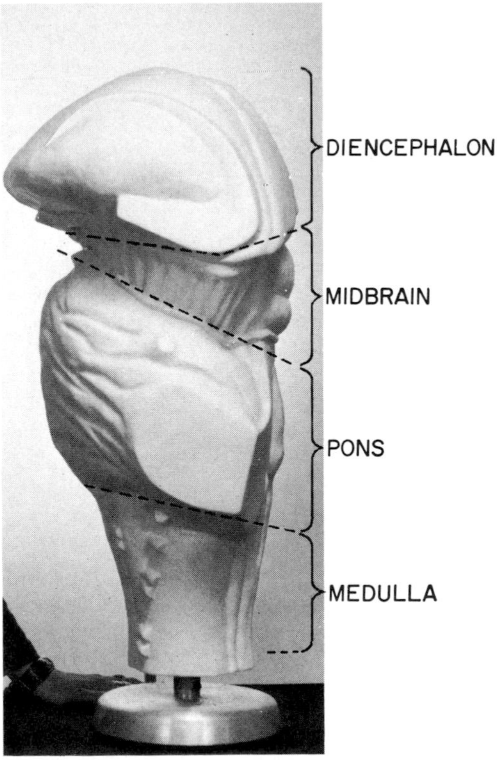

Figure 2–9 The brain stem. This photograph of the oversized Tuft's Brain Stem Model shows the major subdivisions. (From Curtis, Jacobson, and Marcus, 1972.)

DIENCEPHALON

MIDBRAIN

PONS

MEDULLA

motor outflow to the face. The large bulge of the brain stem which is so typical of the pons is made up of fibers coursing down from the cerebrum and
turning and running up into the cerebrum.

The *midbrain* contains the major motor nuclei controlling eye movement.
It includes a huge pair of tracts carrying signals down from the cerebral hemispheres and also contains the sensory tracts which arise in the spinal cord
and continue, with additional fibers added, through the brain stem. The
midbrain exerts control over the state of wakefulness of the entire brain.

The most superior portion of the brain stem is the *diencephalon,* which is
almost completely covered by the cerebrum. It is a paired structure with a
thin fluid space between the two parts. The largest structure within the diencephalon is the *thalamus.* It is the major relay and integration center for all of
the sensory systems, except that of smell. We can "feel" pain (and crude
touch) at the level of the thalamus. This area of the central nervous system,
above all others, is of interest to the practitioner who administers relative
analgesia. Recent experimentation has demonstrated that all sensory tracts
(except those concerned with olfaction) lead into a reticulated area in the

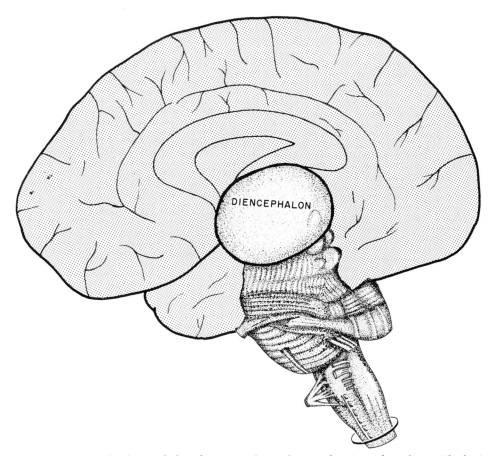

Figure 2–10 The diencephalon shown in relationship to a hemisected cerebrum. The brain
stem has not been dissected. (From Curtis, Jacobson, and Marcus, 1972.)

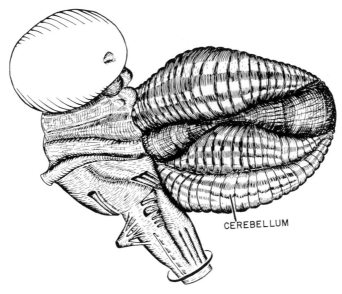

CEREBELLUM

Figure 2–11 The cerebellum and its relationship to the brain stem. These relationships can also be seen in the hemisected brain in Figure 2–5. (From Curtis, Jacobson, and Marcus, 1972.)

thalamus, where they are interrupted by synapses before ascending to the cerebral cortex. The thalamus, then, acts as a relay station for somatic, visceral, visual, and auditory sensations. For our purposes, it is important to stress that all pain sensations must pass through the thalamic area before ascending to the higher cerebral centers for interpretation.

THE CEREBELLUM

The cerebellum has three major connections with the rest of the nervous system. Fibers from the spinal cord carrying information concerning the position of the trunk and limbs enter via the *inferior cerebellar peduncles. The middle cerebellar peduncle* conveys information which has originated in the cerebral cortex. From the cerebral cortex, fibers descend to the pontine nuclei where a synapse occurs. The information is then conveyed from the pontine nuclei to the cerebellum via the middle cerebellar peduncle. Finally, the major outflow from the cerebellum to the thalamus, and eventually to the cerebral cortex, is via the *superior cerebellar peduncles.* It is seen, therefore, that the cerebellum receives, via the inferior cerebellar peduncle, information as to where the limbs are in space, and, via the middle cerebellar peduncle, information as to where they are commanded to be. This information is compared in the cerebellum, and commands are sent out via the superior cerebellar peduncle. The cerebellum also has a strong input from the semicircular canals concerning orientation in space. It is seen, then, that the cerebellum is involved in the unconscious adjustment of the many body muscles to keep us standing up and to provide a background for appropriate and harmonious

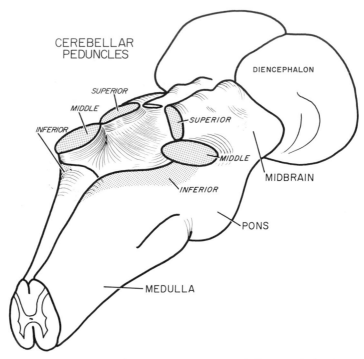

Figure 2–12 The three connections between the cerebellum and the brain stem. (From Curtis, Jacobson, and Marcus, 1972.)

muscle movement. The staggering gait which results from an excessive intake of alcohol is due primarily to the selective alteration of cerebellar function.

THE HYPOTHALAMUS

The hypothalamus is smaller than the thalamus. It forms the walls and the floor of the third ventricle below the hypothalamic sulcus. The hypothalamus is the *most important subcortical center for emotions*. It is also the regulator of homeostatic mechanisms. Through its relationship to the autonomic nervous system and hypophysis it maintains a more or less stable, controlled, internal environment which permits the individual to exist almost in spite of the external environment. It affects body temperature, water balance and neurosecretion, food intake, sleep, and the parasympathetic and sympathetic nervous systems. It affects *cardiovascular reactions in fear, anger, and exercise*. It exerts these powerful influences through the multisynaptic descending autonomic pathways in the lateral margins of the reticular formation as well as by controlling the release of the catecholamines (epinephrine and norepinephrine) from the adrenal medulla.

Norepinephrine causes vasoconstriction of the peripheral vessels, with resultant increased blood flow in the large vessels. The blood pressure and pulse rate rise and the flow of blood in the coronary muscles increases.

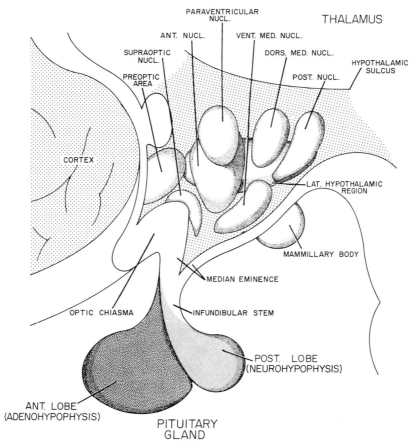

Figure 2–13 The hypophysis and the nuclei of the hypothalamus. (From Curtis, Jacobson, and Marcus, 1972.)

Epinephrine increases the heart rate and the force, amplitude, and frequency of contractions. It also dilates the pupils of the eye and the sphincters of the gastrointestinal system and the urinary bladder, causing voiding and defecation. It inhibits the motility of the gut and causes the bronchial musculature to relax, thereby dilating the bronchial passages. Epinephrine increases oxygen metabolism and the basal metabolic rate. It causes hyperglycemia by triggering an increasing phosphorylase activity, which accelerates glycogenesis in the muscles and liver. In addition, it increases the rate of resynthesis of lactic acid to glycogen, thereby prolonging the contraction of the skeletal muscles.

THE VENTRICULAR SYSTEM

The *ventricles* are structures filled with cerebrospinal fluid; their function is not fully understood. The *lateral ventricles* (the largest) lie in the cerebrum, and are bilateral. They both connect with a single midline structure, the *third*

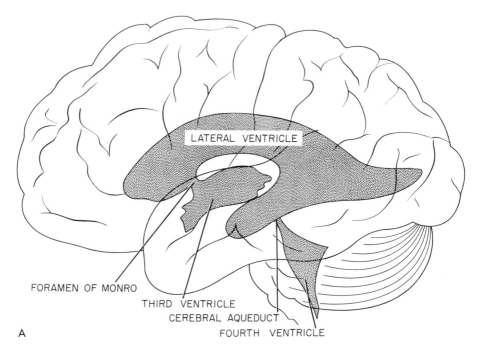

LATERAL VENTRICLE

FORAMEN OF MONRO

THIRD VENTRICLE
CEREBRAL AQUEDUCT
FOURTH VENTRICLE

A

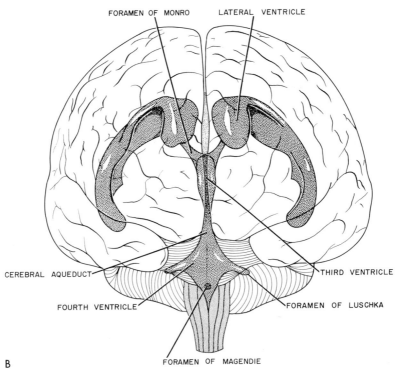

FORAMEN OF MONRO   LATERAL VENTRICLE

CEREBRAL AQUEDUCT   THIRD VENTRICLE

FOURTH VENTRICLE   FORAMEN OF LUSCHKA

FORAMEN OF MAGENDIE

B

Figure 2–14   The ventricular system of the brain. *A*, Lateral, and *B*, anteroposterior views. (From Curtis, Jacobson, and Marcus, 1972.)

ventricle. The third ventricle lies between the two halves of the diencephalon and is connected with a midline structure on the brain stem, the *fourth ventricle*. Cerebrospinal fluid is produced in the lateral ventricles and flows through the third and fourth ventricles. Fluid leaves the system through holes in the roof of the fourth ventricle, flows up around the brain and is reabsorbed by a large venous sinus at the top of the brain. The brain floats in the cerebrospinal fluid surrounding it.

THE BLOOD SUPPLY TO THE BRAIN

The cells of the brain are completely dependent on a continuous supply of glucose and oxygen. They have meager stores of glycogen and do not carry out glycolysis. Brain damage will occur if the oxygen supply is cut off for 4 or 5 minutes or if the glucose supply is cut off for 10 to 15 minutes. The greatest cause of brain damage and neurological disease is the stoppage of blood flow to a region of the brain (a stroke). The cells and axons in the area deprived of blood die and can no longer function.

The brain receives blood from four arteries. Two *vertebral arteries* enter the skull (together with the spinal cord) through the *foramen magnum*. These arteries send branches to the medulla oblongata and the cerebellum. More superiorly, they join to form the *basilar artery* which supplies the pons, midbrain, and parts of the cerebellum. At its superior end, the basilar artery branches to form the *posterior cerebral arteries* which supply the occipital lobes and part of the temporal lobes. This whole system forms the posterior circulation of the brain.

The anterior circulation is supplied by the *internal carotid arteries*. These arteries enter the cranial cavity and almost immediately branch into the *middle and anterior cerebral arteries*. The middle cerebral arteries run laterally through the lateral fissure to supply the lateral surface of the hemispheres. The anterior cerebral arteries run anteriorly and medially to loop over the corpus callosum between the hemispheres, supplying blood to the medial surface of the brain.

The anterior and posterior circulations are connected by the *posterior communicating arteries*. The right and left anterior cerebral arteries are connected by the *anterior communicating artery*. Since the major arteries at the base of the brain are usually interconnected, a failure in blood supply in one of these major arteries will not usually produce a critical decrease in blood flow in the region supplied by that vessel.

The Spinal Cord

The segmental nature of the spinal cord is quite evident upon gross inspection. The nerves which enter and leave the cord do so at regular intervals.

There are two pairs of nerve roots for each segment. While the segmental nature of the spinal cord is evident, the segmental nature of the body regions which it innervates is not. In an earthworm the segment is simply a cylinder

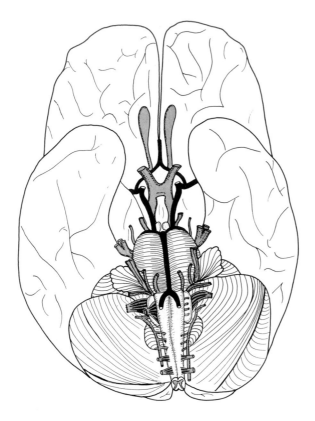

Figure 2–15 The arterial supply to the brain. (From Curtis, Jacobson, and Marcus, 1972.)

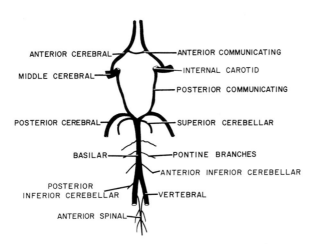

of body wall, and each segment of the worm's spinal cord supplies both sensory and motor innervation to the segment it controls. In human beings the segments are of variable size and shape, yet the principle still holds; each segment of the spinal cord provides both sensory and motor innervation to its own particular segment.

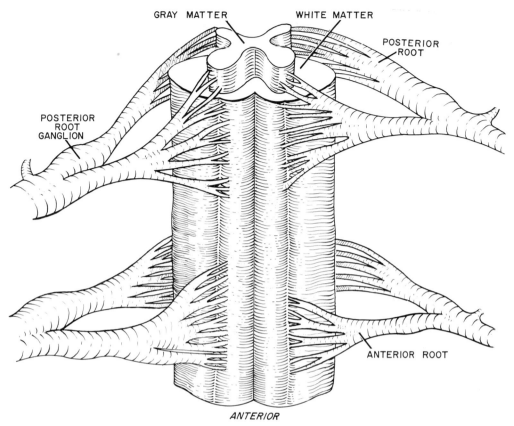

Figure 2–16 A view of the anterior aspect of the spinal cord showing the segmental nature of the spinal cord roots. (From Curtis, Jacobson, and Marcus, 1972.)

In cross section, the spinal cord is found to be composed of two distinct areas, the gray matter and the white matter. The *gray matter* is the central, butterfly-shaped area, which appears gray on gross examination and is composed largely of cell bodies. The cell bodies of the axons which run out to control the muscles are located in the large *anterior horn cells*. Their axons leave the cord by the anterior root. The only way that the muscle at the end of the axon can contract is through stimulation of this anterior horn cell. It is therefore obvious that all motor commands from higher centers, such as the precentral gyrus, are conducted via the anterior horn cells of the appropriate spinal cord segments. The sensory fibers enter via the posterior root and then branch and synapse many times in the gray matter. In some instances a sensory fiber may synapse directly on an anterior horn cell.

The neurons of each segment are organized to give a few stereotyped responses to specific stimuli. The jerking of the knee in response to tapping the patellar tendon is an example of such a stereotyped response.

In addition to its role in segmented responses, the spinal cord also conducts signals to and from the higher centers (brain stem, cerebellum, and cere-

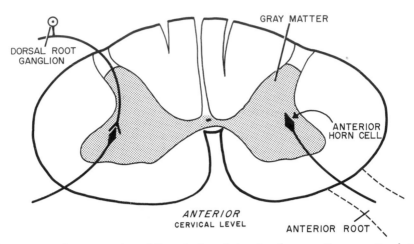

Figure 2-17 A cross section of the spinal cord showing the synaptic connection between a sensory fiber, entering the spinal cord through the posterior root, and a motor fiber, leaving via the anterior root. This particular section is from the neck region. (From Curtis, Jacobson, and Marcus, 1972.)

bral cortex). These *ascending and descending tracts* lie in the lateral spaces surrounding the gray matter. The myelin sheaths of the axons in these areas account for the appearance of the *white matter*. In addition to receiving motor commands from the descending tracts, each segment adds sensory information to the ascending tracts. Most of the axons in the white matter of a segment bypass that segment; they are connecting other segments to the brain.

Each segment of the spinal cord has several functions. It provides a locus for sensory input, a modest integration of information, and motor control of its segment. In addition, it serves as a conduction pathway for ascending and descending tracts.

SENSORY PATHWAYS OF THE SPINAL CORD

The *anterolateral tracts* convey the sensations of pressure and touch; pain from the skin, muscles, tendons, joints, and viscera; warmth and cold; tickling and itching; feelings of muscular fatigue; and sexual sensations. The *posterior white columns* carry impulses concerned with muscle, tendon and joint sensibility; touch and weight discrimination; and perceptual functions such as two-point discrimination and appreciation of vibration and localization.

AUTONOMIC NERVOUS SYSTEM

Much of the effectiveness of the hypothalamus is produced by its innervation of the nuclei in the central nervous system, which form the autonomic nervous system.

The somatic nervous system has its own receptors and effectors which provide cutaneous and motor innervation to the skin and muscles in the head,

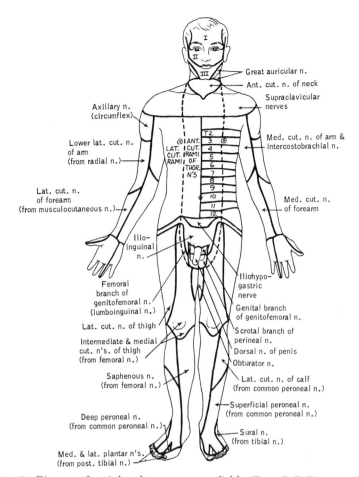

Figure 2–18 Diagram of peripheral nerve sensory fields. (From B. E. Finneson: Diagnosis and Management of Pain Syndromes. Philadelphia, W. B. Saunders Co., 1962.)

neck, and body. The *visceral or autonomic* nervous system also has its own receptors and effectors, which provide visceral motor and sensory innervation to the glands, smooth muscles, cardiac muscles, viscera, and blood vessels. These axons run part of the way with somatic fibers, but they also have separate pathways.

In the somatic nervous system, the efferent neuron is the ventral horn cell. Its axon leaves the central nervous system to innervate a skeletal muscle.

In the visceral nervous sytem two efferent neurons are found: the *preganglionic neuron* and the *postganglionic neuron*. The preganglionic neuron is found in the intermediate horn in the thoracic and lumbar levels of the spinal cord. The axon of this cell leaves the central nervous system via the ventral root and ends in an autonomic ganglion which parallels the spinal cord or is found near the target organ. The postganglionic neuron, or the motor ganglion cell, is located outside the central nervous system and ends in the appropriate gland, smooth muscle, or cardiac muscle.

Reflexes affecting smooth muscle, glands, and the conducting tissue of the heart are called *autonomic reflexes*. The autonomic nervous system innervates those regulators of the body concerned with emergency mechanisms, repair of tissue damage, and the preservation of a constant internal environment (homeostasis). In fear, for example, the following reactions are among those elicited by the autonomic nervous system: an increase in heart rate and blood pressure, dilatation of the bronchi to increase oxygen uptake, and a decrease in coagulation time to reduce the danger of hemorrhage.

The autonomic nervous system is divided into *parasympathetic and sympathetic* systems. The two systems provide dual innervation to glands and viscera and act to produce optimal balance for maintaining the internal milieu under any environmental condition. Following are some examples:

EYE

Parasympathetic: Provide innervation to the muscle and the constrictor of the iris, and permit accommodation for near vision.

Sympathetic: Innervate the dilator muscle of the iris and the levator palpebrae and radial ciliary muscles, producing eye opening (lifting of the lid) and dilation of the pupil for distant vision.

LACRIMAL GLANDS

Parasympathetic: Vasodilation and secretion.

Sympathetic: Vasoconstriction and reduced secretion.

HEART

Parasympathetic: Through axons reaching coronary vessels and atrial musculature, cardiac deceleration is effected.

Sympathetic: Fibers from cardiac nerves enter the cardiac plexus and produce cardiac acceleration.

LUNGS

Parasympathetic: Fibers run in the vagus to the pulmonary plexus in the bronchi and blood vessels, causing constriction of the bronchi and decreased respiration.

Sympathetic: Cause dilation of the bronchi and increased respiration.

ABDOMINAL VISCERA

Parasympathetic: Stimulate peristalsis and gastrointestinal secretion.

Sympathetic: Inhibit peristalsis and gastrointestinal secretion, stimulate secretion from the adrenal medulla, and cause vasoconstriction of the visceral vessels.

PELVIS

Parasympathetic: Fibers supply the uterus, vagina, testes, erectile tissue (penis and clitoris), sigmoid colon, rectum, and bladder. They cause contraction and emptying of the bladder and erection of the clitoris or penis.

Sympathetic: Fibers cause vasoconstriction and ejaculation of semen and inhibit peristalsis in the sigmoid colon and rectum.

CUTANEOUS AND DEEP VESSELS, GLANDS, AND HAIR

Blood vessels receive only sympathetic innervation. Activation of this system produces vasoconstriction (cooling of the skin), sweating, and piloerection.

THE NEURON

The basic functional unit of the nervous system is the neuron. The *neuron doctrine*, as presented by Waldeyer in 1891, described the neuron as having one axon which is efferent and one or more dendrites which are afferent. In addition he noted that the nerve cells are contiguous and not continuous and that all other elements of the nervous system serve to feed, protect, and support them. Although the neurons are not the only cells in the body capable of conducting impulses (muscle cells can also conduct impulses), neurons, when arranged in networks and provided with adequate informational input, can *store information* and *respond in many ways to any stimulus.*

Neurons vary in size and shape and may be unipolar, bipolar, or multipolar. The *most common neuron is multipolar.*

In the adult nervous system the *unipolar cells* are found in the sensory ganglia of the spinal and cranial nerves and in the mesencephalic nucleus of cranial nerve V. In these cells a single process acts as the axon and dendrite. *Bipolar neurons,* which are sensory in function, are found in the retina, rods, and cones, in the olfactory neuroepithelial cells, in the olfactory mucosa in the nasal passages, and in the vestibular and auditory receptors in the inner ear.

Multipolar neurons are found throughout the central nervous system and in the sympathetic ganglia of the peripheral nervous system. They convey both sensory and motor impulses. The multipolar neurons vary greatly in size and in the complexity of their axonal and dendritic fields.

PARTS OF THE NEURON

Each neuron has the following parts:
1. The dendritic zone (dendrite and soma).
2. Axon origin (axon hillock).
3. Axon.
4. Synaptic telodendria.

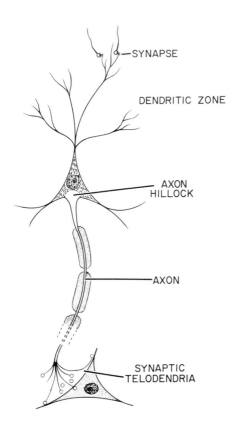

Figure 2-19 Schematic drawing of a multipolar neuron demonstrating dendritic zone (dendrite and soma), axon hillock, axon covered with myelin, and synaptic telodendria. (From Curtis, Jacobson, and Marcus, 1972.)

The dendritic zone receives the input, which converges from many different sources. The action potential originates at the site of the origin of the axon and is transmitted down the axon in an all-or-none phenomenon to the synaptic telodendria, where the impulse is transmitted to the dendritic zone of the next neuron on the chain. The dendrite does not respond in an all-or-none fashion like the axon.

MYELIN

In the nervous system, axons may be myelinated or unmyelinated. The myelin is formed by a supporting cell, which in the central nervous system is called the *oligodendrocyte,* and in the peripheral nervous system the *Schwann cell.* Thus, the myelin sheath is not part of the neuron: it is a covering for the axon. Myelin consists of segments approximately 0.5 to 1 mm. in length. Between these segments are discontinuities in the myelin sheath called the *nodes of Ranvier;* the axon, however, is continuous at the nodes, and axon collaterals can leave at the nodes.

SYNAPTIC TRANSMISSION

Current evidence (McLennan, 1970), based on the presence of (1) a 300 to 400 Å cleft, (2) synaptic vesicles, and (3) an appreciable synaptic delay,

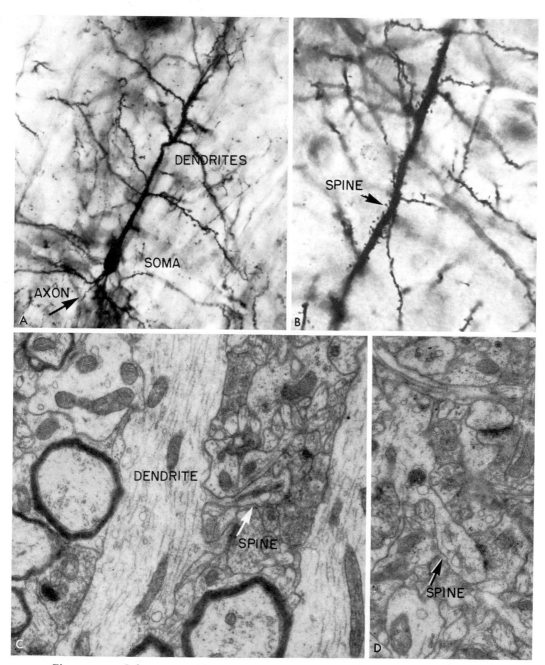

Figure 2–20 Golgi type I cells—neurons with long axons in the motor cortex of the rat. *A*, Entire cell—soma, axon, and dendrite; *B*, dendritic spines; *C* and *D*, electron micrographs of dendritic spines. *A*, Golgi stain, ×100; *B*, Golgi stain, ×250; *C* and *D*, ×30,000. (From Curtis, Jacobson, and Marcus, 1972.)

suggests that synaptic transmission is a chemically and not electrically mediated phenomenon. Various chemical substances have been found which can partake in synaptic transmission. *Acetylcholine* is the best documented transmitter in the central and peripheral nervous systems. Acetylcholine has been isolated in synaptic vesicles and acetylcholine esterase has been found throughout the central and peripheral nervous systems and at postganglionic sympathetic endings.

Catecholamines and 5-hydroxytryptamine have also been linked to synaptic transmission in the central nervous system. *Norepinephrine* has been associated with transmission in the preganglionic sympathetic synapses. *Glutamine, glycine* and *GABA (gamma-amino butyric acid)* have also been shown to participate in nervous transmission.

There is still much uncertainty as to whether these aforementioned substances normally participate in nervous transmission. ATP, substance P, histamine, prostaglandin, steroids, and hormones have also been linked to synaptic transmission. It is still uncertain whether these compounds play a direct role in nervous transmission or if they are just related by their importance to the ongoing functions of the entire body.

RECEPTORS AND EFFECTORS

Each peripheral nerve, whether sensory, motor, or secretory, terminates by arborizing in a peripheral structure.

Effectors

The motor or efferent nerves from the *somatic nervous system* end in skeletal muscles and form the motor end plates. In smooth muscle, cardiac muscle, and glands nerve endings resemble the synaptic endings in the central nervous system. *Visceral motor endings* are seen on muscles in arterioles (vasomotor), muscles in hair follicles (pilomotor), and sweat glands (sudomotor).

Receptors

Sensory endings are found throughout the body and are modified according to the functional specialization of the region. Visceral sensory receptors are similar to somatic sensory receptors associated with the somatic nervous system, except that they are located in the viscera and their accessory organs. The sensory endings subserve pain, touch, temperature, vibration, pressure, heat, cold, proprioception in skin, muscles, and viscera, as well as the specialized somatic and visceral sensations of taste, smell, vision, audition, and balance.

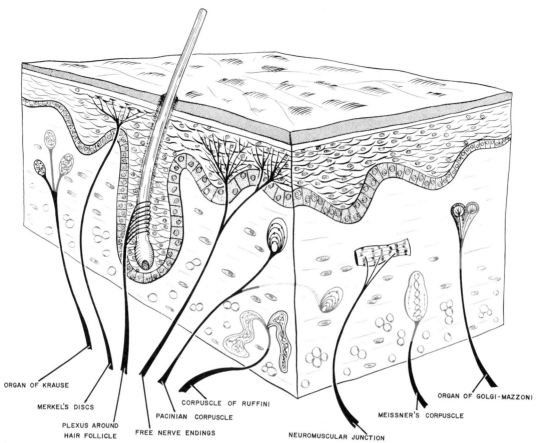

Figure 2–21 Stereogram of the skin, demonstrating sensory receptors and effectors. (After Noback, C. R.: *The Human Nervous System*. New York, McGraw-Hill, 1967.) (From Curtis, Jacobson, and Marcus, 1972.)

Free Nerve Endings

Free nerve endings are formed by sensory fibers which arborize in various tissues, including stratified epithelium, muscle, tendon, connective tissue, mucous, serous membranes, and joints. These receptors are considered to be *pain receptors*, as they are found in tissues where pain is the primary sensation (tooth pulp, dentine, and cornea). Crude touch may also be subserved by these receptors.

Free nerve endings are also found in terminal networks around the disc-shaped tactile cells of Merkel and around the hair follicles in the dermal sheath and outer root sheath. These structures seem to subserve touch.

Encapsulated Sensory Endings

In these endings the nerve is surrounded by a specialized connective tissue capsule of varying thickness. Those include *Meissner's corpuscles, pacin-*

ian corpuscles, muscle and tendon spindles, the cylindrical *end bulb of Krause,* and the *end bulb of Golgi-Mazzoni.*

Meissner's Corpuscles (Tactile). These are presumed to subserve touch. They are found in dermal papillae, being most numerous in fingertips, soles and palms, lips, glans penis, and clitoris.

Pacinian Corpuscles. Pacinian corpuscles are found throughout subcutaneous tissue and are especially numerous in the hand, foot, mammary glands, clitoris, and penis. These corpuscles are pressure receptors.

End Bulb of Krause and End Bulb of Golgi-Mazzoni. These endings are found throughout the body. Many variants of these structures have been identified. They are presumed to subserve heat and cold.

Muscle and Tendon Spindles. The muscle spindles and annulospiral endings in muscles, as well as the tendon spindles and free nerve endings in muscles, are proprioceptive endings which transmit information concerning muscular activity and tendon stretching to the central nervous system.

Supporting Cells

There are billions of neurons in the central nervous system, but the number of non-nervous cells exceed them by five or six times. The *astrocytes, oligodendrocytes, microglia, and ependyma* are the supporting cells or *neuroglia (nerve glue)* of the central nervous system, while the Schwann cells, satellite cells, and fibroblasts are the supporting cells of the peripheral nervous system. These cells thus form the structural matrix of the central nervous system, but they also play a vital role in transporting gas, water, electrolytes, and metabolites from blood vessels to the neural parenchyma and in removing waste products from the neuron. In contrast to the neurons, the supporting cells in the adult CNS normally undergo mitotic divisions.

Astrocytes. Astrocytes form the skeleton of the central nervous system, tend to segregate synapses in the CNS, and help to form a barrier at the inner and outer surfaces of the brain and around the blood vessels. In combination with endothelial cells they help to form the blood-brain barrier.

Oligodendrocytes. These cells form and maintain—and may also digest—myelin.

Microglia. The nerve cells, astrocytes, and oligodendrocytes are ectodermal in origin, whereas the microglial cells are mesodermal in origin. These ovoid cells are the smallest of the supporting cells. They have been called multipotential cells since they appear to be able to act as a phagocyte or to become an astrocyte or oligodendrocyte.

Mononuclear Cells (Lymphocytes, Monocytes, Histiocytes). These cells also seem to act as phagocytes, breaking down the myelin and the nerve cells.

Ependymal Cells. The ependymal cells line all parts of the ventricular system.

Satellite Cells. These are found in sensory and sympathetic ganglia. Functionally, they are similar to astrocytes.

Schwann Cells. The Schwann cell in the peripheral nervous system functions like the oligodendrocyte, forming the myelin and neurilemmal sheath.

NERVE CELL PHYSIOLOGY

Research has demonstrated four very important and interesting properties of nerve cells:

1. There are gross inequalities of chemical concentration between the inside and outside of the cells.

2. The solution inside the cell is electrically negative with respect to the outside solution.

3. Some ions move through the cell membrane more easily than others.

4. The ease with which certain ions move through the cell membrane can vary in time.

These four properties are interrelated and form the basis of all cell function in the nervous system.

THE CHEMICAL POTENTIAL

Cells exist in aqueous solutions. Consequently, it is the *energy of aqueous systems* and their potential for doing work that are of interest to us in the study of cell physiology. The potential factor, called the *chemical potential*, is analogous to all the other potential factors, such as height, temperature, pressure, or voltage. The *capacity factor* is the number of moles involved in the reaction. It is obvious, therefore, that the chemical potential of a simple reactant is primarily a very simple function of concentration.

In the study of the movement of a substance through cell membranes, an important factor is the difference in chemical potential between the inside of the cell and the outside solution. If the substance is moving from a region of low chemical potential to one of high chemical potential we know immediately that energy must be expended. The chemical potential is thus seen to be a potential function. It is expected that energy will flow from a phase of greater chemical potential to a phase of lower chemical potential. The maximum work we can get from a system is equal to the product of the chemical potential times the number of moles involved. If, however, the chemical potential in two phases is equal, no energy will flow; they are in equilibrium.

ELECTRICAL POTENTIAL OF NERVE CELLS

When an electrode is placed inside a nerve axon, the axoplasm is found to be 70 to 90 millivolts (0.07 to 0.09 volt) negative with respect to the bathing fluid. This negative potential is called the *resting potential*. When the distal end of the axon is stimulated by an electric current, the potential suddenly becomes 40 millivolts (mV) positive and just as suddenly (1 to 2 milliseconds) returns to the resting level. This transient change in potential is called an *action potential*.

The action potential always has the same duration and magnitude, no matter where it is measured in the nervous system. When the action potential is measured at several places, each successively farther away from the stimulating electrode, the potential change occurs at successively greater intervals after the stimulus occurs; the action potential is propagated down the axon at a finite velocity. Conduction velocities range from 1 to 100 meters per second.

Since the action potential always has the same magnitude and duration, there must be many "repeater stations" along the nerve. At each of these stations the action potential is renewed.

A single action potential traveling into the central nervous system along a single nerve can inform the system of its presence or occurrence. More complex messages can be carried only by varying the interval between action potentials. The interval between action potentials is the reciprocal of frequency.

The *resting potential* is basically a *potassium equilibrium* potential and as such the cell does not need to expend energy to maintain it. The *action potential*, however, is dominated by the *sodium ion*. The upswing of the action potential represents a brief change in the properties of the cell membrane, so that sodium is the dominantly permeable ion. Since the membrane potential is controlled by the dominantly permeable ion, the potential moves toward a sodium equilibrium potential of +40 to 50 mV. For some reason the increased sodium permeability subsides very soon after its onset and the potential returns to the resting level.

ACTION POTENTIAL PROPAGATION

The mechanism by which the action potential spreads down the axon is simply the spreading of current from the active to the inactive regions. The potential of the active region is very close to the sodium equilibrium potential, whereas the potential of the resting region, a little further down the axon, is close to the potassium equilibrium potential. Ions will flow between these two regions of unequal potential. When the ionic flow crosses the membrane of the resting region, it depolarizes the membrane to threshold, the sodium permeability increases, resulting in further depolarization, and an action potential is generated in the previously resting region.

Refractory Period.   Immediately after an action potential, the axon is incapable of carrying a second action potential. This period lasts for about the duration of the action potential (1 to 2 msec.). This absolute refractory period is followed by a relative refractory period during which a supranormal stimulus is necessary to evoke an action potential. This period lasts for another 2 to 3 msec. These two refractory periods put an upper limit on the nerve's frequency response to about 200 per second.

Local Anesthetics.   Local anesthetics are widely used to block nerve conduction in the peripheral nervous system. Procaine specifically blocks the increase of sodium permeability with voltage. Since the sodium permeability does not increase, the axon remains as a passive cable and will not conduct a nerve impulse. At the same time, the potassium current is reduced; the membrane resistance has increased. Local anesthetics do not change the resting membrane potential.

Local anesthetics affect small nerve fibers before affecting large nerve fibers. Consequently, pain fibers are blocked before motor fibers. As the anesthesia wears off, the small fibers are the last to recover.

REFERENCES

1. American Medical Association: Fundamentals of Anesthesia. Philadelphia, W. B. Saunders Co., 1954.
2. Guedel, A. E.: Inhalation Anesthesia. New York, The Macmillan Co., 1953.
3. Monheim, L. M.: General Anesthesia in Dental Practice. St. Louis, The C. V. Mosby Co., 1957.
4. Ruch, T. C., and Patton, H. D.: Physiology and Biophysics. 19th ed. W. B. Saunders Co., 1965.
5. Curtis, B. A., Jacobson, S., and Marcus, E. M.: An Introduction to the Neurosciences. Philadelphia, W. B. Saunders Co., 1972.
6. McLennan, H.: Synaptic Transmission. 2nd ed. Philadelphia, W. B. Saunders Co., 1970.

RESPIRATION

3

Arthur C. Guyton*

In physiology, the term respiration originally referred to the inspiration and expiration of air. The meaning of this term was broadened by the discovery of carbon dioxide in expired air (Joseph Black, 1757), the discovery and investigation of the properties of oxygen (Joseph Priestley, 1774), and an appreciation of the true objective of the act of respiration (Antoine Lavoisier, 1777). Today the term respiration includes *external respiration*, all the mechanisms and processes involved in the exchange of gases across the pulmonary and capillary membranes; and *internal respiration*, the many reactions by which gases are diffused between the capillaries and individual body cells.

Living systems continually expend energy. This energy is derived within the cells of the body from the oxidation of organic substances to carbon dioxide and other products. The carbon dioxide must be eliminated. The necessary gas exchange occurs in a very simple manner at the cellular level. In single-celled organisms, the individual cell is in contact with its external environment, and by the process of diffusion oxygen and carbon dioxide are exchanged. Of course, as an organism becomes more complex, this simple process is insufficient to meet the demand for oxygen. Consequently, nature has evolved auxiliary means to aid in this process of gas exchange. The air tubes of insects, the gills of fishes, and the lungs of mammals are examples of these auxiliary means. They provide extensive surfaces through which the respiratory gases are easily exchanged. The hemoglobin of man is an example of a specialized chemical compound which facilitates the transportation of oxygen to the tissues.

Since respiration means the transport of oxygen from the atmosphere to the cells and, in turn, the transport of carbon dioxide from the cells back to the atmosphere, this process could be thought of as being divided into four major stages: (1) *pulmonary ventilation*, which means the actual inflow and outflow of air between the atmosphere and the alveoli; (2) *diffusion* of oxygen and carbon dioxide between the alveoli and the blood; (3) *transport* of oxygen and carbon dioxide in the blood and body fluids to and from the cells; and (4) *regulation* of ventilation and other aspects of respiration.

---

*Adapted from Guyton, A. C.: Textbook of Medical Physiology. 5th Ed. Philadelphia, W. B. Saunders Co., 1976.

The gas conduction system comprises the nasal cavity, the pharynx, the larynx, the trachea, and the bronchi and their subdivisions, the bronchioles. As air is conveyed through this system, it is filtered, humidified, and brought to body temperature; that is, it is *conditioned* before it reaches the diffusion surfaces of the lungs and capillaries.

The diffusion or respiratory surfaces of the lung are reached as the bronchioles give off smaller branches called respiratory bronchioles, which in turn divide to form alveolar ducts. The alveolar ducts, which are the last subdivision of the bronchial tree, open out into a number of irregularly spherical cavities called atria. Each atrium opens into a number of irregular chambers, called alveolar sacs, the walls of which are pouched to form alveoli. Each respiratory bronchiole with its dependent alveolar ducts, atria, alveolar sacs, and alveoli constitutes a primary lobule, which forms the functional unit of the lungs. The extremely thin walls of the alveoli contain a rich capillary network, and it is here that the respiratory exchange between the blood and the alveolar air takes place.

PULMONARY VENTILATION

Mechanics of Respiration

BASIC MECHANISMS OF LUNG EXPANSION AND CONTRACTION

The lungs can be expanded and contracted by (a) downward and upward movement of the diaphragm to lengthen or shorten the chest cavity, and (b) elevation and depression of the ribs to increase and decrease the anteroposterior diameter of the chest cavity.

It is readily evident that contraction of the diaphragm pulls the lower boundary of the chest cavity downward and therefore increases the longitudinal length. Upward movement of the diaphragm during normal breathing is caused by simple relaxation of the diaphragm, thus permitting the elastic

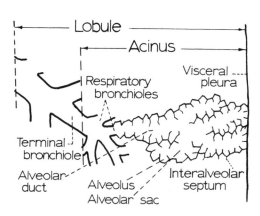

Figure 3-1 Diagrammatic representation of the mammalian respiratory unit. The terminal bronchiole gives rise to 10 to 20 respiratory bronchioles, each of which widens into alveolar ducts with many hundreds of alveoli. The alveolar duct often has several major partitions, the so-called alveolar sacs. Interalveolar septa are shown extending into the sacs; the irregular small spaces thus formed are the alveoli. (From J. Hildebrandt and A. C. Young, *in* T. C. Ruch and H. D. Patton: Physiology and Biophysics. 20th ed. Vol. II. Philadelphia, W. B. Saunders Co., 1965.)

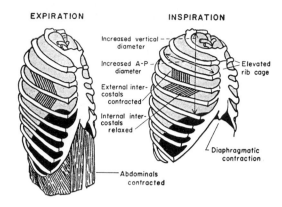

Figure 3–2 Expansion and contraction of the thoracic cage during expiration and inspiration, illustrating especially diaphragmatic contraction, elevation of the rib cage, and function of the intercostals. (From Guyton, 1976.)

recoil of the lungs and pulling the diaphragm upward; in heavy breathing it is also caused by active contraction of the abdominal muscles, which forces the abdominal contents upward against the bottom of the diaphragm.

Elevation of the anterior portion of the chest cage causes the anteroposterior dimension of the chest cavity to increase by the following mechanism: During expiration the ribs extend in a downward direction from the spinal column, but when the sternum is lifted upward, the ribs then extend almost directly forward rather than downward. This makes the anteroposterior diameter of the chest about 20 per cent greater during inspiration than during expiration. Therefore, muscles that elevate the chest cage can be classified as muscles of inspiration, and muscles that depress the chest cage as muscles of expiration.

Normal quiet breathing is accomplished almost entirely by movement of the diaphragm; but during maximal breathing, increase in chest thickness might account for more than half of the lung enlargement.

The Muscles of Inspiration and Expiration

MUSCLES OF INSPIRATION

> Diaphragm
> External intercostals
> Sternocleidomastoids
> Scapular elevators plus anterior serrati
> Scaleni
> Erectus muscles of the spine

MUSCLES OF EXPIRATION

> Abdominals (major muscles of expiration)
> Internal intercostals
> Posterior inferior serrati

THE DIAPHRAGM AND THE ABDOMINAL MUSCLES

Normal *inspiration* is caused principally by contraction of the diaphragm. This muscle is bell-shaped, so that contraction of any of its muscle fibers pulls it downward to cause inspiration.

Ordinarily, expiration is an entirely passive process; that is, when the diaphragm relaxes, the elastic structures of the lung, chest cage, and abdomen, as well as the tone of the abdominal muscles, force the diaphragm upward. However, if forceful expiration is required, the diaphragm can also be pushed upward powerfully by active contraction of the abdominal muscles against the abdominal contents. Thus, all the abdominal muscles combined together represent the major muscles of expiration.

MUSCLES THAT RAISE AND LOWER THE CHEST CAGE

Three different groups of muscles cause inspiration by elevating the entire chest cage. The *sternocleidomastoid* muscles lift upward on the sternum; the *anterior serrati* lift many of the ribs; and the *scaleni* lift the first two ribs. Because the anterior margins of most of the ribs are connected to the sternum, lifting one portion of the anterior chest cage lifts it all.

To cause expiration, the abdominal recti, in addition to helping to compress the abdominal contents upward against the diaphragm, also pull downward on the lower ribs, thereby decreasing the anteroposterior diameter of the chest. Thus, these muscles act as muscles of expiration both by depressing the rib cage and by compressing the abdominal contents upward.

The external and internal intercostals are also important muscles of respiration despite their small size.

Respiratory Pressures

INTRA-ALVEOLAR PRESSURE

The respiratory muscles cause pulmonary ventilation by alternatively compressing and distending the lungs, which in turn causes the pressure in the alveoli to rise and fall. During inspiration the intra-alveolar pressure becomes slightly negative with respect to atmospheric pressure, normally about −3 mm. Hg, and this causes air to flow inward through the respiratory passageways. During normal expiration the intra-alveolar pressure rises to approximately +3 mm. Hg, which causes air to flow outward through the respiratory passageways. During maximum expiratory effort the intra-alveolar pressure can usually be increased to well over 100 mm. Hg, and during maximum inspiratory effort it can usually be reduced to as low as −80 mm. Hg.

FLUID PRESSURE IN THE INTRAPLEURAL CAVITY

The lungs are physically attached to the body only at their hila, whereas their outer surfaces have no attachment whatsoever to the chest wall. However, the membranes of the intrapleural space constantly absorb any gas or fluid that enters this space; this absorption creates a partial vacuum that makes the lungs expand.

The normal pressure of the fluid in the intrapleural space is between —10 and —12 mm. Hg. This negative pressure acts as a suction force to hold the visceral pleura of the lungs tightly against the parietal pleura of the chest wall. When the chest cavity enlarges, this suction causes the lungs also to enlarge. And when the chest cavity becomes smaller, the lungs likewise become smaller. The lungs slide up and down in the chest cavity during respiration, the visceral pleura sliding over the parietal pleura, lubricated by the few milliliters of mucopolysaccharide-containing fluid in the intrapleural space.

The cause of the very negative intrapleural fluid pressure is the continual tendency of the pleural capillaries to absorb fluid from the intrapleural spaces. This is particularly true of the visceral pleural capillaries because these are part of the pulmonary circulatory system and have a very low capillary pressure of about 7 mm. Hg, which causes rapid absorption of fluid.

RECOIL TENDENCY OF THE LUNGS

The lungs have a continual tendency to collapse and therefore to recoil away from the chest wall. This tendency is caused by two different factors. First, there are many *elastic fibers* throughout the lungs which are constantly stretched and are attempting to shorten. Second, and even more important, the *surface tension* of the fluid lining the alveoli also causes a continual elastic tendency for the alveoli to collapse. This effect is brought about by intermolecular attraction between the surface molecules of the fluid that tends continually to reduce the surface areas of the individual alveoli; all these minute forces added together tend to collapse the whole lung and therefore to cause its recoil away from the chest wall.

EXPANSIBILITY OF THE LUNGS AND THORAX: "COMPLIANCE"

The lungs are viscoelastic structures. Therefore, a small amount of intra-alveolar pressure causes them to expand to a certain volume, more pressure causes them to expand to a still greater volume, and so forth. The thorax also has viscoelastic properties, so that the greater the pressure in the lungs, the greater becomes the expansion of the chest. As mentioned previously, the elastic properties of the lungs are caused by the surface tension of the fluids lining the alveoli, and by elastic fibers throughout the lung tissue itself. The elastic properties of the thorax are caused by the natural elasticity of the muscles, tendons, and connective tissue of the chest. Therefore, part of the effort expended by the inspiratory muscles during breathing is simply to stretch the elastic structures of the lungs and thorax.

The expansibility of the lungs and thorax is called *compliance*. This is expressed as the *volume increase in the lungs for each unit increase in intra-alveolar pressure*. The compliance of the normal lungs and thorax combined is 0.13 liter per centimeter of water pressure. That is, every time the alveolar pressure is increased by 1 cm. water, the lungs expand 130 ml.

THE "WORK" OF BREATHING

When the lungs are stretched, energy is expended by the respiratory muscles to cause the stretching. In addition, two other factors that impede the expansion and contraction of the lungs have to be overcome. These are *viscosity of the pulmonary tissues (nonelastic tissue resistance)* and *airway resistance.*

Nonelastic Tissue Resistance. This term simply means that a certain amount of energy is required to rearrange the molecules in the tissues of the lungs and thoracic cage in order to change them to new dimensions. This requires the slipping of molecules over each other, which constitutes a type of viscous resistance.

Airway Resistance. A certain amount of energy is also required to move the air along the respiratory passageways. In normal quiet breathing, this amount of energy is slight, but, when the airway becomes obstructed as a result of asthma, obstructive emphysema, diphtheria, and so forth, the airway resistance may become so greatly increased that a large amount of extra energy must be expended by the respiratory muscles simply to force the air back and forth through the narrow passageways.

THE PULMONARY VOLUMES AND CAPACITIES

1. The *tidal volume* is the volume of air inspired and expired with each normal breath. This amounts to about 500 ml. in the normal young male adult.

2. The *inspiratory reserve volume* is the extra volume of air that can be inspired over and beyond the normal tidal volume. It is usually about 3000 ml. in the young male adult.

3. The *expiratory reserve volume* is the amount of air that can still be expired by forceful expiration after the end of a normal tidal expiration—about 1100 ml. in the young male adult.

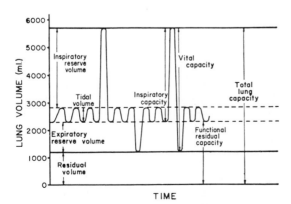

Figure 3–3 Diagram showing respiratory excursions during normal breathing and during maximal inspiration and maximal expiration. (From Guyton, 1976.)

4. *The residual volume* is the volume of air remaining in the lungs even after the most forceful expiration. This volume averages about 1200 ml. in the young male adult. The residual volume is important because it provides air in the alveoli to aerate the blood even between breaths. Were it not for the residual air, the concentrations of oxygen and carbon dioxide in the blood would rise and fall markedly with each respiration. This would be disadvantageous to the respiratory process.

5. *The inspiratory capacity* equals the *tidal volume* plus the *inspiratory reserve volume.* This is the amount of air (about 3500 ml.) that a person can breathe beginning at the normal expiratory level and distending his lungs to the maximum amount.

6. *The functional residual capacity* equals the *expiratory reserve volume* plus the *residual volume.* This is the amount of air remaining in the lungs at the end of normal expiration (about 2300 ml).

7. *The vital capacity* equals the *inspiratory reserve volume* plus the *expiratory reserve volume.* This is the maximum amount of air that a person can expel from his lungs after first filling his lungs to their maximum extent and then expiring to the maximum extent (about 4600 ml.). Other than the anatomical build of a person, the major factors affecting vital capacity are: the position of the person during the vital capacity measurement, the strength of the respiratory muscles, and the distensibility of the lungs and chest cage (compliance).

8. *The total lung capacity* is the maximum volume to which the lungs can be expanded with the greatest possible inspiratory effort (about 5800 ml.).

All pulmonary volumes and capacities are about 20 to 25 per cent less in the female than in the male, and are obviously greater in large and athletic persons than in smaller and asthenic persons.

9. *The minute respiratory volume* is the total amount of new air moved into the respiratory passages each minute. This equals the *tidal volume* × the *respiratory rate.* The normal tidal volume of a young male adult is 500 ml., and the normal respiratory rate is approximately 12 to 15 breaths per minute. Therefore, the minute respiratory volume averages about 7 to 8 liters per minute.

VENTILATION OF THE ALVEOLI

The important factor in the entire pulmonary ventilatory process is the rate at which the alveolar air is renewed each minute by atmospheric air; this is called *alveolar ventilation.* Alveolar ventilation per minute is not equal to the minute respiratory volume because a large portion of the inspired air goes to fill the respiratory passageways, the membranes of which are not capable of significant gaseous exchange with the blood. This is called *dead air space.* On inspiration, much of the new air must first fill the nasal passageways, the pharynx, the trachea, and the bronchi before any reaches the alveoli. Then, on expiration, all the air in the dead space is expired first before any of the air from the alveoli reaches the atmosphere. The volume of air that enters the alveoli with each breath, therefore, is equal to the tidal volume minus the dead space volume. Alveolar ventilation per minute = respiratory rate × (tidal volume − dead space volume). A normal dead space volume is 150 ml.

Alveolar ventilation is one of the major factors determining the concentrations of oxygen and carbon dioxide in the alveoli. The respiratory rate, the tidal volume, and the minute respiratory volume are of importance only insofar as they affect alveolar ventilation.

FUNCTIONS OF THE RESPIRATORY PASSAGEWAYS

The Nose. As air passes through the nose, three distinct functions are performed by the nasal cavities: First, the *air is warmed* by the extensive surfaces of the turbinates and septum. Second, the *air is moistened* to a considerable extent. Third, the *air is filtered.* These are called the *air conditioning functions* of the upper respiratory passageways.

The Cough Reflex. The cough reflex is almost essential to life, for the cough is the means by which the passageways of the lungs are maintained free of foreign matter.

The bronchi and the trachea are so sensitive that any foreign matter or other cause of irritation initiates the cough reflex. The larynx and the carina (the point where the trachea divides into the bronchi) are especially sensitive, and the terminal bronchioles and alveoli are particularly sensitive to corrosive chemical stimuli, such as sulfur dioxide gas and chlorine. Afferent impulses pass from the respiratory passages mainly through the vagus nerve to the

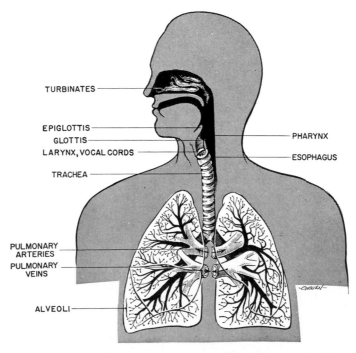

Figure 3-4   The respiratory passages. (From Guyton, 1976.)

medulla. There, an automatic sequence of events is triggered by the neuronal circuits of the medulla, causing the following effects:

First, about 2.5 liters of air is inspired. Second, the epiglottis closes, and the vocal cords shut tightly to entrap the air within the lungs. Third, the abdominal muscles contract forcefully, pushing against the diaphragm while other expiratory muscles, such as the internal intercostals, also contract forcefully. Consequently, the pressure in the lungs usually rises to 100 mm. Hg or more. Fourth, the vocal cords and the epiglottis suddenly open widely so that the air under pressure in the lungs *explodes* outward. This air is sometimes expelled at velocities as high as 75 to 100 miles per hour. Furthermore, and very importantly, the strong compression of the lungs also collapses the bronchi and trachea so that the exploding air actually passes through bronchial and tracheal slits. The rapidly moving air usually carries with it any foreign matter that is present in the bronchi or trachea.

The Sneeze Reflex. The sneeze reflex is very much like the cough reflex except that it applies to the nasal passageways instead of to the lower respiratory passages. The initiating stimulus of the sneeze reflex is irritation in the nasal passageways, the afferent impulses passing in the fifth nerve to the medulla, where the reflex is triggered. A series of reactions similar to those for the cough reflex takes place; however, the uvula is depressed so that large amounts of air pass rapidly through the nose, as well as through the mouth, thus helping to clear the nasal passages of foreign matter.

Artificial Respiration

MANUAL METHODS OF ARTIFICIAL RESPIRATION: THE BACK-PRESSURE ARM-LIFT METHOD

A dozen or more different manual methods of artificial respiration have been advocated and practiced for many years. In general, all depend on a few seconds' compression of the chest to cause expiration, followed in some instances by a few seconds' lifting of some portion of the body to help inspiration. Even with the best of these manual methods a tidal volume of no greater than 500 to 700 ml. can usually be sustained for long periods of time.

The manual method now advocated by the American Red Cross is the back-pressure arm-lift method, which is also called the *Holger-Nielsen method*. This consists of the following maneuvers:

The patient is placed on his face, and his arms are folded in front of his head. The operator kneels in front of the patient's head and performs two operations in rhythmical sequence, approximately 12 to 15 times per minute. First, he places his hands on the back of the patient over approximately the lower half of the scapulae and compresses with about 30 to 40 pounds' pressure. Second, after 2 or 3 seconds he removes this pressure and then grasps the subject under his upper arms and lifts. These two operations cause expiration and then inspiration. The cycle is repeated.

Especially important in any method of artificial respiration is *maintenance of a free airway* through the mouth or nose to the trachea. The tongue of the patient has a tendency to fall into the back of the throat and obstruct the airway. Sometimes it is necessary to pull the tongue forward, and, if available, a special airway device—a curved hollow tube—is inserted through the mouth.

MOUTH-TO-MOUTH BREATHING

A very successful method of artificial respiration is mouth-to-mouth breathing, in which the operator rapidly inspires deeply and then breathes into the mouth of the subject. This method has often been shunned in the past because of the belief that the expired air of the operator would not be beneficial to the subject. This is not true, because normal expired air usually still has an adequate amount of oxygen to sustain life in almost anyone. Additionally, the carbon dioxide in the expired air is sometimes actually desirable because it helps to stimulate the respiratory center of the subject.

MECHANICAL METHODS OF ARTIFICIAL RESPIRATION

Many types of resuscitators are available and each has its own characteristic principles of operation. Basically, they all consist of a supply of oxygen or air, a mechanism for applying intermittent positive and sometimes negative pressure, and a mask which fits over the face of the patient. This apparatus forces air through the mask into the lungs of the patient during the positive pressure cycle and then either allows the air to flow out of the lungs during the remainder of the cycle or pulls the air out by negative pressure.

Earlier resuscitators often caused such severe damage to the lungs because of excessive positive pressures that their usage was at one time greatly depreciated. However, all resuscitators now have safety valves which prevent the positive pressure from rising usually above +14 mm. Hg, and the negative pressure from falling below −9 mm. Hg. These pressure limits are adequate to cause excellent artificial respiration of *normal lungs* and yet are slight enough to prevent damage.

DIFFUSION OF OXYGEN AND CARBON DIOXIDE THROUGH THE RESPIRATORY MEMBRANE (EXTERNAL RESPIRATION)

After the alveoli are ventilated with fresh air, the next step in the respiratory process is *diffusion* of oxygen from the alveoli into the pulmonary blood and diffusion of carbon dioxide in the opposite direction from the pulmonary blood into the alveoli. The process of diffusion is simple, involving merely random molecular motion of molecules, wending their ways back and forth through the respiratory membrane. However, in respiratory physiology we are concerned not only with the basic mechanism by which diffusion occurs but also with the *rate* at which it occurs. We must, therefore, discuss first the physical factors that determine the alveolar concentrations of gases, and secondly, the factors that affect the rate at which these gases can diffuse through the respiratory membrane.

The exchange of respiratory gases through the alveolar epithelium and capillary endothelium takes place with great rapidity. Venous blood enters the lung capillaries with a partial pressure of oxygen below that of alveolar air and a partial pressure of carbon dioxide above that of alveolar air. This blood remains in the alveolar capillaries about 0.7 second, but in this short time it comes to practical equilibrium with the alveolar air. The time required for all the circulating blood to pass through the lungs is approximately 1 minute.

The rate at which gas exchange takes place across the alveolar surface is governed by the following factors:

1. The true partial pressures of the respiratory gases in the alveolar air and the capillary blood.

2. The permeability of the membranes to oxygen and carbon dioxide.

3. The rates of reaction of the different gases with the blood.

4. The area of the absorbing surface.

5. The period of time that the blood is in contact with the respiratory surfaces.

6. The volume of blood exposed to alveolar air at any given time.

THE PHYSICS OF GASES

In order to understand how respired gases and inhalation anesthetics act in the body one must be familiar with the simple properties of gases and liquids. Basic to the discussion is the kinetic concept of fluids. Fluids are composed of particles (molecules) that are in ceaseless motion, continually colliding with each other and with the vessel in which they are contained. The pressure exerted by a fluid is equal to the total impact force of the molecules against the confining wall.

Although the molecules of liquids move around a great deal, they are so close together that they are subject to strong intermolecular attractive forces. Therefore, liquids have a volume independent of the container, and they can exert both pressure and tension in a closed space.

In contrast, the molecules of gases are far apart, and the attraction of one particle for another is very low. Thus, the incessant motion of the particles of a gas causes it to completely fill all the available volume of a container. Gases therefore exert only pressure. The behavior of gases may be explained by simple laws and principles.

Pressure of Gases (Boyle's Law). The pressure of a gas is inversely proportional to its volume (temperature remaining constant). Decreasing the volume of a gas increases the number of particles per unit volume and thus the number of collisions against the walls of the container: the result is an increase in pressure.

The Measurement of Gas Pressure. The pressure of a gas may be indicated by (1) the height to which the gas forces a liquid (water or mercury) in a tube, and (2) the force exerted in terms of weight per unit area (pounds per square inch, grams per square centimeter). Data essential to the measurement of a gas are its temperature, pressure, and volume. Pressure in excess of atmospheric pressure is termed positive pressure; pressure at less than atmospheric pressure is negative pressure. The volume of a gas is usually indicated at standard conditions: 0°C. and 76 cm. Hg pressure. In gas exchange within the body, pressure is also referred to as tension.

Two instruments used in the measurement of gas pressure are:

Manometers.   There are two types, closed and open, each consisting of a calibrated U-shaped tube partially filled with mercury or water.

Pressure Gauges.   In these instruments, the gas exerts a force directly upon a metal diaphragm, which expands and contracts with variations in pressure. These changes are then amplified by a system of levers which control the position of the indicator of a dial. Pressure gauges, which are usually calibrated in pounds per square inch, are suitable for measuring high pressure.

Expansion of Gases (Charles' Law).   The pressure of a gas is directly proportional to its absolute temperature (volume remaining constant). Increasing the temperature of a gas causes an increase in the velocity of the molecules, and thus an increase in the total number of collisions against the walls of the container.

Molecular Weight of Gases (Avogadro's Principle).   At equal temperatures and pressures, equal volumes of gases contain the same number of molecules.

Dalton's Law of Partial Pressures.   In a mixture of gases, each gas behaves as if it alone occupied the total volume and exerts a pressure (its own partial pressure) independently of the other gases present. In any one container having a mixture of several gases, the sum of the partial pressures is equal to the total pressure.

Solubility of Gases (Henry's Law).   The quantity of gas physically dissolved in a liquid at constant temperature is directly proportional to the partial pressure of the gas.

Diffusion of Gases (Graham's Law).   The rate of diffusion of one gas compared to another varies inversely as the square root of their molecular weights. The molecules of a gas or vapor in a closed space distribute equally throughout the space and exert an equal pressure upon all surfaces of the enclosure. The process of distribution of the molecules of a gas in a space is called diffusion.

Pressure Gradient.   A gas or vapor diffuses from an area of higher concentration to one of lower concentration. The difference between the two levels of pressure is called the pressure gradient.

Joule-Thompson Effect.   When a gas passes from a higher pressure to a lower through a porous plug, there is a change in temperature (either a heating or a cooling), depending on the interactions of the molecules of the gas.

Bernoulli's Principle.   The pressure of a fluid in motion through a tube of varying cross sectional areas is least at the narrowest portion, where speed is greatest, and is greatest at the widest portion, where speed is least. Gases behave like fluids but, because they are compressible, they deviate somewhat from this principle.

Liquefaction of Gases.   As a gas is compressed, its molecules are forced into a smaller volume of space. They are thus packed closer together and move faster, so that energy in the form of heat is liberated. Because of the reduction of intermolecular distances, cohesive forces are intensified and, if the compression is continued, condensation occurs and the substance becomes liquid. Certain gases, however, do not liquefy regardless of the pressure applied unless they are cooled. The temperature above which a gas cannot be liquefied by pressure is called the critical temperature.

Differences Between Gases and Vapors. Gases and vapors behave similarly in most respects, the essential difference being that a gas is a vapor existing at a temperature above the critical temperature, whereas a vapor exists at about the critical temperature of the liquid from which it is derived and therefore may be liquefied by pressure without cooling.

Heat Capacity of Gases and Vapors. Gases absorb and conduct heat, their heat capacity varying directly with their molecular weight. The number of calories required to heat a molecule of gas 1°C. is called the molal heat capacity.

PARTIAL PRESSURES

An understanding of partial pressures is an important preliminary to understanding gaseous diffusion from the alveoli to the pulmonary blood, for it is the partial pressure of a gas that determines the force it exerts in attempting to diffuse through the pulmonary membrane.

Figure 3–5 illustrates four separate chambers, each of which has a capacity of 100 volumes of gas. The second chamber is divided by a partition, and 79 volumes of nitrogen at 760 mm. Hg pressure (1 atmosphere of pressure) are placed above the partition and 21 volumes of oxygen at 760 mm. Hg are placed below. Then all the nitrogen in the upper part of chamber 2 is moved to chamber 1, which has a total capacity of 100 volumes. In other words, 79 volumes of nitrogen are expanded to 100 volumes. As this nitrogen is expanded, it can be shown from Boyle's Law that the pressure falls to 79/100 of 760 mm. Hg – that is, to 600 mm. Hg.

The 21 volumes of oxygen at 760 mm. Hg are moved from the second chamber to the third chamber. Here again it can be shown from Boyle's Law

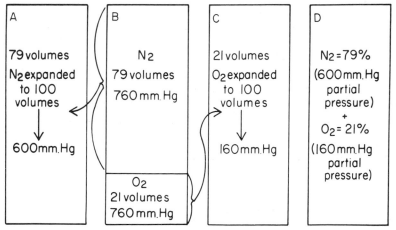

Figure 3–5 Relationship of partial pressures to gaseous percentages in mixtures of gases. (From Guyton, 1976.)

that this expansion causes the pressure of the oxygen to fall to 21/100 of 760 mm. Hg—that is, to 160 mm. Hg.

Finally, the nitrogen in the first chamber and the oxygen in the third chamber are mixed together in the fourth chamber. The original pressure of the nitrogen is 600 mm. Hg, and the pressure of the oxygen is 160 mm. Hg, but the total pressure in chamber 4 after mixing is 760 mm. Hg—the normal atmospheric pressure level. It is obvious that 600 mm. of this 760 mm. Hg results from the presence of nitrogen in the chamber, and 160 mm. results from the presence of oxygen in the chamber. The 600 mm. Hg pressure exerted by nitrogen and the 160 mm. Hg pressure exerted by the oxygen are known as the *partial pressures* of the respective gases in the mixture. The partial pressures of gases in a mixture are designated by the terms P_{O_2}, P_{CO_2}, P_{N_2}, P_{H_2}, and so forth.

From the kinetic theory of gases we know that pressures against any membrane or against any other surface are determined by the number of molecules striking a unit area of the membrane at any given instant times the average kinetic energy of the molecules. Therefore, the partial pressure of a gas in a mixture is in reality the sum of the force of impact of all the molecules of that particular gas against the surface. In other words, in chamber 4 the total force of the nitrogen molecules striking against the chamber walls is sufficient to elevate the mercury in a manometer to a level of 600 mm. The total force exerted by the oxygen molecules striking against the walls of the chamber is sufficient to elevate the mercury in a manometer to a level of 160 mm. With both these gases exerting force against the walls of the chamber at the same time, the mercury is elevated to a total level of 760 mm. Hg.

Molecules in a mixture of gases are constantly striking each other and thereby imparting energy to each other. As a result, each molecule of the mixture, regardless of its molecular weight, has the same kinetic energy as the next molecule. Therefore, the *partial pressure of a gas in a mixture is also a direct measure of the number of molecules of that particular gas striking a unit surface area in a given period of time.*

Because each gas in a mixture exerts its own partial pressure in proportion to the concentration of its molecules, when the gases of a mixture dissolve in a liquid until they come to equilibrium with the gaseous phase of the mixture, the pressure of each dissolved gas is equal to the partial pressure of the same gas in the gaseous mixture. In other words, *each gas is independent of the others in its ability to dissolve in a liquid.* This principle also applies to the solution of gases in blood. Thus, an increase in quantity of carbon dioxide dissolved in the body fluids does not significantly affect the quantity of oxygen that can be dissolved in the same fluids. However, the various dissolved gases often do interfere with the *chemical* reactions of each other.

DIFFUSION OF GASES THROUGH LIQUIDS

The rate of gas diffusion in a fluid depends on:
1. The pressure difference (diffusion gradient).
2. The solubility of the gas in the fluid.

3. The cross-sectional area of the fluid.
4. The distance through which the gas must diffuse.
5. The molecular weight of the gas.
6. The viscosity of the fluid.
7. The temperature of the fluid.

In the body, the last two of these factors (viscosity and temperature) remain reasonably constant and usually need not be considered.

The greater the solubility of a gas, the greater will be the number of molecules available to diffuse for any given pressure gradient.

The greater the cross-sectional area of the chamber, the greater will be the total number of molecules diffusing.

The longer the distance the molecules must diffuse, the longer it will take them to diffuse the entire distance.

The greater the velocity of kinetic movement of the molecules, which at any given temperature is inversely proportional to the square root of the molecular weight, the greater is the rate of diffusion of the gas.

All the factors are expressed in the following formula:

$$DR = \frac{PD \times A \times S}{D \times \sqrt{MW}}$$

DR = Diffusion rate
PD = Pressure difference between the two ends of the chamber
A = Cross-sectional area of the chamber
S = Solubility of the gas
D = Distance of diffusion
$\sqrt{MW}$ = Square root of the molecular weight of the gas

The above formula shows that the characteristics of the gas itself determine two factors of the formula: Solubility and molecular weight. Therefore, the *diffusion coefficient* (rate of diffusion through a given area for a given distance) for any given gas is proportional to $S/\sqrt{MW}$.

If the diffusion coefficient for oxygen is considered to be 1, the diffusion coefficients for the gases of respiratory importance in the body fluids are:

Oxygen	1.0
Carbon dioxide	20.3
Carbon monoxide	0.81
Nitrogen	0.53
Helium	0.95

DIFFUSION OF GASES THROUGH TISSUES

The gases that are of respiratory importance are highly soluble in lipids and in cell membranes. Because of this, these gases diffuse through the cell membranes with very little impediment. The major limitation to the movement of gases in tissues is the rate at which the gases can diffuse through the tissue fluids, not the cell membranes. Therefore, diffusion of gases through the tissues, including the pulmonary membrane, is almost equal to the diffusion rate through water (see Fig. 3–6).

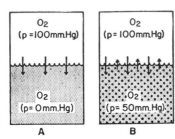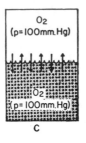

Figure 3-6 Solution of oxygen in water. *A,* When the oxygen first comes in contact with pure water; *B,* after the dissolved oxygen is halfway to equilibrium with the gaseous oxygen; *C,* after equilibrium has been established. (From Guyton, 1976.)

COMPOSITION OF ALVEOLAR AIR

Alveolar air does not have the same concentration of gases as atmospheric air. There are several reasons for this difference. First, alveolar air is only partially replaced by atmospheric air with each breath. Second, oxygen is constantly being absorbed from the alveolar air. Third, carbon dioxide is constantly diffusing from the pulmonary blood into the alveoli. And fourth, dry atmospheric air that enters the respiratory passages is *humidifed* even before it reaches the alveoli. Humidification of the air reduces the oxygen partial pressure at sea level from an average of 159 mm. Hg in atmospheric air to 149 mm. Hg, and reduces the nitrogen partial pressure from 597 to 563 mm. Hg.

RATE AT WHICH ALVEOLAR AIR IS RENEWED BY ATMOSPHERIC AIR

The amount of air remaining in the lungs at the end of normal expiration (*functional residual capacity*) is approximately 2300 ml. Furthermore, only 350 ml. of new air is brought into the alveoli with each normal inspiration. It can thus be seen that the amount of alveolar air replaced by new atmospheric air with each breath is only one seventh of the total, so that many breaths are required to exchange most of the alveolar air. This slow replacement of alveolar air is important in preventing sudden changes in gaseous concentrations in the blood. As a result, the respiratory control mechanism is much more stable in helping to prevent excessive increases and decreases in tissue oxygenation, tissue carbon dioxide concentration, and tissue pH when the respiration is temporarily interrupted.

OXYGEN CONCENTRATION IN THE ALVEOLI

Oxygen is continually being absorbed in the blood, and new oxygen is continually entering the alveoli from the atmosphere. The more rapidly oxygen is absorbed, the lower becomes its concentration in the alveoli; the more rapidly new oxygen is brought into the alveoli from the atmosphere, the higher its concentration becomes. Oxygen concentration in the alveoli is determined by the rate of absorption of oxygen into the blood, and by the rate of entry of new oxygen into the lungs.

CARBON DIOXIDE CONCENTRATION IN THE LUNGS

Carbon dioxide is continually being formed in the body, then discharged into the alveoli. It is also continually being removed from the alveoli by ventilation. The two factors controlling carbon dioxide partial pressure (P_{CO_2}) in the lungs are the rate of excretion from the blood into the lungs, and the rate at which carbon dioxide is removed from the lungs by ventilation.

DIFFUSION OF GASES THROUGH THE RESPIRATORY MEMBRANE

The *respiratory unit* is composed of a respiratory bronchiole, alveolar ducts, atria, and alveolar sacs or alveoli. There are about 250 million alveoli in the two lungs, each alveolus having an average diameter of 0.1 mm. The epithelium of these structures is a very thin membrane, and the alveolar gases are in close proximity to the blood of the capillaries. Consequently, gaseous exchange occurs very readily through these terminal portions of the lungs, which are collectively known as the *respiratory* or *pulmonary membrane.*

FACTORS AFFECTING GASEOUS DIFFUSION THROUGH THE RESPIRATORY MEMBRANE

1. The thickness of the membrane.
2. The surface area of the membrane.
3. Diffusion coefficient of the gas in the substance of the membrane.
4. The pressure difference between the two sides of the membrane.

TRANSPORT OF OXYGEN AND CARBON DIOXIDE IN THE BLOOD AND BODY FLUIDS

It has been pointed out that gases can move from one point to another by diffusion and that the cause of the movement is always a pressure difference from one point to the other. Thus, oxygen diffuses from the alveoli into the pulmonary capillary blood because the alveolar pressure (P_{O_2}) is greater than the pulmonary blood P_{O_2}. The pulmonary blood is then transported to the peripheral tissues. There the P_{O_2} is still lower in the cells than in the arterial blood, causing the oxygen to diffuse out of the capillaries and through the interstitial spaces to the cells.

Conversely, when oxygen is metabolized with the foods in the cells to form carbon dioxide, the P_{CO_2} in the cells is greater than the P_{CO_2} of the tissue capillaries, causing it to diffuse out from the cells to the blood. Once in the blood the carbon dioxide is transported to the pulmonary capillaries from which it diffuses out to the alveoli, since the P_{CO_2} in the alveoli is lower than that in the pulmonary capillary blood.

The transport of oxygen and carbon dioxide by the blood depends on both diffusion and the movement of blood.

UPTAKE OF OXYGEN BY THE PULMONARY BLOOD

The top part of Figure 3–7 illustrates a pulmonary alveolus adjacent to a pulmonary capillary, showing the diffusion of oxygen molecules between the alveolar air and the pulmonary blood. The P_{O_2} of the venous blood entering the capillary is only 40 mm. Hg because a large amount of oxygen was removed from this blood when it passed through the tissue capillaries. The P_{O_2} in the alveolus is 104 mm. Hg, providing an initial pressure difference for diffusion of oxygen into the pulmonary capillary of 64 mm. Hg. The graph below the capillary shows the progressive rise in blood P_{O_2} as the blood passes through the capillary. This illustrates that the P_{O_2} rises essentially to equal that of the alveolar air before reaching the midpoint of the capillary, becoming approximately 104 mm. Hg.

The average pressure difference for oxygen diffusion through the pulmonary capillary during normal respiration is about 11 mm. Hg. This is a "time-integrated" average and not simply an average of the 64 mm. Hg pressure difference at the origin of the capillary and the final zero pressure difference at the end of the capillary, because the initial pressure difference lasts for only a fraction of the transit time in the pulmonary capillary, whereas the low pressure difference lasts for a long time.

DIFFUSION OF OXYGEN FROM THE CAPILLARIES TO THE CELLS

Oxygen diffuses into the tissue cells by a process essentially the reverse of that which takes place in the lungs. The P_{O_2} in the interstitial fluid immediately outside a capillary is low, averaging about 40 mm. Hg, whereas that in the arterial blood is about 95 mm. Hg. Therefore, at the arterial end of the capillary, a pressure difference of 55 mm. Hg exists for diffusion of oxygen.

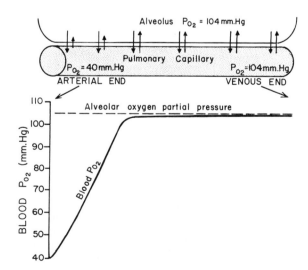

Figure 3–7 Uptake of oxygen by the pulmonary capillary blood. (The curve in this figure was constructed from data in Milhorn and Pulley: *Biophys. J.*, 8:337, 1968.) (From Guyton, 1976.)

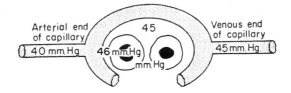

Figure 3–8 Uptake of carbon dioxide by the blood in the capillaries. (From Guyton, 1976.)

DIFFUSION OF CARBON DIOXIDE FROM THE CELLS TO THE TISSUE CAPILLARIES

Because of the continual large quantities of carbon dioxide formed in the cells, the intracellular P_{CO_2} tends to rise. However, carbon dioxide diffuses about 20 times as easily as oxygen, diffusing from the cells extremely rapidly into the interstitial fluids and thence into the capillary blood. In Figure 3–8 the intracellular P_{CO_2} is 46 mm. Hg, while that in the interstitial fluids immediately adjacent to the capillaries is about 45 mm. Hg, a pressure differential of only 1 mm. Hg.

Arterial blood entering the tissue capillaries contains carbon dioxide at a pressure of approximately 40 mm. Hg. As the blood passes through the capillaries, the blood P_{CO_2} rises to approach the 45 mm. Hg P_{CO_2} of the interstitial fluid. Because of the very large diffusion coefficient for carbon dioxide, the P_{CO_2} of venous blood is also about 45 mm. Hg, within a fraction of a millimeter of reaching complete equilibrium with the P_{CO_2} of the interstitial fluids.

REMOVAL OF CARBON DIOXIDE FROM THE PULMONARY BLOOD

When venous blood arrives at the lungs, its P_{CO_2} is about 45 mm. Hg, while that in the alveoli is 40 mm. Hg. Therefore, as illustrated in Figure 3–9,

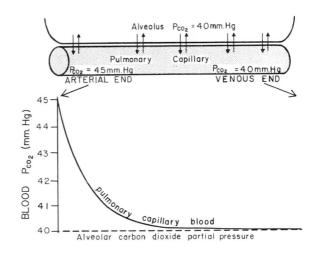

Figure 3–9 Diffusion of carbon dioxide from the pulmonary blood into the alveolus. (This curve was constructed from data in Milhorn and Pulley: *Biophys. J.*, 8:337, 1968.) (From Guyton, 1976.)

the initial pressure difference for diffusion is only 5 mm. Hg, which is far less than that for diffusion of oxygen. However, because the diffusion coefficient for carbon dioxide is 20 times greater than that for oxygen, the excess carbon dioxide in the blood is rapidly passed into the alveoli. The figure shows that the P_{CO_2} of the pulmonary capillary blood becomes equal to that of the alveoli within the first four-tenths of the blood's transit through the pulmonary capillary.

TRANSPORT OF OXYGEN IN THE BLOOD

Normally, about 97 per cent of the oxygen transported from the lungs to the tissues is carried in chemical combination with hemoglobin in the red blood cells, and the remaining 3 per cent is carried in the dissolved state in the water of the plasma and cells. The major function of red blood cells is to transport hemoglobin, which in turn carries oxygen from the lungs to the tissues.

Though hemoglobin is necessary for transport of oxygen to the tissues, it performs still another major function essential to life. This is the function of hemoglobin as an "oxygen buffer" system. The hemoglobin in the blood is mainly responsible for controlling the oxygen pressure in the tissues. Were it not for the hemoglobin oxygen buffer system, extreme variations in the P_{O_2} of the tissues would occur with exercise and with every change in metabolism, blood flow, and atmospheric oxygen concentration.

A person can be exposed to 100 per cent oxygen at normal atmospheric pressure almost indefinitely without developing *acute* oxygen toxicity. However, after a day or so of this exposure, he begins to develop *pulmonary edema* caused by damage to the linings of the bronchi and alveoli. It appears that these local tissues of the lungs are damaged as a result of oxidation of some of the essential elements of the tissues. The reason this effect occurs in the lungs and not in the other tissues is that the lungs are directly exposed to the high oxygen pressure (P_{O_2}), whereas oxygen is delivered to the other tissues at essentially normal P_{O_2} because of the hemoglobin oxygen buffer system. When the P_{O_2} in the air rises above 1500 mm. Hg, this buffer system fails, which then allows the P_{O_2} of all tissues to rise and to cause acute oxygen poisoning.

REGULATION OF RESPIRATION

During exercise and other physiological states that increase the metabolic activity of the body, the respiratory system is called upon to supply increased quantities of oxygen to the tissues and to remove increased quantities of carbon dioxide. The *respiratory center* in the brain stem adjusts the rate of alveolar ventilation almost exactly to the demands of the body so that, as a result, the blood oxygen pressure (P_{O_2}) and the carbon dioxide pressure (P_{CO_2}) are hardly altered even during strenuous exercise or other types of respiratory stress.

THE RESPIRATORY CENTER

The so-called "respiratory center" is a widely dispersed group of neurons located bilaterally in the reticular substance of the medulla oblongata and pons, as illustrated in Figure 3–10. It is divided into three major areas: the medullary rhythmicity area; the apneustic area; and the pneumotaxic area.

THE MEDULLARY RHYTHMICITY AREA

The medullary rhythmicity area is also frequently called the *medullary respiratory center.* It is located beneath the lower part of the floor of the fourth ventricle in the medial half of the medulla. *Inspiratory neurons and expiratory neurons* intermingle in this center. When respiration increases, both inspiratory and expiratory neurons become excited far above normal, transmitting a greatly increased number of inspiratory signals to the respiratory muscles during inspiration and a greatly increased number of expiratory signals during expiration. This discussion is mainly concerned with the factors that increase and decrease the degree of activity of these neurons.

It is in the medullary rhythmicity area that the basic rhythm of respiration is established. In the normal resting person, inspiration usually lasts for about 2 seconds and expiration for about 3 seconds. There is a basic oscillatory circuit located in this center that is capable of causing repetitive inspiration and expiration. However, the medullary rhythmicity area is not by itself capable of giving a normal smooth pattern of respiration when afferent signals

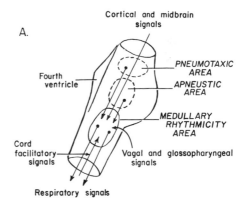

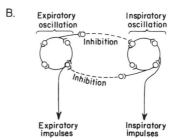

Figure 3–10 *A,* The respiratory center located bilaterally in the lateral reticular substance of the medulla and lower pons. *B,* Theoretical mechanism for the rhythmicity of the respiratory center. (From Guyton, 1976.)

do not reach it from other sources. These signals come from the spinal cord, from the cerebral center and midbrain, from the pneumotaxic area in the upper pons, and from the apneustic area in the lower pons. All of these signals modify the rhythm of respiration and contribute to the normal smooth pattern of respiration.

THE APNEUSTIC AND PNEUMOTAXIC AREAS

These areas are located in the reticular substance of the pons. They are not necessary for maintenance of the basic rhythm of respiration. However, when the apneustic area is still connected to the medullary rhythmicity area but the pons has been cut between the apneustic and pneumotaxic areas, the animal breathes with a pattern of prolonged inspiration and very short expiration, exactly opposite to the normal pattern. This apneustic pattern becomes especially marked when the afferent nerve fibers of the vagus and of the glossopharyngeal nerves have been cut.

If the pneumotaxic area is again connected to the rhythmicity center, the pattern of respiration reassumes its normal rhythm. Stimulation of the pneumotaxic area can also change the rate of respiration.

EFFECT ON THE RESPIRATORY CENTER OF NERVOUS SIGNALS FROM OTHER PARTS OF THE NERVOUS SYSTEM

Respiration is altered by, for example, speaking, suddenly entering a cold shower, being stuck with a pin, or being suddenly subjected to a stressful condition. The changes in respiration result from nerve impulses arriving at the respiratory center from other parts of the nervous sytem.

Impulses from the spinal cord play an important part in keeping the respiratory center active. The overall degree of stimulation of different peripheral sensory receptors throughout the body plays an important role in maintaining normal respiration. For example, when a person's respiratory center has been depressed to the point where respiration has ceased, almost any peripheral stimulus, such as slapping or applying cold water to the skin, can often start respiration again.

THE HERING-BREUER REFLEXES – THE INFLATION REFLEX AND THE DEFLATION REFLEX

There are many receptors in the lungs that detect stretch or compression. Some are in the visceral pleura, others in the bronchi, bronchioles, and the alveoli. When the lungs are stretched, the stretch receptors, especially those of the bronchioles, transmit impulses through the vagus nerves into the *tractus solitarius* of the brain stem, and from there to the respiratory center. These impulses inhibit inspiration, thus preventing further inflation and overdistention of the lungs. During expiration the impulses from these receptors cease, allowing inspiration to begin again. The important effects of the Hering-Breuer reflexes are a decrease in tidal volume and a compensatory increase in

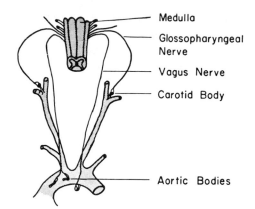

Medulla

Glossopharyngeal Nerve

Vagus Nerve

Carotid Body

Aortic Bodies

Figure 3–11 Respiratory control by the carotid and aortic bodies. (From Guyton, 1976.)

respiratory rate. In addition to altering respiratory rhythmicity, these reflexes also help to maintain the respiratory rhythm.

HUMORAL REGULATION OF RESPIRATION

This refers primarily to the regulation of respiratory activity by *changes in concentrations of oxygen, carbon dioxide and hydrogen ions* in the body fluids. The ultimate goal of respiration is to maintain proper concentration of these substances, since respiratory activity is highly responsive to even slight changes in any one of them.

Carbon dioxide and hydrogen ions exert these effects primarily on the respiratory center in the brain. Oxygen exerts its effect almost entirely on the peripheral chemoreceptors, and these in turn affect the respiratory center.

When all other factors are held constant, an increase in carbon dioxide concentration can increase the rate of alveolar ventilation six- to sevenfold; a decrease in pH (an increase in hydrogen ion concentration) can have the same result. However, under normal operating conditions of respiratory regulation, when all other factors are not held constant, carbon dioxide concentration affects respiration much more than does hydrogen ion concentration.

THE CHEMORECEPTOR SYSTEM FOR CONTROL OF RESPIRATORY ACTIVITY

The chemoreceptors are also sensitive and responsive to changes in oxygen, carbon dioxide and hydrogen ion concentrations. They signal to the respiratory center, helping to regulate respiratory activity. They are located primarily in association with the large arteries of the thorax and neck. Most of them are in the *carotid and aortic bodies* along with their afferent nerve connections to the respiratory center (Fig. 3–11). The *carotid bodies* are located bilaterally in the bifurcations of the common carotid arteries, and their afferent nerve fibers pass through Hering's nerves to the glossopharyngeal nerves and thence to the medulla. The *aortic bodies* are located along the arch of the aorta. Their afferent nerve fibers pass to the medulla through the vagi. Each of these bodies receives a special blood supply through a minute artery directly from the adjacent arterial trunk.

Changes in arterial oxygen concentrations have almost no direct effect on the respiratory center, but when the oxygen concentration in arterial blood falls below normal, the chemoreceptors become strongly stimulated.

DEFINITIONS

Eupnea. Normal breathing.

Tachypnea. Rapid breathing.

Bradypnea. Slow breathing.

Hyperpnea. A rate of alveolar ventilation great enough to cause over-respiration. However, this term is commonly used also to indicate simply a very high level of alveolar ventilation without necessarily implying over-respiration.

Hypopnea. Underrespiration.

Anoxia. Literally, total lack of oxygen; however, this term is more frequently used to mean decreased oxygen in the tissues (the more correct term for which would be *hypoxia*).

Anoxemia. Lack of oxygen in the body fluids. However, the term is generally used to mean reduced oxygen in the body fluids. The better term for this is *hypoxemia*.

Hypercapnia. Excess carbon dioxide in the body fluids.

Hypocapnia. Depressed carbon dioxide. The term *acapnia* is also frequently used to imply hypocapnia, but during life the absolute state of acapnia, with no carbon dioxide in the body fluids, is not possible.

REFERENCES

1. American Medical Association: Fundamentals of Anesthesia. Philadelphia, W. B. Saunders Co., 1954.
2. Guedel, A. E.: Inhalation Anesthesia. New York, Macmillan Co., 1953.
3. Monheim, L. M.: General Anesthesia in Dental Practice. St. Louis, C. V. Mosby Co., 1957.
4. Ruch, T. C., and Patton, H. D.: Physiology and Biophysics. 19th Ed. Philadelphia, W. B. Saunders Co., 1965.
5. Guyton, A. C.: Textbook of Medical Physiology. 5th Ed. Philadelphia, W. B. Saunders Co., 1976.
6. American Heart Association: Standards for Cardiopulmonary Resuscitation (CPR) and Emergency Cardiac Care (ECC). J.A.M.A., 227(Suppl.): 837–866, 1974.

THE PHARMACOLOGICAL BASIS OF INHALATION ANALGESIA AND THE PLANES OF ANALGESIA

4

THE PHARMACOLOGY OF INHALATION ANALGESIA

THE RESPIRATORY CYCLE

Respiration is the means by which gaseous agents are distributed to the tissues to produce analgesia. The variation in pressures within the thoracic cage and lungs as compared to the pressure of the external atmosphere is the factor responsible for the movement of gases. The pressure within the thoracic cage is a negative one, which tends to pull the parietal pleura away from the visceral pleura, thereby creating a negative pressure within the lungs and causing air or gas to rush into the lungs until the pressure is equalized. As the thoracic cage is expanded, the volume of the lungs increases owing to an increase in this negative pressure.[15] The inspiratory effort is due mainly to nervous impulses that stimulate the contraction of the diaphragm and inter-costal muscles. In actual function, however, a great many factors enter into the respiratory picture, which are integrated through various nerve pathways, as discussed in Chapter 3.

Nitrous oxide and oxygen administered through a nasal inhaler pass through the nasopharynx and oropharynx, down the trachea into the right and left bronchi and on to the alveoli of the lungs. The gases are then transferred across the lung alveoli into the blood plasma and red cells of the circulatory system. In this phase, i.e., in external respiration, the process is much the same as in breathing atmospheric air. It is in the phase of internal respiration that the analgesic agent has its effect.

Alterations in Internal Respiration

The exact mechanism[21] by which anesthetics produce a reversible de-pressing action on the brain is not known. A basic assumption must be made that every cell in the body requires adequate oxygen for the continuance of its

79

normal function. The exact manner in which blood cells utilize oxygen is extremely complex and is not yet fully understood. What is known, however, is that during the oxidative process many different compounds are formed. At each link in this complex chain of compounds, oxygen transfer is mediated by an enzyme. If one of these enzymes is altered in any manner, a modification of oxygen transfer ensues. Thus a cell can be temporarily deprived of its ability to function normally even in the presence of a metabolic supply of oxygen. It could be postulated that nitrous oxide acts by combining with the cellular lipoids, and thereby alters one or more of the many enzymes involved in the complicated oxidative process. It is important to stress here that in the administration of analgesia, oxygen utilization by the cell is *never* arrested, but only slightly diminished.

The cells of the body differ in their degree of reaction to oxygen reduction. Nerve cells react most readily to the slightest change in the partial pressure of oxygen. It has been found that the more recent the phylogenetic development of a tissue, the more sensitive is that tissue to alterations in oxygen consumption. The cerebrum, as the most recent and highly developed segment of the brain in the evolutionary process, reacts most rapidly to changes in oxygen supply. The blood supply to the brain through the carotid artery exceeds that of any other part of the body. Although the brain represents only 2 per cent of the total body weight, it receives 33 per cent of the output of blood from the left ventricle of the heart. The cells of the brain also have a greater proportion of lipoid content. Anesthetic agents can act as such because they perfuse nerve tissue sooner than the tissues of other vital organs.

Although nitrous oxide enters the body by inhalation through the lungs, it is conveyed to the tissues by the blood. It is a true anesthetic agent, and its distribution to the brain is dependent on the volume of blood supplied to the organ and on the lipoid content of its component cells.

The action of nitrous oxide on the central nervous system is a readily reversible one.[20] If metabolic oxygen has been provided, the cells of the central nervous system are restored to normal function immediately after cessation of inhalation of nitrous oxide. The circulation time of the blood carrying the gas from the lungs to the brain and back to the lungs is approximately 30 seconds.

THE NERVOUS SYSTEM

Physiological studies of the anesthetic state received great impetus from the work of French, Verzeano, and Magoun,[4] who demonstrated a centrally located area in the brain stem which appears to be essential to the maintenance of the conscious, alert state and which has been shown to be particularly sensitive to depressant drugs. Using auditory and sciatic stimulation, these investigators showed that ether or pentobarbital sodium blocked impulses propagated through the reticular system, while the lateral sensory pathways continued to conduct with unimpaired intensity.[4] Similarly, Arduini and Arduini[1] found that potentials in the reticular system showed a much greater susceptibility to alteration by metabolic changes and by depressant and excitant drugs than did potentials in the other direct afferent pathways. Finally, procaine has been shown to have a demonstrable effect on activity in the reticular system.[1] These studies strongly suggest that the modification of neural transmission through the reticular system is of major importance in the production of the anesthetic state.

It is well known among anesthesiologists that during the induction of anesthesia a stage is reached in which the patient retains auditory perception after the ability to perceive painful stimulation is lost. *Anesthetic drugs seem to have a selectivity for the neural mechanisms subserving pain perception at dosages that may leave other perceptions relatively unaffected.*

As part of a long-term investigation of the nervous mechanisms subserving the pain process, Haugen and Melzack[8] studied the effects of analgesic mixtures of nitrous oxide and oxygen on responses in the medial and lateral pathways in the cat brain stem evoked by stimulation of a pain source. The tooth pulp was selected as a recognized source of the sensation of pain, and potentials evoked by stimulation of the tooth pulp in cats were traced into the trigeminal root and the midbrain and thalamus. The areas of the midbrain responding to the electrical stimulation of tooth pulp were differentiated into five functional groups on the basis of anatomical location, response latency, and behavior during repetitive stimulation at various frequencies. Nitrous oxide was selected as the anesthetic agent because of its analgesic action in concentrations having ample oxygen to obviate hypoxia and because it can be administered and withdrawn from the experimental animal without the delay noted with fat-soluble agents or the barbiturates.

The results of this study are as follows:

1. No effect was observed on the potentials in the trigeminal lemniscus.
2. A significant diminution of responses was observed in the trigemino-

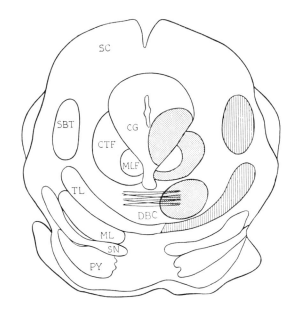

Figure 4–1 Brain stem areas conducting impulses from tooth pulp. Vertically hatched areas are the classic pain pathways, the spinobulbothalamic tract *(SBT)* and the trigeminal lemniscus *(TL)* adjacent to the medial lemniscus *(ML)*. Dotted areas are three additional regions from which tooth pulp impulses have been recorded: one in the central gray *(CG)*, one in the central tegmental fasciculus *(CTF)*, and one in the reticular substance lateral to decussation of the brachium conjunctivum. Section is at the level of the superior colliculi *(SC)*. (After B. Melzack, W. A. Stotler, and W. K. Livingston, *J. Neurophysiol.*, 21:353–367, 1958.)

bulbothalamic path, the dorsal secondary trigeminal pathway, the central gray area, and the reticular formation.

3. Nitrous oxide seemed to have a selective action on that part of the pattern most closely related to pain perception, for that was the portion where potentials were abolished.

THE CHOICE OF AN ANALGESIC AGENT

Dental practitioners have always been interested in the control of pain and fear. In medicine many of the procedures that cause pain are surgical procedures, which are almost invariably done in a hospital. A general anesthetic is usually employed, and during this procedure analgesia is merely a brief stage through which the patient passes on his way to the stage of surgical anesthesia. For this reason, analgesia as a distinct entity has been largely overlooked in hospitals. Recently, however, through attempts to maintain patients in lighter planes of anesthesia, the value of the stage of analgesia in general surgery has been recognized and explored. It is interesting that neurosurgery and open heart surgery are being performed with the patient in the maintained analgesic stage, although the agents used are different from those employed in dentistry.[6]

The dentist rarely treats matters of life or death. His patients are usually ambulatory and in fairly good health, and the choice of an analgesic medium to best fulfill his objectives must be governed by these circumstances. There must be no danger of morbidity or mortality, and the conditions under which the medium is administered should allow for quick recovery, ease of application, and minimal side effects.

To begin the search for an analgesic agent, it is necessary to establish the meaning of the term:

An *analgesic* is a substance which raises the pain reaction threshold without loss of consciousness.

A *good analgesic* is a substance which not only raises the pain reaction threshold without loss of consciousness, but in addition improves the patient's mental and emotional attitude toward the experience.

In keeping with these requirements, an ideal analgesic for the ambulatory dental patient must meet the following criteria:

1. It must be safe, nonexplosive, pleasant smelling.
2. Fear and anxiety should be diminished.
3. It should obtund pain.
4. Some degree of amnesia should result.
5. It should produce a state of euphoria.
6. The method of administration should be convenient and uncomplicated.
7. There should be rapid onset of effect, ease of maintenance, and rapid reversibility.
8. Side effects should be minimal.
9. There should be no development of tolerance.
10. There must be no danger of addiction.
11. It should have universality of application.

12. The frequent use of premedication should not be necessary.

13. There should be a wide range between the concentration inducing the onset of analgesia and that inducing the onset of unconsciousness.

Choice of an analgesic agent will also be influenced by the answers to the following questions:

1. Is the patient normal, or is he handicapped physically, mentally, or emotionally?

2. Does treatment require completion in one visit?

3. Is the primary objective the development of the patient into a good dental patient on a continuing basis?

A comparison of the pharmacology of the inhalation analgesic agents must lead to the irrefutable conclusion that nitrous oxide stands out above all others as the drug of choice.[9] Four agents are here chosen for comparison.

Fluothane

Fluothane has a low analgesic potential during the conscious phase. It is 100 per cent potent and has a 0 to 4 per cent range between the concentration inducing the onset of analgesia and that inducing respiratory and cardiovascular collapse. It is also very costly and requires a highly trained anesthesiologist for its administration. Fluothane can thus be eliminated as an analgesic agent, although it is an excellent anesthetic agent.

Ether

Ether is an excellent analgesic agent, but it is explosive and has a sharp, irritating odor. The range between the concentration inducing analgesia and that inducing respiratory arrest is 1 to 10 per cent. Ether increases salivation and is often followed by nausea. It is eliminated rapidly through the lungs, unchanged. In the lighter planes of anesthesia it has no apparent transient effects on any of the vital systems.

Trichlorethylene

Trichlorethylene is an excellent analgesic and is most selective for the fifth cranial nerve. It, too, increases salivation and may cause nausea. In the usual mixtures it is nonexplosive but has an irritating odor. The range of concentration from that inducing analgesia to that inducing respiratory and cardiovascular collapse is from 2.5 to 5 per cent. In higher percentages it may damage the vital organs.

Nitrous Oxide

Nitrous oxide is equivalent in its analgesic potential to 10 to 15 mg. of morphine and is also ataractic in nature. It is nonexplosive, rarely produces nausea, and has a bland, pleasant, nonirritating odor. The least potent of the four drugs under discussion, nitrous oxide has a 15 per cent potency. Because of this, the gas was originally discarded for anesthetic use during major surgery. Yet this very lack of potency represents its major value when used as relative analgesia on ambulatory dental patients. With adequate oxygenation it does not have the power to produce respiratory or cardiac collapse. Its range of concentration from that inducing analgesia to that inducing unconsciousness may run from 5 to 80 per cent, which is indeed an extremely wide range. Because of its rapid elimination from the lungs in an unchanged state, nitrous oxide permits rapid ambulation of the patient. Finally it is a relatively inexpensive drug and requires only a simple gas machine for its administration.

Our evaluation of the four agents leaves no room for doubt that nitrous oxide is the agent of choice by a great margin for the dentist using an inhalation analgesic on ambulatory patients.

Relative analgesia with nitrous oxide is a chemically induced, altered psychological state which eliminates the fear and pain of the dental experience. It results from the psychological and physiological effects of low alveolar concentrations of nitrous oxide. Relative analgesia may also be defined as an *altered state of consciousness* in which fear and anxiety are obliterated and cerebral interpretation of pain stimuli modified.

THE ANALGESIC ACTION OF NITROUS OXIDE

The analgesic action of nitrous oxide derives from a fortunate combination of properties: its low boiling point, its stability in living tissue, and its great solubility in body fluids. Nitrous oxide boils at −89.4°C., and other things being equal the boiling point determines the rate of diffusion and the rate of elimination of a particular inhalation agent; of course, the faster the rate of elimination, the more rapidly the patient recovers consciousness. Because of its low boiling point and its high molecular activity at body temperature, nitrous oxide rushes out of the blood and lungs at a tremendous rate when the nasal inhaler is removed. Ether, in contrast, requires a much greater time for elimination because of its higher boiling point and the fact that, unlike nitrous oxide, its elimination is delayed by its union with various lipoid tissues in the body. Moreover, because nitrous oxide is soluble in the body fluids, it is transported in a manner similar to the transportation of food and oxygen. In this way it is readily absorbed and eliminated.

Arterial blood normally carries about 18.5 per cent by volume of oxygen. Nearly all of this oxygen is united with hemoglobin in the form of oxyhemoglobin, which acts as a storehouse from which oxygen is liberated into the bloodstream in its travel through the tissues. The tissues absorb oxygen from the serum; the serum is, therefore, the medium of exchange between the air and the hemoglobin in the lungs and between the hemoglobin and the tissue cells throughout the body. It contains a small amount of oxygen, 0.24 per cent by volume. Our body cells therefore live in an environment of 0.24 per cent of oxygen, much as do fish, which derive their oxygen supply from water carrying a similar low percentage of oxygen.

Although the air we breathe contains about 80 per cent nitrogen and 20 per cent oxygen, the blood takes up only 1.7 per cent by volume of nitrogen. This is, however, seven times as much as the volume of oxygen carried by the blood serum. From this 1 to 7 mixture in the serum, the body cells have no difficulty in obtaining plenty of oxygen for normal oxidation or combustion.

On the other hand, it has been shown that blood serum dissolves 26 per cent by volume of nitrous oxide. This means that the solubility of nitrous oxide in blood serum is about 15 times that of nitrogen. This greater solubility of nitrous oxide in the body fluids helps to explain the difference in effect on the central nervous system between nitrous oxide and nitrogen. Since nitrous oxide is able to reach the body tissues more easily, we can begin to understand why a mixture of 80 per cent nitrous oxide and 20 per cent oxygen can produce anesthesia, whereas the same proportion of nitrogen and oxygen (as it exists in air) has no anesthetic effect whatsoever.

It was formerly thought that nitrous oxide was not a true anesthetic agent, that it created its effect by the exclusion of oxygen. This theory is obviously not valid to anyone who has administered nitrous oxide either as general anesthesia or as analgesia. It is self-evident to the initiated that a good analgesic state may be induced in many individuals with a mixture of 90 per cent oxygen and 10 per cent nitrous oxide.

Quantitative Measurement of Nitrous Oxide Analgesia.   The analgesic action of nitrous oxide was first demonstrated quantitatively by Seevers and his co-workers.[19] In their study of changes in the pain reaction threshold by means of a specially devised needle algesimeter, the optimal concentration of nitrous oxide with retention of ability to cooperate was found to be 35 to 40 per cent. A later study by Chapman, Arrowood, and Beecher[2] revealed that 20 per cent nitrous oxide is as effective an analgesic as is 15 mg. of morphine sulfate.

In 1948, Sonnenschein and his associates[22] undertook a further study on the mechanism of nitrous oxide analgesia. The purposes of this study were to determine (1) the quantitative aspects of analgesia, and (2) the relationship between the analgesia and induced general psychomotor performance.

Nitrous oxide was administered with oxygen by means of a nasal inhaler, with constant flow at atmospheric pressure from standard anesthesia equipment; the Millikan oximeter was used to determine the level of oxygen saturation. The pain threshold was determined by electrical stimulation of the tooth pulp through a metal filling. Psychomotor activity was measured by means of the Johnson code—various sets of nonsense words with respective letter codes. The subject was to associate the proper set of words with the correct letter code.

Sensory Effects.   To evaluate sensory effect two threshold readings were taken. The first was a just perceptible sensation, not painful in itself; the second was that point at which the sensation merged into true pain. Readings were taken under nitrous oxide inhalation with the following concentrations of oxygen: 10, 20, 33, and 40 per cent. It was the general observation of the subjects that the influence of the gas caused a change in the quality of the pain so that, with increasing concentrations of the gas, it became increasingly difficult to denote the point at which the sensation became true pain. *The el-*

ement of noxiousness of the stimulus decreased, and the sensation became somewhat more diffuse. In other words, the subject's interpretation of the painful stimulus as such became more difficult. His attitude toward the noxious stimulus was changed: he was less concerned with it.

Psychomotor Effects.   These tests demonstrated that, as the concentration of nitrous oxide was increased, there was a concomitant decrease in psychomotor performance. The subject was less and less able to concentrate and he felt remote from his surroundings. Nitrous oxide was used in 10 to 33 per cent concentrations.

Conclusions

1. Nitrous oxide has a definite analgesic action in small concentrations (10 to 20 per cent).

2. In this range, too, the ability to concentrate is decreased, as is the ability to interpret painful stimuli as such.

3. A rise in pain reaction threshold is associated with a decrease in psychomotor performance.

4. It is most certainly not true that any of these results is due to anoxemia, since they all were evident in the presence of an arterial oxygen saturation of 95 to 100 per cent.

The Pharmacology of Nitrous Oxide.[3]   No known *chemical reaction* involving nitrous oxide occurs on its inhalation. Its pharmacologic actions occur mainly in the central nervous system and are mild.

Elimination.   The elimination of nitrous oxide takes place largely through the lungs. A small amount of excretion occurs also through skin, sweat glands, urine, and intestinal gas.

Cerebrospinal Fluid.   There is no change in the composition or volume of the cerebrospinal fluid attributed to nitrous oxide.

Cough Reflex.   When used as general anesthesia, nitrous oxide causes the cough reflex to be suppressed only to a moderate extent. When used as relative analgesia, there is no suppression of the cough reflex.

The Circulatory System.   Nitrous oxide does not cause any change in *heart rate* or *cardiac output*, nor any changes in *arterial pressure* or *venous pressure*. Cutaneous *venodilation* does occur, and this effect has been used to facilitate venipuncture when veins are not visible before induction. The *blood volume and composition* are not changed except after more than 24 to 48 hours of continuous administration in concentrations greater than 25 per cent nitrous oxide. Under these conditions the white blood count is decreased. It returns to normal upon cessation of administration of nitrous oxide.

The Respiratory System.   The *sensitivity of the nasolaryngotracheal area* is markedly reduced, and the *sense of smell* is decreased. The latter effect has made nitrous oxide popular as an induction agent with the use of more irritating anesthetic agents. Nitrous oxide is much less toxic than other inhalation anesthesia drugs.

The Gastrointestinal System.   Esophageal, gastric, and intestinal peristalses are not affected, and gastrointestinal secretions continue. Gas in bowel may be replaced by nitrous oxide as a result of the denitrogenation process. The hepatic and pancreatic functions are unaffected.

The Genitourinary System.   There is no change in kidney function, ureteral peristalses, bladder tone, or urine formation, nor any effect on the genital organs.

Metabolism.   Nitrous oxide does not appear either to stimulate or to depress metabolism, as is evidenced by oxygen uptake.

Toxicity of Nitrous Oxide.   Nitrous oxide will depress the bone marrow and the white cell count after prolonged administration. This depressant effect has been utilized in the treatment of leukemia. However, no evidence is available at present to show that life was prolonged. After cessation of administration of nitrous oxide, the white cell count returns to its former value. There is no evidence that any toxic property of this gas becomes manifest during its use as an anesthetic or analgesic agent. The above depressant effects are noted *only* after continual administration for 48 hours.

The classic work of C. B. Courville gave proof that any brain damage following nitrous oxide anesthesia was due to concomitant asphyxia or hypoxia and not to any toxic effect of nitrous oxide itself.

THE PLANES OF ANALGESIA

Guedel[7] divided inhalation anesthesia into four stages: the first stage — analgesia; the second stage — delirium (excitement); the third stage (which is divided into four planes) — surgical; and the fourth stage — respiratory paralysis.

This division of anesthesia into four stages and the division of the third or surgical state into four planes does not show any divisions of the first stage, the stage of analgesia. When surgical anesthesia (stage 3) is the objective, stage 1 is a very short, very fleeting phase of the administration, the stage being bypassed very rapidly. Quite understandably the anesthetist has no interest in lingering at this point. Should, however, one's objective change, should the operator become interested in keeping his patient in the analgesic stage, a new vista emerges. It is then seen that the stage of analgesia has much greater length and breadth than was formerly realized. Since we now wish to keep the patient in this stage, and not go beyond it, we induce what is called the *maintained analgesic stage.*

The maintained analgesic stage may be divided into three planes: plane 1 and plane 2 constitute the stage of relative analgesia and plane 3 is the stage of total analgesia (Fig. 4–2). Table 4–1 delineates the signs and symptoms of the planes of analgesia and the average doses that will produce them. It should be stressed that this table applies only to the reactions of a patient who has been trained in the use of analgesia and who does not breathe excessively through the mouth. The dosages to be used and their effects on a patient who is taking analgesia for the first time present a unique problem which is explored in Chapter 6. Excessive oral respiration would obviously dilute the analgesic effect at any given dose level.

In latter years it has become more and more obvious that Guedel's clas-

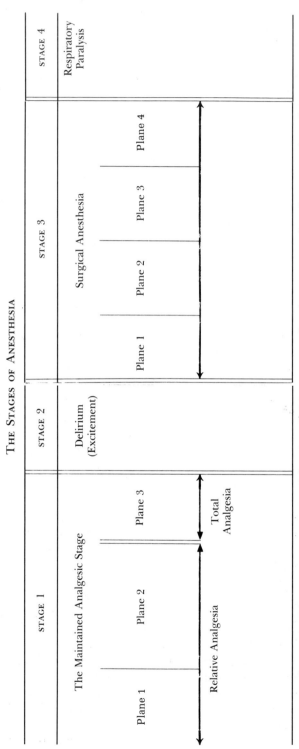

Figure 4-2   Schematic representation of the relation of the maintained analgesic stage to the other stages of anesthesia.

sification of the four stages of anesthesia does not hold true for many drugs now used for inducing general anesthesia and that there may be a fourth plane somewhere between the so-called stage of analgesia and the stage of excitement which holds great promise for clinical application by those trained in its use. It is called the plane of amnalgesia by Klock and Tom.[11] Although there are no obvious indications to let the operator know when his patient is passing from one plane to another, a little experience with relative analgesia soon teaches the dentist to judge the stage his patient is in at a given moment. This holds true because the dentist quickly learns to evaluate the level of analgesia by the patient's ability to maintain an open mouth without the use of mouth props, the degree of contraction of the orbicularis oris, the movements of the tongue against the instruments being used in the oral cavity, the frequency of eyewinking as compared to the normal rate, and the degree of relaxation of the mandible. He can also gain additional insight into the patient's status by noticing the "look" in his eyes, the position of his hands, and the general appearance of relaxation of his body. After a short exposure to the clinical application of analgesia, the dentist can derive a clear and distinct impression of the sum total of these signs by just a glance and the response of the oral tissues. It becomes almost instinctive to "sense" at what level his patient is. Further evaluation of the analgesic level can be based on the lucidity and rapidity of response, or lack of response, to the dentist's queries.

DENTAL ANALGESIA: THE STAGE OF RELATIVE ANALGESIA

In the stage of relative analgesia the patient's threshold to pain, cold, warmth, and light touch is raised. Although the special senses may be partly obtunded and a sensation of numbness is described, superficial and deep reflexes remain active, and the sensorium remains clear. Consciousness is impaired only to a slight degree. These changes may be demonstrated by placing the patient in the analgesic state and then stimulating the skin with a sharp instrument. There is a quick withdrawal from the stimulus. However, depending on the degree of analgesia relative to the intensity of the stimulus, the patient may not interpret the stimulus as painful. Although it may evoke a reflex and the subject is aware of being stimulated, the reaction to and the interpretation of the severity of the pain are dulled. Pain relief of this sort without abolition of reflexes is inadequate for major surgery, but it is highly suitable for most dental operations, especially when the fear-eliminating properties of this stage are kept in mind.

Since nitrous oxide was first used by Horace Wells in 1844, it has been the anesthetic of choice in the dental profession. The flexibility of control, the ease and rapidity of induction, and the quick recovery with no after-effects when this agent is the analgesic has made it particularly valuable and suitable for dentistry. The subjective symptoms depend upon the depth of analgesia, the patient's mental attitude, and the technique of administration.

TABLE 4-1   The Planes of Analgesia

PLANE	AVERAGE DOSES	RESPIRATION	GENERAL MUSCLES	EYE	PULSE RATE	BLOOD PRESSURE	PATIENT MAINTAINS AN OPEN MOUTH WITHOUT MOUTH PROPS	PATIENT FOLLOWS DIRECTIONS	DEGREE OF AMNESIA	EFFECT ON PAIN	EFFECT ON FEAR	APPEARANCE OF PATIENT	SUBJECTIVE REACTIONS
1	*Continuous flow* (open air valve) 3 liters O_2 2-4 liters N_2O *Intermittent flow* (closed air valve) 10-15% N_2O 90-85% O_2 at 1-2 mm. pressure	Normal	Normal	Pupils normal and contract normally to light; conjunctiva sensitive	Normal	Normal	Yes	Yes	Very slight	Marked elevation of pain reaction threshold	Diminution to complete elimination	Normal; relaxed; a fully conscious patient	A feeling of relaxation; may experience tingling in fingers, toes, lips, or tongue
2	*Continuous flow* (open air valve) 3 liters O_2 4-8 liters N_2O *Intermittent flow* (closed air valve) 15-25% N_2O 85-75% O_2 at 2-3 mm. pressure	Normal	Normal	Pupils normal; rate of winking reduced; a relaxed, dreamy, far-away look	Normal	Normal	Yes	Yes, but more slowly	Moderate to complete	Pain reaction markedly reduced or eliminated	Elimination	Relaxed; euphoric; less aware of his immediate surroundings and less concerned with activity around him	May feel a warm wave suffuse entire body; humming, droning, or vibratory sensation; a feeling of headiness, lethargy or drowsiness; voice becomes "throaty"; a feeling of euphoria, safety; thoughts may wander beyond treatment room

3	Continuous flow (open air valve) 3 liters O₂ N₂O 6-10 liters N₂O (closed air valve) 3 liters O₂ 4-8 liters N₂O *Intermittent flow* (closed air valve) 25-50% N₂O 75-50% O₂ at 2-3 mm. pressure	Normal	Usually normal; sometimes rigid mandible or rigid body	Very hard stare; angry or very sleepy look; eyes may close; eyeball may become eccentric	Normal	Normal	No. mouth tends to close; may open if operator presses on lower lip, but immediately closes again	Most usually not	Complete	Pain reaction eliminated	A short exposure (1-2 min.) to this plane is useful for controlling extreme fear; longer exposure brings many patients into a state of fear and then excitement	Begins to assume appearance of unconsciousness; totally unaware of his surroundings; jaw may become rigid; body may stiffen	May have hallucinatory dreams; experience fear, a feeling of falling, a fear of dying with inability to do anything about it

The Signs and Symptoms of Relative Analgesia

What does a patient look like and what does he feel when in the stage of relative analgesia? A patient in this stage is conscious, and his facial expression is that of a conscious individual. His respiration is normal and smooth, and his muscles are relaxed. The pupils are normal and they contract normally to light. The conjunctiva is sensitive, there is no rolling of the eyeballs, the eyelids do not resist opening, and they wink when touched. The patient's pulse rate is normal, as are his blood pressure and the color of his skin.

After breathing nitrous oxide and oxygen for 30 to 40 seconds, the patient may become aware of first the taste of the gases and then the odor. The odor of nitrous oxide may best be described as a mild ethereal odor. Its mildness and lack of irritating qualities make it pleasant and easy to take for most people, a fact of tremendous importance to the dentist, because it means more ready acceptance of analgesia by the patient, especially when first introduced.

The first subjective symptom may be a tingling sensation in the toes, the fingertips, or the tip of the tongue. Often a patient will describe a tingly or numb sensation in the lips. These symptoms are due to vasomotor excitation. Although they are fairly characteristic of the light analgesic state, not all of these symptoms are necessarily present at each administration. Then, too, the patient may not always be able to clearly distinguish them, especially when he has gone deeper into the analgesic stage. Operators new to the use of analgesia often use the absence of these symptoms as an indication that the analgesia is too light. The reverse may be true, however, for the patient may already be in the deep analgesic state. The best procedure when in doubt is to begin work on the patient. Since we are treating a conscious patient, his reaction, verbal or physical, will indicate his status.

The patient may experience diaphoresis as a result of a psychic disturbance during the state of altered consciousness. If desired, this can be prevented by premedication with belladonna.

As the patient gets deeper into the analgesic stage, he may feel a warm wave suffuse his entire body. He has a feeling of lethargy. Very often he experiences a humming, droning, or vibratory sensation throughout his body, somewhat like the soft purring of a motor. At this time, the patient may also describe a feeling of headiness or drowsiness, similar to light intoxication. His voice becomes throaty, losing its natural resonance. Normally the voice is projected through the head and nose; under analgesia the voice seems to acquire a peculiar, characteristic throaty tone.

Although the patient under analgesia is not unconscious, he is not fully awake. He knows something is going on about him, yet he is less aware of his surroundings and less concerned with what is taking place than normally. In spite of himself, he begins to experience a feeling of relaxation. He has a feeling of well-being, of safety, of euphoria. There is a feeling of being in a friendly atmosphere and of having a friend at hand should there be the need of one. He feels warm and comfortable, as if he were in a pleasant dream. Words reach him as from a great distance. He may hear the doctor ask a question, yet he may not readily respond because he thinks, "I know the doctor is asking me a question, but I can't be bothered answering. I feel too good to bother answering."

As the deeper phase of the relative analgesic stage is attained, pain disappears but recognition of touch and pressure is still present. Sounds come to the patient distinctly but more distantly. Sudden loud noises may bring him out of his pleasant euphoric state. If he attempts to lift his arm or leg, it will feel heavy and cumbersome, and he cannot fully control its movements. His thoughts very often wander far afield. He may engage in philosophical thoughts or mull over religious problems. He may attempt to solve some of the world's problems and be anxious to impart this knowledge to the doctor upon awakening. Usually, however, he is unable to do so; his memory of the immediate past is dim.

Relative Versus Total Analgesia

A clearer understanding of the stage of dental analgesia that should be administered fixes more clearly in the mind of the operator the limits within which he must work in order to avoid light anesthesia and the excitement stage. A drastic change in the idea of what should be the main reason for the use of analgesia in the practice of dentistry has contributed most to present-day success. It has long been known that nitrous oxide in analgesic doses reduces or eliminates pain. What was not so well understood was its potential for changing the emotional status of the patient in the dental chair. In the earlier literature, this characteristic was rarely mentioned, and then only as a minor or insignificant fact. In latter years, stressing the far greater importance of inducing a state of well-being, euphoria, and lessened fear and anxiety has led to the greatest change in approach to the patient and to the greatest degree of success in the application of analgesia to the practice of dentistry.

When the raising of the patient's pain reaction threshold was the primary objective, the operator reasoned that he could eliminate more pain by putting his patient deeper into the analgesic state. Thus, he aimed toward the plane of total analgesia. At this point, the line between analgesia and the excitement stage or light anesthesia is thin or perhaps nonexistent. At this point, too, the operator finds his patient teetering between being conscious and cooperative and being unconscious. Here nausea is far more likely to occur, the patient finds it difficult to keep his mouth open, and the cough reflex becomes a matter of concern. And most importantly, it is here that fear is generated!

In contrast, when elimination of the patient's fear is a main objective, the operator has an entirely different picture and a completely different patient. He will not seek total analgesia but will keep his patient in the planes of relative analgesia. The patient will be conscious of, but less aware of and less concerned with, what happens around him. He keeps his mouth open and complies with directions; the cough reflex is not suppressed, but fear, pain, and anxiety are gone. The patient can alter the rate and depth of his breathing voluntarily, or he may dilute his symptoms by reverting to mouth breathing. In the planes of relative analgesia, nausea is rare, and slipping into the excitement stage or anesthesia is virtually impossible.

The difference between relative analgesia and total analgesia can be clarified further on a quantitative basis. When the dentist wishes primarily to eliminate pain and to work toward total analgesia, he may start the administration with 25 per cent nitrous oxide and increase to 80 per cent nitrous oxide. The dentist whose main objective is the elimination of fear of the dental experience may start with 5 per cent nitrous oxide and increase toward 35 per cent with an average operating dose of 10 to 20 per cent nitrous oxide.

At this point, the reader may question the reasons for stressing the difference between the planes of relative analgesia and total analgesia. Why is it so important? Why not attempt to gain the plane of total analgesia? It is true that achieving the plane of total analgesia would eliminate the pain reaction completely, as has been mentioned. In the process, however, an instrument of an entirely different nature is being employed. This instrument is not as easily mastered by the average dental practitioner and is not as universally accepted by patients. It is also *much less effective in eliminating fear of the dental experience.* It is true that the attainment of complete analgesia and amnesia all the time is impossible with the use of relative analgesia. Yet, in return for giving up this objective, the dental practitioner gains an instrument of much greater value.

From a clinical point of view, it could be stated that the instrument called relative analgesia functions up to the point at which the patient closes his mouth and does not hear or obey a direction to open his mouth.

Table 4–2 shows the comparative signs in the patient in relative analgesia and in the patient too deep in analgesia (light anesthesia). The patient entered this latter stage because the operator was aiming at the plane of total analgesia. A careful perusal of this table will explain why many such dentists have discarded the use of analgesia. The patient was always slipping beyond relative analgesia and passing into light anesthesia or the excitement stage. Of course, there could be no harm to the patient, but the relatively inexperienced operator drew rapidly away from what seemed to him to be an uncontrollable situation.

Relative Analgesia Versus General Anesthesia

Whenever a new instrument is devised, it is but natural to compare it with established instruments that are used for the same purpose. In the early evaluation of relative analgesia, the premise was that analgesia was being used mainly to eliminate physical pain. It was then immediately compared to general anesthesia and to local anesthesia with regard to its physical pain-eliminating properties. The reasoning went thus: Analgesia does not put a patient completely to sleep; therefore it is not as good as general anesthesia. Analgesia does not numb as completely as local anesthesia; therefore it is not as good as local anesthesia. If it is not as good as either of these two instruments, why use it at all?

Of course, the fallacy in this reasoning lies in the failure to realize that analgesia has uses which cannot be fulfilled with either general or local anes-

TABLE 4–2   Signs of Relative Analgesia Versus Light Anesthesia

	RELATIVE ANALGESIA	LIGHT ANESTHESIA
Respiration	Normal, smooth	Superficial slow breathing, often irregular
	Inspiration of normal duration	Prolonged inspiration
	No phonation	Phonation due to reflexes of pain
	No holding of breath or grunting	Holding of breath, grunting
General muscles	No movements, muscles relaxed	Purposeful movement or rigid muscles
	Facial expression of a conscious individual	Facial expression of pain or semiconsciousness
	Nausea extremely rare	Nausea more frequent
	Purposeful but delayed resistance as result of trauma	Reflex or purposeful resistance as result of trauma
Eye	Pupils normal, contract normally to light	Pupils large, contract to light actively
	Conjunctiva sensitive	Conjunctiva sensitive
	No rolling of eyeballs	Eyeballs roll quite rapidly
	Eyelids do not resist opening, wink when touched	Eyelids resist opening, wink when touched
Pulse rate	Normal	Accelerated
Blood pressure	Normal	Normal
Color of skin	Normal	Pink or no change normally
		In anemics, no color change
		In plethorics, slight cyanosis

thesia. In addition, its synergistic action with local anesthesia enhances the value of the latter.

For both general anesthesia and analgesia we use the same gases and sometimes the same gas machines. We also use a modified form of the first stage of anesthesia. These similarities have given rise to a great deal of confusion between the two instruments. In reality, the only points which general anesthesia and relative analgesia have in common are the machines and the gases. From there on they are entirely different and distinct instruments. Their use involves different techniques and different approaches to the patient. Their objectives and their place in the practice of dentistry are radically different.

It might be well at this point to state the vast differences between analgesia and general anesthesia with nitrous oxide and oxygen from the clinical point of view. The first and most obvious difference is the fact that under general anesthesia we are dealing with an unconscious patient, whereas with analgesia we treat a conscious patient, a patient who is able to converse with the operator and who can and will follow the operator's directions, a patient whose protective reflexes are functioning fully. This may be a superfluous statement to one who has had experience with analgesia or general anesthesia, but the novice is somewhat unsure as to how deep in anesthesia his patient should be. The fact that in analgesia we deal with a conscious patient is of extreme importance. It means that the patient can cooperate with the operator. He can expectorate, if necessary, although this is not encouraged, as will be explained in a later chapter. The cough reflex and swallowing reflex are present at all times, so that throat curtains or mouth packs are unnecessary.

Also contraindicated are such things as restraining straps or pharyngeal airways. Mouth props are also entirely unnecessary; the patient in the analgesic state keeps his mouth open by himself. If he closes his mouth and does not open upon direction of the operator, he is too deep in relative analgesia. This is a very simple but highly important point. Its importance lies in the fact that any operator, new or initiated, can easily determine when his patient is getting beyond the planes of relative analgesia. He has but to ask his patient to open his mouth. If the patient does not respond, he is approaching total analgesia.

Finally, with analgesia we do not, and should not, hold the nasal inhaler against the patient's face. This is often done in administering general anesthesia to eliminate atmospheric air. In analgesia, however, we do not operate with a leakproof system. Since the patient's mouth is open and no mouth inhaler is used, there is always a certain amount of mouth breathing. Holding the nasal inhaler against the patient's face not only is uncomfortable to the patient but is poor procedure from a psychological point of view.

When general anesthesia is administered, the volumetric flow of nitrous oxide to the lungs is high. With relative analgesia we use low volumes of nitrous oxide with percentages of oxygen as high as 95 per cent. That eliminates any possibility of personality change, brain damage, or fatality. There has never been a fatality with the use of nitrous oxide and oxygen for analgesia. This statement is based on the experience of dentists who have reported their use of analgesia and on the experience of the author, which comprises well over 150,000 administrations over a period of 35 years, in addition to postgraduate teaching of the administration of analgesia to thousands of dentists in the past 27 years. This experience has served to affirm that the administration of analgesia is a completely safe procedure.

During anesthesia the operator must be guided only by the signs observed in the patient. During analgesia, since the patient is conscious and can answer questions put to him, we can ask him to tell us his symptoms. By the way he answers, by the rapidity or slowness with which he responds, or by his failure to respond, we can very easily ascertain at what level of analgesia he is.

The administration of anesthesia is usually a one-time procedure; very seldom is a series of administrations necessary. On the other hand, the administration of analgesia, once it is introduced to the patient, becomes a routine procedure, routinely used at almost his every visit to the dentist.

The administration of anesthesia, being an infrequent and special event and being most often associated with oral surgery, creates a certain amount of emotional tension and apprehension in the patient. Analgesia, which becomes routine after the initial introductory administration and which may be used for all dental procedures, eliminates nervous tension, apprehension, and fear.

For the administration of anesthesia, special preparation of the patient is necessary. He very often requires premedication, he must be given directions about eating, he must empty his bowels and his bladder. For analgesia no such routine directions are indicated, although in infrequent cases, directions on eating are necessary. This is explained in the section on nausea and vomiting (Chap. 7). In addition, analgesia acts as its own premedication after the initial exposure.

After the administration of anesthesia, a time-consuming period of recuperation is necessary. After analgesia, with few exceptions, one to three minutes of oxygenation is all that is required for the patient to get out of the dental chair and go about his business, fully recovered.

General anesthesia is used mainly for oral surgery to eliminate the fear and pain of the particular procedure, whereas analgesia is useful in every branch of dentistry, without exception. It may be used for every dental operation to eliminate the fear of dentistry by reducing mental and physical pain to a minimum.

Table 4–3 summarizes the distinct differences between relative analgesia and general anesthesia with nitrous oxide and oxygen. In clinical applications

TABLE 4–3 Clinical Differentiation Between General Anesthesia and Relative Analgesia

GENERAL ANESTHESIA	RELATIVE ANALGESIA
1. Patient is unconscious.	1. Patient is conscious.
2. Protective reflexes absent.	2. Protective reflexes functioning fully.
3. Some risk entailed.	3. No fatality on record.
4. No air admixed.	4. Air admixed.
5. Operator must be guided solely by signs observed in the patient.	5. Operator may be guided by signs and symptoms.
6. Usually a one-time procedure.	6. Used routinely at almost every visit.
7. An infrequent, special event: Generates a degree of fear and apprehension.	7. Eliminates fear and apprehension.
8. Special preparation of patient is necessary: a. Premedication. b. Fasting preoperatively. c. Emptying of bladder and bowels.	8. No special preparation of patient: a. Premedication rarely used. b. Fasting preoperatively rarely necessary. c. No need to empty bladder or bowels.
9. Time-consuming period of recuperation is necessary.	9. Recuperation requires only 1 to 3 minutes of oxygenation.
10. Used mainly for oral surgery to eliminate fear and pain.	10. Used in every aspect of dental treatment to eliminate fear of the dental experience, and reduce pain, anxiety, and discomfort to a minimum.
11. Necessary adjuncts: a. Mouth props. b. Restraining straps. c. Throat packs. d. Pharyngeal airways.	11. No adjuncts necessary: a. Patient maintains an open mouth. b. Excitement stage is never reached. c. Cough reflex, swallowing reflex in full function. d. Laryngospasm impossible.

the difference is so great that one could be expert in the administration of general anesthesia and yet not be proficient in the administration of relative analgesia. Conversely, every dentist can easily become proficient in the use of relative analgesia without becoming an expert in anesthesia. However, whether the dental practitioner administers general anesthesia or relative analgesia, he must have a proper background in the basic physiology and psychology involved.

Relative Analgesia and Local Anesthesia

What is the proper relationship of nitrous oxide and oxygen analgesia to local anesthesia? Analgesia is not, and was never meant to be, a substitute for local anesthesia. Since the first procaine injection by Guido Fischer in this country in the early part of this century, local anesthesia has proved to be a powerful tool in the improvement and execution of dental procedures. It would be difficult to visualize the practice of dentistry today without the use of local anesthesia. But the value of local anesthetic injection is enhanced, for both the dentist and the patient, by the use of analgesia. It also permits of fewer injections. It is no secret that millions of people fear that needle, even though the actual physical pain involved is minimal. This fear is completely controlled when the patient is under analgesia at the time of the injection.

If we adopt as our creed that we will make the chain of painlessness as complete as possible for every dental operation, we will not be content to say: "I get along very well with only an injection." The operator may be completely satisfied, but is the patient of the same mind? This chain of painlessness must contain links that will eliminate the fear of pain as well as the pain itself.

Although there are procedures in dentistry that require the use of local anesthesia, analgesia alone can suffice in many cases in which local anesthesia is now used. Analgesia permits of greater freedom of action in many cases. A situation frequently encountered is that of a patient with four comparatively simple cavities to prepare, one in each quadrant of the mouth. Should this patient insist on local anesthesia for all operative work, four visits would often be required. With analgesia, it would be a simple matter to complete all four preparations at one sitting. Not only is the proper use of analgesia a time saver without equal, but when local anesthesia is desired and indicated, the use of a synergistic combination with analgesia permits an ideal psychosomatic solution to the problem.

Relative Analgesia and Intravenous Sedation

These two modalities can be used synergistically so that the following advantages may accrue:

1. The patient is under nitrous oxide analgesia during the insertion of the needle, thus controlling the pain and fear of the injection.

2. Nitrous oxide tends to inflate cutaneous vessels, thus facilitating venipuncture.

3. When nitrous oxide analgesia is administered, less of the intravenous drug is required.

4. Towards the end of the procedure, whenever possible, the administration of the intravenous drug may be stopped and the patient maintained only with nitrous oxide analgesia. This would result in a shorter recovery period.

Introducing analgesia into a dental practice is not merely adding another instrument; it means much more. Because of its special potential for eliminating fear, it acts as a catalytic agent, or filter. All dental procedures are processed *through* analgesia. The result is a better way of practicing dentistry, better for the patient and far better for the dentist.

The Benefits of Relative Analgesia in Dental Practice

Most laymen, when thinking of the dentist's work, think only of the pain and discomfort endured because of tooth reduction. It is common knowledge, however, that the occasions for pain, fear, and discomfort during dental treatment occur during procedures other than tooth reduction. The use of analgesia is invaluable to an even greater extent in these situations, because there is no other method in use today that serves so well the purposes of both the dentist and the patient.

BENEFITS TO THE PATIENT

First and foremost, relative analgesia *eliminates the fear* of the dental procedure. This is the most important result and should be the most important objective. Keeping this in mind permits the operator to properly evaluate the success of analgesia with his patients. All the other many advantages of analgesia stem from this one all-important characteristic.

By eliminating fear and relaxing the patient, a high proportion of the *pain* involved in dental procedures is also *eliminated*. A patient who is tense and afraid and anticipates pain will feel pain to an exaggerated degree. It is no overstatement to say that more than 50 per cent of all pain involved in dentistry is eliminated by doing away with fear, anxiety, and anticipation of pain.

To state that the main objective of analgesia is to eliminate fear does not in any way detract from its second most important goal—the elimination or dulling of physical pain. It does away completely with the pain of many procedures and is partially effective in others. Even when it is partially effective, patients do not seem to mind the pain as much; many have described their feelings:

I know this is hurting me, but imagine how much greater the pain would be without analgesia.

I feel some pain, but I don't seem to mind it.

I feel as if there were a buffer between the drill and my tooth.

I feel as if somebody else's tooth is being drilled.

Another benefit is the dulling of associated unpleasant stimuli. For example, bone is an excellent conductor of sound and the noises created by dental instruments are magnified as they are transmitted throughout the cranium.

Most people intensely dislike the sounds and vibrations of dental instruments, and fearful people translate these sound stimuli into pain stimuli. Under analgesia, *sounds and vibrations of burs, wheels, and stones are dulled,* and they are not translated into pain sensations. Moreover, because the patient *is less aware of his surroundings,* he is not fearful of the manipulations of the dentist or of the sight of surgical instruments, blood, injection procedures, and so on.

Another extremely important and useful property of analgesia is its ability to *eliminate or greatly reduce the memory of pain.* Thus, although a patient may have experienced some pain, when he is brought out of the analgesic state he may have completely forgotten it, or he may not remember its full intensity. This is of great importance, especially in treating the child-patient. It permits analgesia to be its own premedication. Once the patient discovers what analgesia can do for him in the dental chair, he does not fear the subsequent visit, nor does he feel as though he had undergone an ordeal at the end of any one visit. Thus analgesia performs its functions *before, during,* and *after* each dental experience.

Nitrous oxide in anesthetic doses does not induce muscular relaxation. However, in the stage of relative analgesia the *patient exerts less conscious control over the movements* of the mandible, tongue, orbicularis oris, and head. Mental relaxation produces muscular relaxation.

A fearful patient tends to become more tense and afraid (and thus less cooperative) as the length of the operation increases. *The patient under analgesia has no idea of the lapse of time.*

Because fear and pain are controlled, *the patient will more readily present himself for treatment,* and will be more eager to complete his treatments. The tendency to stay away when the recall date comes due is lessened. The patient becomes highly cooperative, and consequently his dentition is maintained at a much higher level of health for a much longer span of time.

BENEFITS TO THE DENTIST

By securing all the above benefits for his patient, the dentist finds that important dividends fall to him. In former years, before the popularization of Freudian thinking and our greater understanding of the term "psychosomatic," we were wont to label many of our patients as cranks or hypochondriacs, uncooperatives, or untouchables. As we know today, such classification was an admission of failure on our part. We felt ourselves unable to cope with them, that they were impossible to care for, that we would do the best "under the circumstances." Or we would send them elsewhere. The overwhelming majority of these people were relegated to this category because they were fearful. Being fearful, they reacted in an exaggerated fashion to many procedures which we regard as minor. To the dentist with a busy practice, such patients are great time-wasters. They usually do not keep appointments on time, and they readily break appointments. Yet, in most cases these individuals want their oral condition cared for. Their behavior is based on fear of the dental experience.

Once this fear is removed with analgesia the transformation is almost magical. These individuals become excellent patients. They present themselves on time and are highly cooperative in the dental chair. The operator finds that he saves much time, both with the fearful patient and with the good patient.

The so-called untouchables, having done without dental care for a very long time, usually have badly deteriorated dentition. This is our problem. We earn our livelihood by practicing dentistry, and these people have a great deal to be done. Once fear is removed, we find our patients more ready to accept our diagnosis and prescription.

The gagging patient often presents a difficult problem. The impulses provoking this reflex may result from tactile, visual, acoustic, olfactory, or psychic stimuli. In dental practice, gagging may be a problem during the taking of impressions and roentgenograms and in routine operative procedures because of the copious amounts of water necessary today with high-speed handpieces. Analgesia causes sufficient *depression of the gag reflex* to control the situation at all times.

Patients introduced to analgesia are highly enthusiastic recommenders. A patient whose fear has been removed suddenly, after living in fear of the dentist for many years, cannot stop talking about it to his friends and neighbors. He recommends his dentist highly to all who will listen, and justly so.

Let us not overlook the physical and mental benefits to the dentist. A relaxed and fearless patient means a more relaxed and more efficient operator who can perform faster and better dentistry with less physical and emotional strain on himself. In this way, the dentist's maximal efficiency is extended over many more years of practice.

REFERENCES

1. Arduini, A., and Arduini, G.: Effects of drugs and metabolic alterations on brain stem arousal mechanism. J. Pharmacol. Exp. Ther., 110:76, 1954.
2. Chapman, W. P., Arrowood, J. G., and Beecher, H. K.: Analgesic effects of low concentration of nitrous oxide compared in man with morphine sulfate. J. Clin. Invest., 22:871, 1943.
3. Eastwood, D. W. (Ed.): Clinical Anesthesia. Clinical Use of Nitrous Oxide. Philadelphia, F. A. Davis Co., 1964.
4. French, J. D., Verzeano, M., and Magoun, W. H.: Extralemniscal sensory system in brain. A.M.A. Arch. Neurol. Psychiat., 69:505, 1953.
5. French, J. D., Verzeano, M., and Magoun, W. H.: Neural basis of anesthetic state. A.M.A. Arch. Neurol. Psychiat., 69:519, 1953.
6. Greenfield, W.: Broader concepts and applications of inhalation analgesia. J. Amer. Anal. Soc., 2:6, 1964.
7. Guedel, A. E.: Inhalation Anesthesia. New York, The Macmillan Co., 1953.
8. Haugen, F. P., and Melzack, R.: Nitrous oxide effects on responses evoked in brainstem. J. Amer. Soc. Anesthesiol., 18:183, 1957.
9. Jaffe, M.: Choosing an inhalation analgesic through pharmacological comparison. J. Amer. Analgesia Soc., 2:4, 1964.
10. Johnson, H. M., and Paschal, F. G.: Psychobiology, 2:193, 1920.
11. Klock, J. H., and Tom, A.: Nitrous Oxide Amnalgesia. North Conway, N.H., Reporter Press, 1965.
12. Langa, H.: Analgesia for modern dentistry. N.Y.J. Dent., 27:228, 265, 1957.
13. Langa, H.: Nitrous oxide-oxygen analgesia for modern dentistry. Dent. Dig., 66:126, 1960.
14. Millikan, G. A.: Oximeter, instrument for measuring continuously oxygen saturation of arterial blood in man. Rev. Scient. Instr., 13:434, 1942.

15. Monheim, L. M.: General Anesthesia in Dental Practice. St. Louis, The C. V. Mosby Co., 1957.
16. Monheim, L. M.: Local Anesthesia and Pain Control in Dental Practice. St. Louis, The C. V. Mosby Co., 1957.
17. Peterson, C. G.: Neuropharmacology of procaine; central nervous actions. Anesthesiology, 16:976, 1955.
18. Rothchild, H.: The physiological basis of analgesia. New York Dent. J., 32:164, 1966.
19. Seevers, M. H., et al.: Analgesia produced by nitrous oxide, ethylene and cyclopropane in normal human subject. J. Pharmacol. Exp. Ther., 59:291, 1937.
20. Seldin, H. M.: Practical Anesthesia for Dentistry and Oral Surgery. Philadelphia, Lea & Febiger, 1947.
21. Shipper, P. E.: The mechanism of nitrous oxide analgesia. J. Amer. Anal. Soc., 2:4, 1964.
22. Sonnenschein, R. R., Jamison, R., Loveseth, L. J., Cassels, W. H., and Ivy, A. E., et al.: A study on the mechanisms of nitrous oxide analgesia. J. Appl. Physiol., 1:254, 1948.

PAIN AND THE PSYCHOLOGICAL BASES OF FEAR OF THE DENTAL EXPERIENCE

5

PAIN

Although always a subject of human curiosity, pain was not analyzed systematically until the middle of the nineteenth century, when Ernst Weber succeeded in drawing a distinction between pain and the sense of touch. Weber reasoned that heat, cold, and pressure are specific stimuli resulting in particular sensations, whereas pain has no specific stimulus but rather is much like hunger or nausea.

The theory of specific nerve energies, formulated in 1880, postulated that each quality of sensation depends on the stimulation of distinct nerve fibers and that these fibers constitute a pathway between receptor organs and the brain. This concept enlisted influential supporters for a time, but it was soon undermined by the report of Goldscheider. Failing in his efforts to elicit a pure pain response in the skin, this investigator concluded that sufficient stimulation of any sense would result in pain.

The situation remained clouded until in 1894 Van Frey demonstrated pain spots in the skin. Following his lead, investigators eventually proved pain to be a special sensation with its own receptors and pathways. Over the past three decades, there has been an enormous increase in the scientific study of pain. From it has evolved a concept in which pain is seen as an extremely complex experience and, most importantly, one that is subject to modification.

DEFINING PAIN

With the development of special instruments that permit the measurement of pain, attention was drawn to the perceptual aspect of pain, as opposed to the concept of pain as an emotional response. As this aspect was explored, it soon became evident that individual reactions to pain and the capacity to endure pain vary widely and, again most importantly, can be modified to a considerable extent. Not only emotional states but also religious

103

beliefs and strong feelings can be the dominant factors in the perception of pain.

Since emotions have an effect on reactions to pain, pain reactions can be modified by conditioning. This aspect of pain reaction is of tremendous importance to the dentist, for it provides him with an additional approach to the problem of eliminating fear of pain during the dental experience. By influencing this factor, as well as the reactions in smooth muscles, glands, and skeletal muscles, he can radically change not only an individual's perception of pain but also his attitude toward it.

Perhaps this human phenomenon can be understood more clearly in terms of the dissociation of the perception of pain from the reaction to pain. For example, most of us are familiar with the indifference to injury often shown during the excitement of games or in the heat of an argument. Similarly, reports from the battlefield recount the heroic unselfishness of men who, completely unmindful of their own injuries, have performed almost impossible feats. Likewise, during certain religious and mystical practices, persons have appeared to be insensible to pain. And during parturition, women who have confidence in their physician or who want very much to bear a child are more indifferent to pain than those who have no confidence in their physician or who do not want a child. The pain experience, therefore, involves not only the perception of pain but also a pattern of reaction that varies greatly in both a physiological and a psychological sense.

Such variations in the response to pain demonstrate the fundamental error of those investigators who held that for any given stimulus of a certain strength a corresponding response must follow. The relationship between a pain stimulus and the subjective response is not simple, but rather it is influenced by conditioning, by the neural processing of the stimulus, and by the psychologic reaction.

To almost all who have been subjected to protracted, severe pain, the pain is regarded as a pernicious and punishing affliction. Thus it is not surprising that the word pain is derived from the Latin *poena*, a penalty or punishment. In the writings of many ancient peoples, pain is described as a curse of the gods on those who had displeased them.

In attempts at defining pain, a stumbling block has been that pain is interpreted according to the training and attitude of the investigator. The physiologist interprets pain as a sensation much like seeing or hearing. The biologist recognizes pain as a warning signal that alerts an organism to harmful stimuli. The sociologist sees pain and anticipation of pain as instruments of learning and social preservation. The psychologist notes the conversion of a neural impulse into a sensory experience. To the sufferer, however, pain is a debilitating ordeal.

Although pain is a universal experience, and everyone knows what is meant by it, the subjective nature of this sensation makes it uncommonly difficult to define. Definitions of the sensation of pain seem to tell us only what we already know—that pain is unpleasant. Many efforts to define pain are merely descriptions of the anatomy and physiology involved. Yet such attempts may bring us closer to a satisfactory definition of pain. Monheim has described pain as "an unpleasant sensation created by a noxious stimulus which is mediated along specific nerve pathways into the central nervous system, where it is interpreted as such."[22]

Because noxious stimuli disturb the equilibrium of an organism, they are highly motivating in and of themselves. That is, no learning is necessary for an organism to react to them. The resultant behavior is typically avertive. Pain stimuli, the most important of the noxious stimuli, usually take precedence over other stimuli. We know that pain is induced by various kinds of noxious stimuli—mechanical, thermal, chemical, and so on—but we do not know the means by which they excite a receptor.

In an attempt to get at the two-sided nature of pain, Bishop offered the following observations:

> Pain is what the subject says hurts. You can't get behind that. It consists, however, of two phenomena: A. *Pain as a subjective experience*, repeated as a *sensation* referred specifically to some part of the body sufficiently unpleasant to be designated as painful by the subject. This unpleasant sensation will of course vary with emotional state, anxiety, anticipation of disaster, etc. It may be due to activation of any modality of sense, and possibly to none. B. *Pain as a physiological process*, with a subjective evaluation in addition to perception, is a result of stimuli to sensory nerve endings or pathways of two types of fibers: certain small myelinated fibers causing pricking pain on adequate stimulation, and unmyelinated fibers causing burning pain. Both pass up the lateral columns of the cord after synapse in the substantia gelatinosa.

Descriptions of subjects' reactions to pain, although useful in determining the presence or absence of pain, are likewise unsatisfactory as definitions of pain. What we are after is a definition of the experience of pain, and not of its outward manifestations.

So it is that, although everyone knows from personal experience what pain is, no one has been able to define it to the satisfaction of others. Yet a comprehensive definition of pain could open the way to new methods of relieving pain and of dispelling many human fears.

THE MEASUREMENT OF PAIN

Experiments devised to measure pain have been difficult to evaluate owing to the fundamental difference in the reaction to experimental pain as opposed to pathologic pain. In experiments, the subject realizes that the pain, although unpleasant, presents no danger to him, that there is no threat to his bodily integrity. In contrast, the man suffering from peptic ulcer is only too conscious of the source of his pain and of the accompanying tissue damage, and his sensitivity to the painful stimuli is correspondingly greater than that of the subject to whom a stimulus of equal strength is applied experimentally.

In designing experiments for the measurement of pain, methods were required which would eliminate errors stemming from the problems mentioned in the foregoing discussion. That is to say, investigators were faced with the necessity of eliminating personal bias, both on their part and on the part of the subject; of providing the subject with criteria for evaluating his pain; and of facilitating communication between the investigator and his subject. To meet these goals, new methods have been based on the following concepts:

1. Two qualitatively similar pains can be quantitatively compared.

2. A pathologic pain can be compared in this way with a simultaneously occurring experimental pain.

3. An increasing experimental pain can be objectively measured.

4. An accurate end point can be subjectively established for the point at which pathologic pain and experimental pain reach equal intensity.

5. By inference, the measure of the experimental pain at this end point is the measure of the pathologic pain of unknown intensity.

On the basis of these criteria, equipment was designed to produce pain, to measure it, and to adjust the strength of the stimulus. The subject controls the equipment; he is instructed to initiate the stimulus and then to terminate it when he feels that the pain induced is equal to his pathologic pain. Such methods as these have led to the development of the concept of pain threshold.

The Pain Threshold

There is a point at which pain first barely becomes perceptible. This point is known as the pain threshold, and it is calculated in terms of the lowest intensity of noxious stimulus that will evoke it. In experiments the subject must tell the investigator when this point is reached. For this reason only a conscious and willing person can be the subject of pain threshold studies. Nevertheless, animal studies of pain, in which their presumed reactions to pain are used as a guide, have yielded useful data.

That pain is ever a "pure" sensation at the conscious level is doubtful. The neural impulses released by the noxious stimulus are "processed" at the level of the spinal cord and at higher levels. This activity is itself a part of the pain reaction. Yet, fundamental to most investigations in experimental pain is the concept that the pain threshold represents a pure perception of pain. It is also held that the pain threshold is much the same in all subjects and in the same subject at all times. Currently, these concepts are widely regarded as true, and yet they cannot be accepted as the whole truth.

THE PAIN REACTION

Pain is a phenomenon of the central nervous system, and it is becoming increasingly evident that the cortex is more involved in the consciousness of pain than had been previously considered. In this regard, the action of analgesics in raising the pain reaction threshold is quite possibly a result of their effect on the mental state of the subject. Preoccupation with pain tends to lower the pain reaction threshold; environmental distractions, mood changes, and interference with mental processes tend to raise the pain reaction threshold. As Bishop put it:

> It is not clear in view of the obvious central effect of drugs whether they have any effect on the periphery in ordinary analgesic dosage, nor is it always clear whether the increased perceptual threshold under drugs is in effect a result of changed mental attitude, lack of attention, interest, or less careful discrimination.

We may, therefore, conceive of any rise in the pain reaction threshold in analgesia as being secondary to changes in the mental state.

That emotion or distraction can dilute or even block the perception of pain has long been common knowledge. It has been demonstrated in hypnotic suggestion and hysteria that, although there is no change in the peripheral pain apparatus, there is no pain reaction to noxious stimuli. Current evidence supports the view that analgesics afford relief from pain by their action on the reaction component of pain and that there is little relationship between a rise in the pain threshold and relief from pain.

A characteristic of sense organs found in pain spots is that even a single brief stimulus has a persistent after-effect. For example, a single electric shock to such nerve endings sets up in the fiber a repetitive series of nerve impulses. This is unlike the situation in other kinds of nerve fibers, in which a single shock sets up but a single impulse.

FACTORS PERTINENT TO THE CONTROL OF PAIN

The foregoing has brought to us a body of knowledge which permits a more effective approach to the problem of controlling pain:

1. It is known that pain is not always perceived after injury even when the victim is fully conscious and alert. Thus a knowledge of pain perception goes beyond the problem of pain itself. It helps us to understand the enormous plasticity of the nervous system and how each of us responds to the world in a unique fashion.

2. Research has shown that pain is much more variable and modifiable than many believed in the past.

3. There is much evidence that pain is not simply a function of the amount of bodily damage. The amount and quality of pain one feels are also determined by his previous experiences and how well he remembers them, by his ability to understand the cause of the pain and to grasp its consequences. Even the significance of pain in the culture in which one has been raised plays an essential role in how he feels and responds to it.

4. Fear plays a great part in determining how much pain one feels. Obstetricians have demonstrated that fear increases the amount of pain felt during labor and birth.

5. Early experience has a tremendous influence on the perception of pain.

6. There is a considerable body of evidence that people attach different meanings to wounds and that these meanings have a powerful influence on

pain reaction to these wounds. Indeed, it is altogether possible that a wound that produced intense pain reactions in a man could under different circumstances produce an entirely different reaction. Consider, for example, the experience of Dr. Henry K. Beecher during World War II. Beecher found that in combat hospitals, only one of three severely wounded soldiers required morphine to relieve his pain. Most of these extensively wounded men denied any pain or explained that their pain was so slight that they did not need any medication. These soldiers were obviously not in shock, nor were they incapable of feeling pain, for as Beecher observed, they complained as vigorously as normal men at an inept venipuncture.

Following up this experience on his return to clinical practice, Beecher observed the reactions of a group of civilians who had undergone major surgery that produced wounds comparable to those suffered by the soldiers. When these men were asked whether they wanted morphine for their pain, four of five appealed for an injection to relieve their intense pain.

On the basis of this experience, it was determined that there is no simple, exclusive relationship between a wound in itself and the amount and quality of pain. Other factors play a role, and among them is the *significance* of the wound: To a soldier, a serious wound may mean release from the battlefield with the knowledge that he has done his job; he may experience relief and euphoria. To the civilian, major surgery may be a catastrophe threatening not only himself but also the well-being of his family; he may well be depressed and experience intense pain. This study rejects the notion that the more severe the wound, the more intense the pain.

7. Preoccupation with pain tends to heighten the experience of pain. By the same token, any activity that demands prolonged concentration or causes excitement can diminish or completely block out the perception of pain. This phenomenon is seen almost daily in athletic contests in which players sustain injuries without even noticing them.

8. The mere anticipation of pain intensifies the experience of pain. In this regard, it should be noted that morphine relieves pain when the patient is anxious but has no apparent effect once his anxiety has been dispelled.

THE PSYCHOLOGY AND PHYSIOLOGY OF PAIN

We now believe that the same injury can produce different reactions in different persons or in the same person at different times. As the foregoing observations indicate, the higher functions of the brain can modify the patterns of neural impulses stimulated by an injury. To explain this phenomenon, we must assume that such higher functions as emotions, thoughts, and concentration represent the actual activities of nerve impulses. Indeed physiologists have amassed much evidence to support this marriage of psychological and physiological processes.

Only a short time ago it was believed that, on external stimulation of the skin, a neural impulse was conveyed directly to the appropriate area of the cerebral cortex to produce the sensation (touch, pain, and so forth) indicated by the particular stimulus. Recently, however, physiologists have shown that systems of nerve fibers travel from the higher areas of the brain to connect with the message-carrying pathways in the spinal cord (Fig. 5–1). Electrical stimulation of these cerebral areas can modify or completely suppress a message, preventing it from ever reaching the brain. In fact, a completely different message may reach the brain.

It is possible that these nerve fiber systems furnish the mechanism through which the higher brain centers modify or suppress neural impulses after an injury. It is also possible that this can be accomplished at every junction in the central nervous system at which impulses are passed from one neuron to the next. On the basis of this theory, it can be visualized how psychological events influence the experience of pain.

Pain receptors are believed to be branching networks of fibers whose receptive areas overlap one another so that, when the skin is injured at a single point, two or more networks transmit a series of impulses along the nerve fibers that lead to the spinal cord. The spinal cord then receives a pattern of neural impulses, rather than a single train or series. As the pattern of impulses passes from the sensory fibers to the neurons of the spinal cord, the pattern can be altered and its duration diminished by interference from other stimuli.

In the spinal cord, the neural impulses ascend to the brain, some to the thalamus and others to the reticulated cells of the lower brain. Thus a new pattern of sensory impulses is formed, and this pattern proceeds through

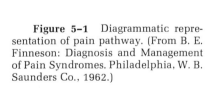

Figure 5–1 Diagrammatic representation of pain pathway. (From B. E. Finneson: Diagnosis and Management of Pain Syndromes. Philadelphia, W. B. Saunders Co., 1962.)

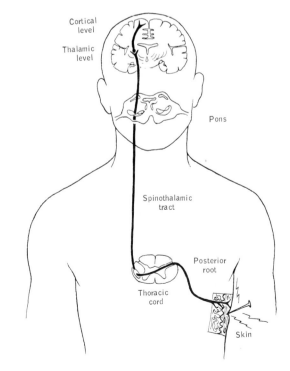

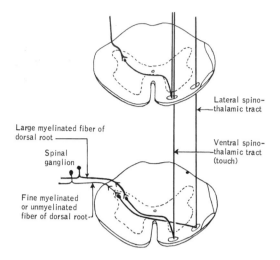

Large myelinated fiber of dorsal root

Spinal ganglion

Fine myelinated or unmyelinated fiber of dorsal root

Lateral spino-thalamic tract

Ventral spino-thalamic tract (touch)

Figure 5–2 Formation of the spinothalamic tracts. (From B. E. Finneson: Diagnosis and Management of Pain Syndromes. Philadelphia, W. B. Saunders Co., 1962.)

various routes to the higher brain. The electrical activity along three of these routes, including the spinothalamic tract (Fig. 5–2), is diminished by those analgesic agents, such as nitrous oxide, which inhibit pain without disturbing other senses such as sight and hearing.

Dramatic support for the concept of various levels of awareness of sensation was presented by Cannon, who reviewed the evidence for the thalamic control of emotion. He noted that in emotional reactions patients who have lost voluntary control of one side of the face show the same response in both sides of the face, whereas those who have suffered unilateral thalamic injury can voluntarily control both sides of the face but register emotion on only one side. Moreover, he found that the thalamus is the site at which dull sensations can be translated into intense sensations. Once released from cortical control, it is apparent that the thalamus is the site of control of the emotional component of pain and other sensations. As Cannon states:

> Just as the cortex cannot cause, so likewise it cannot prevent, those stormy processes of the thalamus that increase the blood sugar, accelerate the heart, stop digestion, or produce the other disturbances characteristic of great excitement. When an emotion is repressed, therefore, it is repressed only in its external manifestations.

For just this reason the emotionally upset person is beyond the logic of argument, a fact that should be borne in mind by the dentist who is tempted to reason with a distraught patient.

CONCLUSIONS OF IMPORTANCE TO THE DENTIST

THE PAIN MECHANISM

This consists of two phases: pain perception and pain reaction.

Pain Perception. Pain perception is the neural mechanism involving stimulus, impulse, and reception. When a pain stimulus reaches threshold intensity at the pain receptor ending, the environmental change causes a wave of excitation (an impulse) to travel along the peripheral nerve toward the brain. Pain perception depends on the intactness and normal functioning of the neural structures and varies very little from one individual to another. Disease or trauma of the neural structures will alter perception. From a clinical viewpoint pain perception is a physiological mechanism the importance of which lies solely in producing the reactive phase of the pain process.

Pain Reaction. Pain reaction is of great clinical importance to the dentist. It is the end result of the perception—the interpretation each individual makes of the pain impulse. Pain reaction occurs in the higher brain centers and involves complex neuro-anatomical and physiopsychological factors, which are modified by the stored information in the brain, i.e., by the subject's past experiences and his general attitude toward them. Consequently pain reaction is a definite clinical entity that varies a great deal from individual to individual. It manifests itself in many ways: crying, withdrawal, wincing, wringing of hands, perspiring, tapping of feet, humming, tachycardia, increased respiratory rate, extra heart beats, and elevated blood pressure. Factors such as emotional status, will, attitude, environment, fear, and apprehension all influence the type of response.

THE THALAMIC AREA

The tracts of the pain fibers enter the thalamic area, and it has been demonstrated that decerebration below the thalamus produces an ineffectual response to pain. In recent years increasing importance has been given to that part of the brain stem called the reticular formation. This reticular center appears to act as an arousal center, a driving force, a spark plug for cortical and thalamic activity. Animal experimentation has demonstrated that a lesion in or isolation of this reticular area prevents an animal from being roused from a sleeping state by a stimulus which would ordinarily produce pain. However, if the reticular center is left intact and if the pathways conducting pain are surgically separated, the same painful stimulus will rouse the animal.

Anesthesia. Many authorities today believe that a general anesthetic produces its effect by depressing the activity of the arousal area, thus eliminating cortical response even though the cortex may still be receiving pain impulses. It has been demonstrated that nitrous oxide depresses the functioning of this reticular activating center.

States of Feeling. The thalamic area is thought to be concerned also with states of feeling, or emotion.

Relative Analgesia. If the thalamic area governs states of feeling and acts as an arousal center and as a relay station for pain stimuli going to the cerebral cortex, then it can be understood how nitrous oxide can produce the following effects by a depressive action on the functioning of this area:

Amnesia. Stimuli have difficulty reaching the cerebral cortex with any continuity because of the depression of the arousal center.

Disorientation. Normally, there is a constant interaction between the sensory areas of the brain and the reticular center. Interference with this normal interchange results in confused brain activity.

Greater Pain Tolerance. Clinically a rise in pain threshold means a rise in pain *reaction* threshold. Depression of the arousal center depresses cortical activity and response, thus allowing the subject to remain in a dreamy state.

Diminution of Fear. Less awareness, disorientation, amnesia, and altered interpretation of pain stimuli create a euphoric state.

This discussion explains why the use of inhalation analgesia with nitrous oxide presents the dentist with a patient who is conscious but not fully alert, who is disorientated relative to activity around him, who loses his fear and his concept of the passage of time, and whose thoughts may wander and focus on events outside the dental treatment room. The use of local anesthetic agents eliminates pain perception; the administration of general anesthesia eliminates pain reaction completely. Inhalation analgesia provides an extremely effective, additional approach to the control of fear, pain, and discomfort during dental treatment.

PSYCHOLOGICAL BASES OF FEAR OF THE DENTAL EXPERIENCE

The reciprocal nature of fear and pain demands that the dentist combine psychological conditioning with the use of nitrous oxide and oxygen. Because they have been trained to accomplish this, many thousands of dental practitioners in the United States are now using relative analgesia successfully. Although no pretense is made here that the dentist should function as a psychiatrist, it is essential that he learn about the basic psychological factors involved in treating the oral tissues, for success in treatment necessitates an understanding of the whole patient: his fears, his motivation, his sense of values, and his background.

As we have noted, Monheim has defined pain as "an unpleasant sensation created by a noxious stimulus which is mediated along specific nerve pathways into the central nervous system, where it is interpreted as such."[22] To date, this is the best definition of a sensation which has been almost impossible to define. We know that an individual's reaction to a painful stimulus depends on factors other than the strength of the stimulus. We have also come to realize that past experiences having symbolic meaning can alter the degree of pain experienced during dental treatment and hence can affect the patient's attitude and opinion relative to his dentist. It is therefore imperative that the dental practitioner understand some of the basic psychological elements that influence the patient and his reaction to dental treatment. As Fox points out:

> There is no fine dividing line between the sciences. The physiologist has to be concerned with physics and chemistry; the sociologist with psychology and anthropology; and the psychologist with sociology, biology and even political science and economics. The dentist should have some knowledge of these subjects so that he may more effectively treat and diagnose. Some dentists possess the type of personality which almost immediately relaxes the patient and allays fear. Others seem to create hostility and tension. Through clinical observation it is well known that a patient who is tense and anxious will actually experience more pain.[9]

THE ORAL CAVITY AND PERSONALITY[2]

Erikson states that "psychological phenomena have undergone an evolutionary history similar to that of biological structures. Biological and psychological phenomena are closely interrelated, for there has been a simultaneous development of physiological structure and of psychological endowment."[7] He sees in each man's psychogenic life cycle a repetition of his phylogenetic evolutionary history. Although organically, the newborn baby is the same as his prenatal counterpart, psychologically he is already endowed with personality.

Bodily experiences and sensations are the first "social" experiences of the newborn child. These experiences remain imprinted in his mind and affect his future emotional development. The initial emotional experiences center in the areas of the body with which early life experiences are begun and they become closely associated with these areas, thus making them highly significant emotional zones. The first three or four months of life are concerned with the intake of food and air, with perception of light and sound, and so forth. Since the intake of food is the most important and most regular of the conscious activities of the infant, he makes primary contact with the outer world through the sucking activity of his mouth. At this very early age he associates the oral zone with discomfort and the ability to relieve it. The effects of these early associations serve as nuclei around which will be constructed many elaborations of personality and object relations. If we, as dental practitioners, can accept and realize this, we will not then be surprised or amazed that the oral zone should be so heavily invested with emotional content for the rest of life. Belmont has said:

> The early oral activities of the child are of great potential psychological significance; for they play an integral role as the precursors of the child's later pleasure-seeking orientations, his emotional relationships with outside objects and as the beginnings of a means of differentiating himself from the outside world.[2]

Embryological Derivation

Ribble has summarized the *embryological derivation* of the parts of the mouth in a way that makes it easier to understand why so many functions are fused in the first oral activity:

> The lining of the oral cavity is developmentally a part of the skin which has become folded in to form a pouch. This indicates that the mouth is fundamentally an organ of *touch*. Its nerve supply comes directly from the brain through five different cranial nerves. In the first weeks of foetal development, nose and mouth are one cavity, separated from the digestive tract by a membrane which later breaks through and disappears. Thus it is seen that in the beginning, the mouth is a large pocket just beneath the brain, with which it is connected much more closely than with the stomach.
>
> The hard palate, which will later separate the nose and the mouth, begins to develop at about the sixth week of intrauterine life. This structure is char-

acteristic of sucking animals (mammals) and plays the important role of dividing the mouth into an eating and breathing cavity. It might be compared with the diaphragm, another structure peculiar to mammals, which divides the body into the chest, or breathing compartment, and the abdomen, or digestive apparatus.[24]

During the time that the mouth and nose form a single cavity, the tongue begins to develop. At first, it is located directly above the main artery to the head, suggesting that its first function has to do with pumping blood toward the brain. From this position, it migrates upward into the floor of the mouth and begins to take on new functions. Its first activity is an upward pumping, directly the reverse of sucking, and this action is sometimes seen in premature babies and in infants with Down's syndrome, who constantly protrude and retract the tongue. This pumping action brings it back and forth across the sensitive hard palate and in all probability constitutes the first direct tactile experience of the individual.

The rich supply of cranial nerves to the tongue reflects its proximity to the brain during developmental life. These nerves, along with those that supply the diaphragm and the sensory lining of the mouth, are all correlated in the sucking reflex, and around this important mechanism the sensory life of the infant develops. Bonnard submits that, for the infant, the primal psychological role of the tongue is that it gives "tactile proof of not being wholly deserted, in that there was still one faithful and responsive companion" whom the child can summon at will.[3]

The Beginnings of Perception

At birth the infant can perceive only those sensations that originate within his body, for until now he has been protected from outside stimuli. The oral zone seems to be the first to evidence a response to stimulation—a turning of the head toward the stimulus and a snapping movement of the mouth.

The environmental changes undergone at birth are drastic; in effect, an infant is transformed from a water animal to a land animal. During fetal life the oral cavity, larynx, and adjoining structures are bathed in amniotic fluid. After birth the air rapidly dries these mucosal surfaces. This condition (dryness of the mouth, throat, and nasal passages) creates a sensation of thirst, which is relieved when the infant sucks the mother's milk through the nipple.

The act of sucking and deglutition is the infant's first coordinated muscular action. The muscles of the mouth, then, are the first to be brought under control, and the mucosal surfaces of the oral cavity are the first to be used in tactile perception. For these reasons, no doubt, nature has endowed the oral cavity with the capacity to react to the sensations of touch, taste, temperature changes, pain, and smell and with the ability to react to all the sensations involved in the act of deglutition.

In this manner the oral cavity serves as a bridge between the perception of inner sensations and reactions to outside stimuli. As Spitz says, "It is the cradle of all external perception and its basic model; it is the place of transition for the development of intentional activity, for the emergence of volition from passivity." No wonder, then, that this primal cavity is associated with many strange experiences both pleasurable and unpleasurable. Since the earliest sensory experiences take place here, the imprint of these experiences remains in the unconscious throughout life.

The Infant

The eruption of the deciduous teeth, between the ages of five and eight months, suddenly changes the sensations in the mouth. These changes are thought to affect the developing personality. It is common knowledge that during teething, a baby may be irritable and fretful and may not eat well. Erikson has presented the dilemma in which the child finds himself at this critical transitional stage:

> It is, of course, impossible to know what the infant feels as his teeth "bore from within"—in the very oral cavity which until then was the main seat of his pleasure—and what kind of masochistic dilemma results from the fact that the tension and pain caused by the teeth, those inner saboteurs, can be alleviated only by biting harder.[7]

Just what this can mean to the very young child, we are left to discover from direct observations and the results of psychiatric investigations in older children and adults. We do know that, with the advent of teething, the child progresses from a passive receiver to one who actively takes and holds. Just as he has learned to use his hands and eyes to deal with objects in his immediate surroundings, the child now gains more active control of his mouth, biting and grasping the objects at hand. These very activities, however, are those most likely to precipitate the reaction of weaning, a process that to the child seems to be a punishment, a rejection by the mother who gratifies his needs. Now the child simultaneously experiences pain, anger, and hurt, and these feelings are intimately associated with the mouth. Here, then, the situation is compounded, for "a social dilemma [is added] to a physical one. For where breast feeding lasts into the biting stage, it is now necessary to learn how to continue sucking without biting, so that the mother may not withdraw the nipple in pain or anger."[7] Or, as Belmont put it, "Here we have a situation in which the mouth has taken on the qualities of aggression and active acquisition and at the same time becomes the site of potential deprivation, hurt, and suffering—the biting must be controlled and limited."[2]

Given these circumstances, it follows that the child's later personality is considerably influenced by events during this period. Should he encounter heavily charged episodes during this period of development, the course of his personality development may be altered, having lifelong effects, as may be seen in the influence of this period on dreams, fantasies, and the patient-dentist relationship. With respect to the latter, Belmont advises that:

> With the very young child, in a way that we adults tend to forget and cover over, much is made of the biting, hurting, prehensile grasping functions of the teeth. Children have many aggressive fantasies involving teeth and, ac-

companying these, they have fantasies of retaliation and reparation. The child in the dentist's chair, in many instances, finds himself the victim of his own projected aggression, in addition to the realistic traumatic effect of dental procedures. These oral fantasies and the realistic traumatic aspects of the dental experience are very much intertwined and interrelated.[2]

The Child and Adolescent

After the second deciduous molars erupt, and the child has his full set of primary teeth, there is a lapse of approximately four or five years until the first permanent molars begin to appear. Usually this period is one in which oral experiences are less influential, although the child may suffer traumatic experiences such as tonsillectomy, painful caries, or filling procedures. Then, at about the age of six, the child once again undergoes the loss and eruption of teeth, during which a host of reactions may be engendered, depending on the circumstances. To appreciate the child's response, it is again necessary to recall his vulnerability and the intensity of his reactions. He may suffer shameful embarrassment and humiliation from the loss of his teeth and be painfully uncertain whether he will ever grow new teeth. During this period, too, he is often given graphic descriptions of the results of neglect of his teeth. His reactions to these can only be guessed at.

In adolescence, as the youth becomes more concerned with his physical appearance, there is a renewed concern with his teeth. White, healthy teeth are attractive and instill a sense of pride in appearance, whereas yellow, uneven, or poorly cared for teeth cause embarrassment and a loss of self-esteem.

The Adult

As the adolescent grows into adulthood, the condition of his teeth may be regarded as a symbol of his general state of health. And as he grows still older, he may recall his parents' attitude when they first got dentures. They may have viewed the loss of their teeth as a landmark on the road to old age, for it is true that many lose their teeth at an age when they are particularly vulnerable to this idea. Moreover, the significance attached to the loss of teeth takes other and more varied forms. Belmont states that:

> A great deal has been learned about the unconscious meaning of teeth for the patient from the analytic investigation of dreams. Their loss may be feared as indicating deterioration, death, abandonment, deprivation, mutilation, castration and decay. It may also be desired in dreams as a representation of the wish to be infantile once again and cared for at the breast of a protecting mother. Ultimately, the tooth dream seems to relate back to the basic feelings deriving from the infant's oral relation to the mother, but these feelings and symbols are overlayed by and condensed with affects and symbols associated with later stages in the hierarchy of the psychosexual development of the individual. Depending on the circumstances associated with the dream, a lost tooth may equally readily represent the relinquished nipple or lost genital; a cavity lined with tooth-like projections may refer equally to the mouth or vagina dentata. In the unconscious it is not too difficult to interchange the two.[2]

Lack of understanding of the emotional values associated with the oral zone, and of the reasons that so much fear seems to be evidenced upon treatment, has kept millions of people from having sorely needed dentistry performed. It has also prevented active patients from having all necessary work completed. It has made the dentist's daily task, an extremely difficult one at best, even more trying and more difficult. It has created misunderstandings between patient and dentist, since both parties approach each other with different attitudes. The patient's thoughts are primarily conditioned by anticipated painful experiences. The dentist, on the other hand, may be thinking primarily in terms of the difficulty of the work to be performed and of the time necessary to do the work well.

REACTIONS TO STRESS

The Reaction of the Patient

Recently there have been efforts to study the physiologic response to emotional stress induced by dental treatment. The first problem was to find a reliable method of appraising stress in the dental patient. Ship and White set out to study the relationship between routine dental procedures and physiologic stress by using adrenal cortical activity as a measure.[27] This was determined by measuring changes in the eosinophil levels in peripheral blood. They observed the eosinophil responses of healthy adults during the performance of many common dental procedures.

In 1939 Dalton and Selye showed consistent reductions in circulating eosinophilic leukocytes in the peripheral blood as a result of various alarming stimuli. These included surgical trauma, insulin hypoglycemia, hemolysis, hemorrhage, cold, epinephrine, labor, eclampsia, cesarean section, fever, electroshock, coronary occlusion, congestive heart failure, muscular activity, and anoxia. They demonstrated that the magnitude of the eosinopenic response varied directly with the degree of stress. Many other investigators demonstrated that the emotions could play a large role in the eosinophil response to stress.

Ship and White evaluated three interdependent conditioning factors with respect to their roles in the production of eosinopenia following dental treatment: pain, tissue insult, and the emotions (anxiety, apprehension, and fear). Here are the results of their study:

1. All dental procedures caused significant stress responses in subjects compared to responses in controls.

2. Stress responses to various operative dentistry procedures were not significantly different from responses to the relatively innocuous interview, radiographic and oral examinations, or prophylaxis appointments.

3. Local anesthesia produced no stress reduction in operative dentistry.

4. Barbiturate premedication produced only a slight reduction in the stress reaction to operative dentistry.

5. The stress reaction to oral surgical procedures was greater than the re-

action to all other procedures tested. Here barbiturate premedication reduced stress by 26 per cent.

6. *Anxiety, fear,* and *apprehension* during the course of dental treatment appeared to be the primary factors involved in the stress-inducing aspects of dentistry.

In another carefully controlled study, the response of the adrenal cortical mechanism was observed in dental patients who were undergoing procedures in oral surgery. The criterion used here was the level of the plasma steroids. The results of this study showed that the *psychic trauma* of anticipating oral surgery was the most significant stimulus to the adrenal cortex. In other words the anticipation of pain, the fear of pain, caused great chemical changes in the patient's body.

We must face the fact that people feel more than they think, that pure, undiluted rational thinking does not exist. Emotions vary and modify all our thoughts. This holds true even in the most logical, the most intellectual, individual. Fear seems to overpower rational thinking when pain is anticipated, especially in the average individual's relation to the dental experience. In fear, the autonomic nervous system — the instrument of the emotions — is activated, as is the cerebral cortex. If we are to judge by the millions of people who do not apply for dental treatment, as well as by the highly irrational fear of many of those who do apply, the obvious conclusion is that the autonomic nervous system gets the upper hand over the cerebral cortex far too often.

ANXIETY AND FEAR

Since the utilization of relative analgesia has as its primary objective the elimination of fear and anxiety, we should discuss, to some limited extent, the basic psychology and physiology involved. Dental practitioners are particularly concerned with these emotions and their covert and overt manifestations, because they have to deal with them in their daily work. In addition, the successful clinical application of relative analgesia depends on an appreciation by the dentist of the presence of fear and anxiety in his patient and on his ability to cope with their manifestations.

Most authorities on the subject agree that there is a difference between anxiety and fear. *Fear,* they say, is attached to an *external object* or situation. One man may fear another, or he may fear a wild animal. A child might have fear of punishment by a parent or teacher. And, sadly, a child may fear the dentist. Fear, therefore, is a reaction to an *external danger.*

Anxiety, on the other hand, seems to be generated by an *internal threat,* a feeling that all is not well, that some terrible event is about to happen. Anthropologists and psychologists tell us that primitive man experienced fear but not anxiety. His evolutionary development was not such that he could cope with abstract ideas. He could fear external threats such as wild beasts but, when he did experience sensations akin to fear within himself, he externalized them by attaching his fears to something in his environment. So it would seem that the experiencing of anxiety is yet another price that the human being has had to pay for the greater development of his cerebrum.

Unfortunately, the human being is physiologically unable to distinguish between anxiety and fear; that is, anxiety is accompanied by physiological changes that are appropriate for mobilizing against an external threat, but are most often inappropriate to situations arousing the anxious state. The acutely anxious patient, with a rapidly pulsating heart, dilated pupils, and deep respirations, is reacting physiologically as if his body had to prepare itself to meet some immediate external physical danger. Should this state continue, as in chronic anxiety, functional and organic changes may take place, especially in the cardiovascular and gastrointestinal systems.

Anxiety results from the inability of the individual to cope with daily life situations. When he continues to experience anxiety, and when his emotional system fails to adjust itself properly to the total sensory input, he experiences *stress*. Susceptibility to stress is determined by heredity, early conditioning, fatigue, and general health.

The dentist sees many of the common signs and behavior of anxiety in his dealings with his patients: the subject who is alert to an exaggerated degree, who is restless and talks too much, who is overly eager to obey, who answers questions almost before they are put to him. Such outward manifestations are, of course, obvious to the dentist, but he should also appreciate what may be going on inside the patient. Some of the common symptoms of anxiety are apprehension, mental and muscular tension, and palpitation. When these symptoms are prolonged, the patient suffers chronic fatigue and cannot sleep well.

The anxious and fearful patient is difficult to treat. As has been mentioned, anxiety, fear, and apprehension appear to be the primary factors in the stress-inducing aspects of the dental experience. Relative analgesia is the most effective instrument for dealing with this situation, and it is almost universally acceptable to patients when properly introduced.

CONTRIBUTING FACTORS

It is imperative to solve the problem of fear of the dental experience (Fig. 5–3). So long as it continues to exist, it acts as a main deterrent to the practice of dentistry, diluting the efforts of the dental profession toward the dissemination of knowledge concerning its technical improvements and pain-eliminating procedures (Fig. 5–4). It prevents the major portion of the population from applying for treatment, thus denying them the high level of oral health which is their due and which we are capable of giving them.

That fear of the dental experience does exist to a great degree cannot be denied. One has but to ask any dental practitioner, patient, or potential patient. And this is so despite the great improvements in techniques and instruments. Local anesthetic injections are far more effective than they were even a decade ago. Modern high speed cutting instruments with water and air coolants greatly reduce pain stimuli and the time required to do dental work.

Why, then, this irrational fear of the dental experience? There are many possible explanations. The oral zone is not only the earliest and most important organ of aggression in animal evolution, it is also the first area in the in-

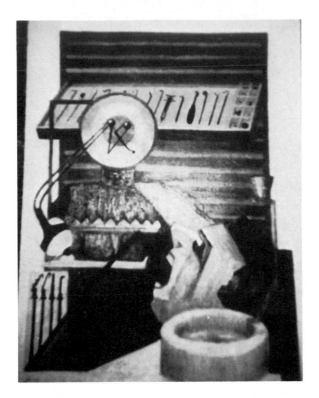

Figure 5-3 An unknown artist's concept of fear of the dental experience.

fant to become sensitive to pain and touch. The importance of the oral zone in this regard is suggested by the fact that the first cranial nerve to be myelinized is the trigeminal or fifth, which supplies the jaws and teeth. Those who lean toward Freudian theory explain the fear of dental treatment by emphasizing the erotic importance of the oral zone and its important linkage to the id of the individual, so that the manipulations of the dentist may assume the significance and severity of much more dire and foreboding acts.

Early conditioning also plays a very important part. If a child is surrounded by people who look upon dental treatment with a certain amount of dislike or trepidation, he will most likely react to dentistry in similar fashion. Should this child hear other members of his family give gruesome descrip-

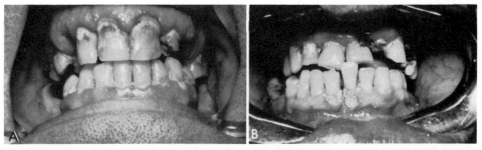

Figure 5-4 Two patients who suffered destruction of oral health due to fear of the dental experience.

tions of their "horrible" experiences in the dental chair, he will immediately attach special significance to the dental chair and to dental pain. He will thus be adversely conditioned, a problem patient before he ever visits the dentist. This same child may grow up to be a highly intelligent individual, yet still retain his irrational fear of the dental experience. He may know, intellectually, that having his oral condition treated is not a matter of life and death, just as he knows that the actual physical pain will be fully controlled. Nevertheless, knowing all this, he may still approach the visit to the dentist with extreme apprehension and fear.

Jokes and cartoons about the dentist can still be considered factors in prolonging that unholy trinity of "pain-fear-dentist." These seemingly harmless carry-overs from preanesthesia days continue to do great harm.

The nature of dental treatment is also a factor. Dental treatment is repetitive; rarely can the necessary work be done in one or two sittings. If fear of dentistry is not eliminated at the outset, it increases in geometric proportion as time goes on.

Fear of the unknown seems to be inherent in human nature. This is a factor to be considered when initiating a child to dental treatment.

The Reaction of the Dentist

Eradication of fear of the dental experience is a pressing problem for other reasons, too. These pertain to the economics of practice and to the health and well-being of the dentist himself. For example, the preparation of an occlusal cavity on a lower molar may take only a few minutes with modern cutting instruments, *if* the work is done on a fearless, cooperative patient. The same procedure could take a half hour or more when the patient is fearful.

The dental practitioner has only his time and skill to purvey. If he has to expend 30 minutes on a 2 minute procedure he has lost income. Conversely, if he is able to convert a half hour procedure to one that takes 2 minutes through effective control of the patient's reactions, he has automatically increased his income.

As dental practitioners we all have certain aims in life. Some of these may be conscious, others subconscious. We would like to be as successful as possible, and to achieve a certain degree of financial independence. Furthermore we would like to achieve this in as short a period of time as possible. We do not mind hard work, but we would prefer that this work extract from us a minimum of physical and emotional energy. Working daily in a pleasant, relaxed atmosphere is extremely important. Fatigue, tension, hurry, worry, and indecision are the greatest enemies of serenity and good health. All the courses we take in order to improve our technique are futile and meaningless if we find ourselves at the end of the working day so unnerved, so incapacitated that we cannot practice dentistry with a sense of pleasure and gratification and of accomplishment.

When we deal all day long, day after day, with people who are tense, afraid, and in pain, we cannot help but absorb some of that tension into our own system, no matter how relaxed we may be. The morbidity and mortality rates from heart disease are unusually high among dentists and physicians because they are subject to their own inner tensions and because they seem to acquire and absorb the stresses and strains of their patients. Anxiety and tension are infectious!

It is common knowledge that a variety of traumatic factors in daily life increase arterial pressure in susceptible people. What then is more important than to begin treatment of a patient by so modifying his treatment and his reaction to it that he is put to a minimum of stress and strain? The dentist himself will then have less to absorb. As Weiss and English put it:

> The psychiatrist listens to complaints of patients, absorbs their hostilities and aggressions, and puts up with their infantile demands. With many psychiatrists this is easier because in their training they have gained insight into their own emotional needs and can look upon those of the patient more realistically. No one has full insight into his own emotional problems. The dentist is subjected to many of the same attitudes, feelings, hostilities and demands as is the psychiatrist, but he has not been trained to recognize or handle them as objectively. It is extremely difficult to remain emotionally neutral to the emotional fluctuations of a patient. The dentist is engaged in an occupation in which the complete elimination of pain and discomfort is an impossibility. This is difficult for the dentist as well as for the patient. If the dentist has an unconscious emotional conflict as most people do, then the infliction of pain on others may be accompanied by guilt and self-reproach. At the end of the day he may feel fatigued, depressed and uncomfortable, as a result of his own unconscious feelings about the infliction of even unavoidable pain.
>
> The dentist is also exposed to the reactions of patients who present open or concealed hostility to his procedures. This adds more to his own problems. Few of us are well enough integrated and composed to withstand frequent over-reaction to pain by patients, day after day. Since dental treatment is repetitive it is essential for the dentist to develop a good interpersonal relationship between the patient and himself. To do this he should have some knowledge of personality types.[31]

Understanding his patient will also facilitate the introduction of the patient to relative analgesia.

IMPLICATIONS FOR THE DENTIST

The oral zone is related symbolically or directly to all the major passions and instincts: to self-preservation, to hate, and to love. It possesses a tremendous emotional potential, which may explain some of the "exaggerated" and strange reactions to what we know are relatively mild dental procedures. Ryan[25] suggests that the dentist keep these facts in mind when making diagnoses and planning treatment. He does not suggest that the dentist function as a psychiatrist, but that he adopt the psychosomatic point of view. While urging this approach as an extremely valuable adjunct to dental treatment and diagnosis, he warns against its use as a substitute for dental procedures. When this approach is employed in making a diagnosis, we find ourselves considering the psychological and emotional implications of our treatment as well as making use of the x-ray, the mouth mirror, and the explorer.

The Training of the Dentist

The undergraduate dental student practices technique during the first half of his educational career on a docile mannikin head. When he is faced with his first live patient he is very often astounded at the different role he must now play. Up to this point he had been asked to fulfill only the role of a technician; now he discovers that he has to play many parts. It is the author's belief that the practice of modern dentistry requires the possession and exercise of more varied attributes than are called for in any other profession.

Although dentistry is a young profession, it has made tremendous strides in its century of existence. Modern dentistry requires not only that the dentist be a technician, but also that he possess the abilities of an artist, a sculptor, a ceramist, that he be a diagnostician, radiologist, surgeon, anesthetist, and psychologist. A dentist who has been in practice for a number of years has developed a degree of manual dexterity that permits him to speak of certain procedures as "simple preparations." In truth these procedures are not simple; even were they to be done on a typodont tooth placed on a table, their proper execution would require a high degree of skill and a good deal of knowledge. However, the dentist works on living teeth with sensitive dentine and live pulps, set in living bony structures and surrounded by delicate soft tissues. If to this picture a moving tongue in a mobile head is added, it can easily be seen why dentistry is no simple task.

The work of a dentist would be difficult enough if he merely had to concern himself with the technical problems involved in the performance of dental procedures. The task, however, is made even more difficult by the fact that he has to deal not only with the pain involved but also with the fear and anticipation of that pain on the part of the patient.

About 125 years ago, dentistry established its own schools, independent of schools of medicine. Both good and bad results followed this schism. My feelings are that this independent road permitted a faster development of dentistry, although it had to go through a period of technical development before it began to encompass the biological aspects of treatment.

Today, at the undergraduate level the basic sciences are taught in equal degree to dental students and medical students. And, I think the time is drawing near when the dental student will receive instruction in the psychology of dental treatment. It is in the schools of dentistry that the future dental practitioner should be made aware of the great importance of treating the whole patient, of treating his psyche as well as his body. He must be taught the relationship between the construction of a successful set of dentures and the establishment of proper rapport between the patient and himself. He should be shown how the acceptance of a prescription often depends on his understanding of the individual with whom he is dealing, and why control of fear before and during surgical intervention makes for fewer untoward postoperative sequelae.

I concur with Giddon[11] when he says that the undergraduate curriculum would then have to include such subjects as control of fear and pain, normal development of personality and its adjustment to crisis situations, the influence of anxiety, and the basic psychological processes of learning and conditioning. It would also include the study of abnormal growth and development and abnormal psychological and social factors and their manifestations in behavioral problems. With this knowledge imparted to him at an early stage in his career, the graduate could then start the practice of dentistry with a greater appreciation of the value of history-taking and with the ability to treat successfully patients of every kind and to make better diagnoses and prognoses.

It is heartening to learn that this concept is now beginning to be more fully appreciated and implemented, as is evidenced by the following thoughts, pronounced by a psychiatrist[35] at a plenary session on comprehensive pain and anxiety control held by the American Association of Dental Schools:

"Pain is an inevitable and frequently devastating part of human experience. Yet, despite the truly important advances recorded in recent years in the control of pain, much remains to be understood about this intensely personal and highly variable phenomenon. In order to diagnose and effectively control pain, then, the dentist must have an understanding of the many social, cultural, and psychological variables which affect the patient's perception of and reaction to pain. In addition, he should be aware of certain behavioral principles which he may utilize in controlling reaction to pain.

"The word 'pain' is derived from the Latin 'poena' meaning penalty, implying somehow that discomfort is a result of or at least meaningfully related to sinfulness and wrongdoing. Hence, the guilt so often associated with pain and illness in our culture. Similarly, 'mal de dent,' the French term for toothache, characterizes 'mal' from the Latin 'malum,' or evil.

"There are several major reasons why dentists should be concerned with effective pain control. First, it is a well established fact that the fear of pain and the anxiety attached to it are major barriers to the seeking of care. Second, pain is a frequent presenting symptom for many patients, as much as 75 per cent in some medical outpatient departments and, if we can accept a growing feeling among psychiatrists, rapidly becoming today's major conversion symptom. The days of paralysis or hysterical blindness are over. Pain is now the major conversion symptom. I think that is why you are seeing it in the temporomandibular joint syndrome. Third, prevention of pain is an important motivating factor for seeking of care and should be the major goal of all health personnel.

"The observations of psychodynamics involved in pain and pain relief by clinicians skilled in observing real-life behavior of patients are worthy of more attention. Of particular note is their clinical observation that pain may arise from disturbed emotions as well as from disordered tissues and can serve many meanings for the patient.

"In this regard it has been suggested that pain frequently becomes the sufferer's major preoccupation of defense against the stresses of life and that not all patients who are relieved of their pain are uniformly grateful.

"Psychiatrists have also noted that relief of psychogenic pain without relief of the underlying psychological conflicts or tensions may precipitate depression and other psychiatric symptoms.

"A major contribution to the understanding and review of the factors affecting response to pain has been the more complete identification and classification of some of the social and behavioral variables which may enter into this response.

"It is abundantly clear that factors such as age, the situation, perceptual and cognitive set (i.e., expectations, early experience, past experience, cultural view of pain and illness), socioeconomic class, personality characteristics, and emotional state may all affect the response to pain. Consideration of such variables can provide a broad conceptual framework from which to approach research and teaching in this field.

"Until recently there was little compatibility between those who thought of pain in a physiological sense and those who thought of it in a psychological sense. Now this is beginning to change, as indicated by such emerging theories within physiology as the gate control theory.

"There are a number of issues which underlie some of the problems in the field and which may well be responsive to the contributions of the behavioral sciences.

"First it is best not to try to distinguish arbitrarily between physiological and psychological components of the pain experience, but rather to focus on the multi-dimensional aspects of the total pain experience. It is now clear that there are at least three levels in this response — absolute threshold, the sort of anything-at-all initial sensation, pain threshold level or onset of perceived pain, and the pain tolerance level or limit of the ability to endure.

"The second issue surrounds our changing knowledge concerning the stability of the pain threshold level. For a long time it has been assumed that variations in pain response were a function of changes in pain tolerance levels and that pain threshold was relatively uniform.

"This position has recently been challenged by Dr. Samuel Dworkin of Columbia University, School of Dental and Oral Surgery, who has found that both pain threshold and pain tolerance are diminished in a dental setting where the pain experience has an important contextual meaning.

"Third, if we are to fully understand pain it is important to distinguish between pain studied in the laboratory and that experienced in the clinical setting.

"Beecher, Lasagna, Sausen and others feel that pain can only really be understood in the clinical setting, since the laboratory experiment lacks the anxiety and the threat of the former. In Shore's laboratory, when the experimenter turned the painful stimulus on himself, he found it to be less painful in every case than that reported by the subject. Indeed, his cognitive set of what to expect may well have reduced his perception of the stimulus as painful.

"Finally, it is felt that anxiety is the crucial variable in the study of pain, a fact long appreciated by practitioners. The greater the anxiety, the less the tolerance for pain. Many of the techniques used by physicians and dentists to alleviate pain include a large element of anxiety reduction. Unfortunately, there is limited correlation between psychological and physiological measures of anxiety and relatively little relation between these and pain threshold levels, although there is some correlation with pain tolerance levels.

"One of the problems here is that anxiety, like pain, is itself a multi-dimensional concept which, depending on how it is viewed, may have characteristics of a state, a process, or a trait variable, each of which is measured in a different way.

"Although it is true that most psychological techniques serve to raise tolerance levels rather than threshold levels, this is probably of little concern to the patient or to the practitioner.

"The problems of pain, stress, and fear are inextricably intertwined in the dental situation. So, in spite of remarkable improvements in dental anesthetics and techniques, the prospect of a visit to the dentist still evokes fear in many people. Too little attention has been placed on efforts to understand and alleviate the psychological discomforts of dental treatment. Among the procedures suggested for coping with the stress of dental treatment are:

1. Distraction and displacement away from the threat.

2. Verbalization or communication with others about the threat.

"Much of the value of individual and group psychotherapy comes from the ability to ventilate one's feelings to meaningful others. Unfortunately, it is difficult to communicate how one feels with a rubber dam and a mouthful of instruments.

"Still other patients attempt to manipulate the threat through establishing control over it, either through some sort of advance information or preparation or control. It is too bad that we haven't got a way of letting the patient control what goes on or somehow indicate to the dentist what is going on, because this would immediately move his pain threshold higher.

"Affiliation is another common coping mechanism. When people feel threatened, they prefer to be with friends. By establishing a close relationship with a doctor, nurse, friend, or even a fellow patient, one may feel that he is not entirely alone.

"Further procedures which one may utilize in dealing with pain and stress include some that have been part of the armamentarium of helpers and healers since ancient times—reassurance, support, suggestion, reward. Even Pavlov's dogs and Miller's rats responded differently to pain when they were rewarded at the same time the pain was presented as a stimulus. How they work is an appropriate endeavor for behavioral science reseach.

"Another time-honored method for managing pain involves the use of placebos, especially where anxiety and apprehension are significant.

"In an extensive review of a number of studies, it was found that placebos are effective in about 35 per cent of patients. Paradoxically, only 3.2 per cent of patients with laboratory-induced pain experienced relief from placebos.

"Closely related, of course, is the clinical use of hypnosis, which it is claimed is effective in about one-third of patients.

"The basic mechanism of hypnotic relief of pain consists not of some special technique but of suggestions of relief given in a close, trusting, interpersonal relationship—nothing that any of you cannot give.

"As you all realize, the high effectiveness of hypnosis in children is that they are easily suggestible and when one looks at the kind of relationship between doctor and patient, it is indeed a reinforcing relationship for a dependency kind of thing, and under those circumstances, a close relationship can result in suggestions of relief which will work.

"To these must be added the coping mechanisms of desensitization, relaxation, and biofeedback which have arisen directly from recent work in the field of applied behavior analysis or behavior modification."

Dr. Baldwin concluded his lecture with a plea for the inclusion of the behavioral sciences in the research efforts on pain and anxiety control particularly in conjunction with the physiologist and pharmacologist. He stressed the need to teach this material in the dental schools.

Treating the Whole Patient

The dentist cannot successfully treat the mouth without treating the whole patient; he cannot disregard the rest of the patient's body or his state of mind. The clinical application of this principle may be relatively new, but the concept itself is very old indeed. Dunbar[6] points out that:

> Nearly half a millennium B.C. Socrates came back from army service to report to his Greek countrymen that in one respect the barbarian Thracians were far in advance of Greek civilization. *They* knew that the body could not be cured without the mind. This is the reason why the cure of many diseases is unknown to the physicians of Hellas, because they are ignorant of the whole.

It was Hippocrates who said, "In order to cure the human body, it is necessary to have a knowledge of the whole of things." And Paracelsus wrote, "True medicine only arises from the creative knowledge of the last and deepest powers of the whole universe; only he who grasps the innermost nature of man, can cure him in earnest." Socrates concluded, "Just as you ought not to attempt to cure eyes without head, or head without body, so you should not treat body without soul."

Today we are aware of the tremendous chemical changes that take place in the body as a result of stress and emotional tension. We know of the changes that take place in salivary output, in the adrenal glands and blood vascular system, in the lining of the stomach, and we are fully aware of the relationship between these changes and the causation of diseases such as peptic ulcer, coronary diseases, hypertension, mucous colitis, and some arthritic conditions. We, as dental practitioners, know full well the relationship between emotional tension and the causation of oral pathosis. Forces as powerful as these cannot be considered lightly by the dentist, for all too often the prospect of dental treatment brings them into play. The dentist must attempt to recognize and understand the fear reaction in his patient and to consider its elimination a primary and integral part of his treatment.

The Management of Patients with Certain Psychological Traits

Nearly every dental patient is interested in the esthetic result of treatment. There are some, however, who value this end to such a degree that they may lead the dentist into fabricating reconstructions that are not functionally correct and that will not endure for a reasonable length of time. Usually these patients are *narcissistic*. Never doubting their self-importance, they are at the same time not quite sure of themselves, constantly needing reassurance and praise. If the dentist allows such a patient to force him into a course of action that he knows is not proper, both parties will come to grief. I find that such persons can be handled more effectively by patient explanation and a good deal of praise and by listening attentively; in short, by catering to their most important motivating drives.

Certainly every dentist has had at least one patient who exhibits the following characteristics. He is neat and well mannered and agrees with everything you say. He keeps his appointments on time and seldom changes an appointment. In fact, he may be greatly upset if you should have to change one of his scheduled appointments. Such an individual must have everything explained to him in great detail. And, because of his compulsive nature, all recommendations must be made very carefully, for he will remember and follow them exactly. I recall an instance in which I was teaching a young man how to brush his teeth properly, explaining and demonstrating the technique of massaging the gingival tissue and then eventually ending up on the tooth structure. It would seem that the explanation was not sufficiently clear, for the patient did not understand that the massaging action of the brush should commence on the gum tissue about one-eighth of an inch from the free margin of the gingiva. On the contrary, he had initiated the action in the areolar tissue of the mucobuccal fold. When he returned one week later, his oral tissues were terribly scarified and inflamed. He had continued to follow my supposed instructions even though the results were so painful and so obviously harmful. Properly instructed, such patients will conserve their dental work for long periods of time, because they follow the dentist's advice relative to maintaining a high level of oral hygiene.

As has been mentioned, the mouth plays an important role in the emotional development of an individual. It is therefore a frequent focus of psychosomatic complaints by the *hysteric* patient. When such patients are of the opposite sex, the dentist should be on his guard, for hysterics are romantics who fall in and out of love very easily. They have an unconscious wish for love which may cause them to interpret certain remarks by the dentist as a sexual advance.

Some patients seem to enjoy pain. Too many of this type do not present themselves for treatment, but those who do can be recognized by their soft-spoken, gentle manner and their feeling of inferiority. They may come an hour early for their appointment and are extremely cooperative during painful procedures. Because of their *masochistic* tendencies, they do not present a great problem for the dentist.

Women who are approaching menopause may create many problems for the dentist. The approach of menopause can represent a threat to their self-esteem, and the emotional turmoil engendered may focus on the oral zone and generate various phobias and psychosomatic symptoms which are very difficult to treat properly. *Glossodynia* is a frequent symptom, which they interpret as carcinoma. Their symptoms and fears may create enormous problems for the dentist, especially when he is constructing a removable appliance. They must be authoritatively assured that they do not have cancer, and that their oral condition will not cause death.

The patient who exhibits *bruxism* is most often troubled by inner tensions and frustrations. He may present an outward façade of calm that hides his inner rage. He may speak in a calm, deliberate voice, even when he is telling you how much pain you have given him during treatment. The absence of head or body movements during dental treatment should not be construed by the dentist as signs of painlessness.

All who practice dentistry have had to deal with the perennially *dissatisfied patient*. Whatever is done for him meets with complaints and carping, and the more we try to please, the less favor do we find in his eyes. Since these people dislike themselves, they cannot like anyone else. The taking of the history of such a patient frequently reveals that his last several dentists failed to satisfy him because they were either too careless, cold, and indifferent or too friendly or mercenary. The history may also reveal that he was equally dissatisfied with his physicians. It is therefore best to be on guard when a new patient commences to criticize the previous dentist and his work. Despite his criticisms, remain calm and be a patient listener. Perhaps the only time such a patient will be satisfied is when the dentist loses his temper, for then the dissatisfied one has again proved that he was right, that no dentist wants to help him, that none cares about him and his needs.

Land has estimated that one of every 10 dental patients has a severe *overlay of emotional illness*.[15] But they are not difficult to treat, and they are greatly appreciative of any help given. The best approach is kindness and gentleness, with the development of a good dentist-patient relationship.

Many dental patients have somatic symptoms, yet no organic disease can be found despite a painstaking and thorough investigation. Of particular interest to the dentist are such symptoms as bruxism, ptyalism, drying of the mouth, excessive smoking, temporomandibular joint pain and noise, burning or tingling sensations in or around the tongue, tics, tongue thrusting, fingersucking, and the biting of the tongue, lip, cheek, nails, or objects such as a pipe or pencil. There is evidence, too, that severe psychological or physiological stress is implicated in recurrent aphthous stomatitis, acute dental caries, and periodontal diseases.

A patient who is anxious to an inordinate degree will fear the simplest of dental procedures; for example, a mandibular block may produce anxiety bordering on severe panic in the disturbed patient. In anticipating such reactions, it is well to remember that emotional reactions have long been associated with changes in the moisture of the mouth and throat, as demonstrated by the early experiments of Pavlov in which the relationship of salivary gland secretion to psychological states was established. Emotional excitement, apprehension, fear, and anger often seem to produce a dryness of the mouth.

Emotional disturbances are so common in the general population and show themselves so clearly in the dental treatment situation that the family dentist is often the first to observe evidence of severe emotional difficulties. The most frequently observed symptoms in emotionally disturbed dental patients are depressed mood, crying, anxiety, obsessions, phobias, irritability, guilt feelings, desperation, and lack of confidence. Usually, only the degree and duration of the distress are significant, since we all experience these same symptoms at one time or another. In any event, building the proper dentist-patient relationship is essential, and the use of relative analgesia with nitrous oxide and oxygen helps immeasurably to treat these patients effectively.

Many people are so overwhelmed by inner conflicts that they *begin to lose contact with reality*. They may become obsessed with their hair, skin, or teeth. Since they do not care for their teeth or oral tissues, they frequently present with periodontal disease and caries. Patience and sympathy go a long way in treating such patients.

It cannot be overstressed that the use of nitrous oxide and oxygen as relative analgesia is highly effective in treating all kinds of patients, whether they be normal or emotionally disturbed. Because relative analgesia has a favorable psychological effect as well as a physiological effect, treatment is more effective, more efficient, and less traumatizing for both the dentist and the patient.

Conclusions

Psychology is most certainly not an exact science, but the dentist can gain much from the information the psychologist has developed relative to the oral zone. A better understanding of the mouth as the primal cavity and a clearer understanding of the influence of the development of the oral cavity on the development of the human being and his personality can assist us immeasurably in treating the whole human being, instead of just his mouth.

If the dentist is thinking primarily in terms of the difficulty of the work to be performed and the time required to do it, consideration of the patient's physical and mental pain will be secondary. As a result, when the patient has been presented with an excellent diagnosis and prescription, he may answer "I will think it over, Doctor" or "I will speak to may wife" or "I cannot afford it." Any of his answers may be legitimate, but very often they are the result of fear of the dental experience.

The dentist, by recognizing the possible existence of this fear in his patient and by acknowledging its existence as a substantial factor in his estimation of the dentist-patient relationship, will have much greater success in handling his patient. The first thought in the dentist's mind when he greets a new patient should be, "I must do everything in my power to relax this individual and to allay his fears." If he practices this with each patient, he will find that in the process he himself has developed greater composure and serenity.

Being friendly and congenial does not take too much effort. Lord Chesterfield once said, "The Art of pleasing requires only the desire." It is amazing what a desirable reaction this produces in the patient, and in the doctor, too. To be a good listener certainly requires little effort. It is an art, but a passive art. If you show the patient that you are giving him your undivided attention, you not only flatter him but also learn a great deal about his main complaints and the main reasons for his being in your chair. Remembering his name also makes him feel that you are interested in his particular case and that you understand his particular problems.

The physical set-up (décor, and so forth) of the office is very important.

Cleanliness and neatness of all personnel in the office and orderly arrangement of all equipment generate a feeling of confidence in the patient. The personality of the dental assistant is also of prime importance, for he or she is usually the first to meet the patient, and the doctor is very often judged by the impression he (she) makes on the patient.

The psychosomatic approach in dentistry not only is scientific but in the end is also extremely rewarding. By allaying fear in the patient, the dentist finds that his daily task is lightened and his own tensions are lessened, that he saves time and thus is more productive with less strain on himself. This means a great deal to his patients as well as to his own family. He will also find that he encounters fewer untoward postoperative sequelae.

In this regard it is worth noting that the dentist and the patient apply different criteria in evaluating a dentist's work. When a dentist describes a colleague as being a good dentist he usually means that he is a good technician, one who turns out a gold inlay or gold crown whose margins are perfect and whose anatomical carvings are perfect; his dentures are beautiful and function well. When, on the other hand, a patient says that his dentist is a good dentist he means much more than that. He means not only that his dentist produces good work, but that he is highly pleased with the *way* in which he produces it.

Thus, as dental practitioners we are successful and attract patients in direct proportion to our sympathetic handling of them, as well as to the quality of the work performed. A "light hand" is a description of long standing, but it means much more than just having a light, delicate touch. It means that the patient knows that his dentist is keenly aware of the delicacy of the tissues being treated and is doing everything possible to minimize pain and trauma. It means that the patient feels that his dentist is sympathetic and kind and that he is doing everything in his power to relax him and allay his fears and apprehensions. It is not sufficient, today, to be a good technician. We must earn our patients' respect as a "good dentist." We must earn it, because our success in this venture brings tremendous benefits not only to our patients but to ourselves as well.

In the effort to control fear, pain, and discomfort, all modalities at our command should be employed. The *proper chairside manner* goes a long way toward relaxing the patient and allaying his fear. Elimination of conductivity in the peripheral nerve (*local anesthesia*) is one of our most important and basic approaches to solving the problem. Complete elimination of the pain reaction (*general anesthesia*) is of tremendous value when indicated. The use of the *intravenous route* for the production of both analgesia and general anesthesia has opened yet another pathway for the dentist. And lastly, the use of nitrous oxide as *relative analgesia* has proved itself to be a multifaceted medium through which the dental practitioner can filter all his procedures so that not only are fear and pain controlled, but the efficacy of other media is enhanced.

Of course, in choosing a particular medium for control of fear, anxiety, discomfort and pain, the dentist must first ask himself or herself several important questions:

1. *What are the dentist's own background and training in the use of a particular modality?* It is self-evident that the administration of general anes-

thesia requires much more training and experience than does a technique in which the patient is conscious throughout the procedure and has all his protective reflexes functioning fully.

2. *Who is the patient ?* Is he a so-called normal individual, or is he physically, mentally, or emotionally handicapped?

3. *What is the dentist's primary objective in treating this particular patient?*

a. Is completion of the treatment at this one visit an absolute necessity?

b. Is this an emergency procedure?

c. Is the dentist desirous of transforming this patient into a good, cooperative dental patient on a continuing basis?

REFERENCES

1. Beecher, H. K.: Measurements of Subjective Response. New York, Oxford University Press, 1959.
2. Belmont, H. S.: The development of the oral cavity as related to the development of the total personality. J. D. M., 19:86, 1964.
3. Bonnard, A.: The primal significance of the tongue. Int. J. Psychoanaly., 41:301–307, 1960.
4. Brenner, C.: An Elementary Textbook of Psychoanalysis. New York, International Universities Press, 1955.
5. Brown, N. O.: The Psychoanalytical Meaning of History, New York, Random House, 1959.
6. Dunbar, F.: Emotions and Bodily Changes. New York, Columbia University Press, 1954.
7. Erikson, E. H.: Childhood and Society, New York, W. W. Norton & Co., 1950.
8. Finneson, B. E.: Diagnosis and Management of Pain Syndromes, Philadelphia, W. B. Saunders Co., 1962.
9. Fox, L.: The control of pain and apprehension and use of local anesthesia in periodontics. Dent. Clin. N. Amer., July, 1961.
10. Gardner, E.: Fundamentals of Neurology. 5th ed. Philadelphia, W. B. Saunders Co., 1968.
11. Giddon, D. B.: Patient management—psychologic. Anesthesia Progress, 13:207–209, 1966.
12. Hart, H. H.: Practical psychiatric problems in dentistry. J. Dent. Med., 3(No. 4): 1964.
13. Isaacson, R. L. (Ed.): Basic Readings in Neuropsychology. New York, Harper & Row, 1964.
14. Land, M.: Oral behavior and the emotions as a factor in diagnosis. New York J. Dent., 36:310, 1966.
15. Land, M.: Mangement of emotional illness in dental practice. J. Amer. Dent. Assoc., 73:631, 1966.
16. Landa, J. J.: The Dynamics of Psychosomatic Dentistry. New York, Dental Items of Interest Publishing Co., 1953.
17. Livingston, W. K.: What is pain? Sci. Amer., 188:59, 1953.
18. Lorand, S.: On the meaning of losing teeth in dreams. Psychoanal. Quart., 17:529, 1948.
19. Lorand, S., and Feldman, S.: The symbolism of teeth in dreams. Int. J. Psychoanaly., 36:145–161, 1955.
20. Meares, A.: The Management of the Anxious Patient. Philadelphia, W. B. Saunders Co., 1963.
21. Melzack, R.: The perception of pain. Sci. Amer., 204:41, 1961.
22. Monheim, L.: General Anesthesia in Dental Practice. St. Louis, C. V. Mosby Co., 1957.
23. Ranson, S. W., and Clark, S. L.: The Anatomy of the Nervous System. 10th ed. Philadelphia, W. B. Saunders Co., 1959.
24. Ribble, M. A.: The Rights of Infants. New York, Columbia University Press, 1943.
25. Ryan, E. J.: Psychobiologic Foundations in Dentistry. Springfield, Ill., Charles C Thomas, 1946.
26. Shannon, I. L., et al.: Stress in dental patients. (Reprinted from the Journal of Oral Surgery.) Anesthesia and Hospital Dental Service, Jan., 1963.
27. Ship, I. I., and White, C. L.: Physiologic Response to Dental Stress. Bethesda, Md., National Institute of Dental Research. National Institute of Health, March, 1960.

28. Solomon, A. L.: Analgesia and anesthesia, a comparison. J. Amer. Anal. Soc., 3:4, 1965.
29. Spitz, R.: The Primal Cavity, Psychoanalytic Study of the Child. Vol X. New York, International Universities Press, 1955.
30. Watson, L. E.: Lights from Many Lamps. New York, Simon and Schuster, 1951.
31. Weiss, E., and English, O. S.: Psychosomatic Medicine. Philadelphia, W. B. Saunders Co., 1957.
32. Wenger, M. A., et al.: Physiological Psychology. New York, Henry Holt & Co., 1956.
33. Whittaker, J. O.: Introduction to Psychology. Philadelphia, W. B. Saunders Co., 1965.
34. Wyburn, G. M.: The Nervous System. New York, Academic Press, 1960.
35. Baldwin, D. C.: Contributions of the behavioral sciences to comprehensive pain control. J. Amer. Anal. Soc., 11:15–18, 1973.

THE INTRODUCTION OF ANALGESIA

6

Formerly, the concept that proper technique and equipment were all that was necessary to obtain good results with analgesia was accepted almost without question. The dentist was advised that all he had to do was to set the rate of flow and the proportions of gases at certain readings on the gas machine flowmeters and good analgesia would result. Today it is known that even with perfect technique, if the dentist is unable to overcome the patient's initial fear of this unknown procedure, failure may follow. There must first be instilled in the subject a feeling that the dentist is sympathetic and kind, that he is confident in himself and of analgesia. *The fear of the instrument itself must first be eliminated.*

The advantages of using analgesia in the practice of dentistry are many, but they cannot be brought to fruition until the procedure has been success-fully introduced to the patient. For this reason, it is highly important that the dentist accept the basic premise that analgesia is used primarily to eliminate fear of the dental experience. It is an almost universal truth that the patients who are most afraid of dental treatment are precisely those who are most afraid of analgesia. Few patients will accept analgesia without some trepidation; most will mentally resist it or be hesitant to try it. Even though the patient has im-plicit confidence in his dentist, fear of the unknown remains a potent factor. Yet this fear will be mixed with a great desire to try analgesia when the dentist has held out to the patient the significant possibility that by overcoming his fear of analgesia he will overcome all his fears of the dental experience.

This is certainly a strong incentive, for although fearful, such patients want very much to have their dental health restored. They are truly desirous of having a sympathetic dentist lead them toward this end. It is therefore in-cumbent upon the operator to help them gently over the primary hurdle. Not everyone, of course, fears analgesia but, since it is difficult to make this ap-praisal at the outset, a greater degree of success is obtained when it is as-sumed that fear is always present.

Under analgesia subjective symptoms vary with the individual patient. In the introductory stage he will probably be conscious of exhilaration and of a sensation of warmth throughout the body. This may be followed by a feeling of lassitude and a sense of remoteness from what is going on around him. Such a state is quite pleasant *if the patient resigns himself to it.* If, on the other hand, he makes an effort — inevitably unsuccessful — to keep control of

135

his faculties, he may become worried by his inability to do so. Relaxation becomes impossible, and an unsuccessful administration results. This is why such great care is needed in introducing analgesia. The subject must be taught to accept the sensations.

Once elimination of fear is accepted as the primary reason for using analgesia, the necessity and importance of a carefully planned psychological introduction to the patient is readily understood. This planned introduction is important for several reasons, not least among which is that an initial failure seldom gives the dentist an opportunity to try again with the same patient.

Stressing the importance of the introduction does not signify a difficult or lengthy procedure. On the contrary, the dentist carries this procedure through but once with each patient, and it does not take more than 5 to 10 minutes of his time. This investment of time is more than compensated for by the many time-saving benefits of using analgesia at each subsequent visit.

Success is highly rewarding for the dentist. It is a never-ending source of pride and gratification to be able to treat successfully a patient who has been burdened with a lifetime fear of the dental experience. The patient is now under treatment in the dental chair, fully cooperative, but his thoughts have wandered beyond the confines of the dental treatment room! When this ideal is attained, the subject is truly in a semihypnotic state. Moreover, after once having accepted the experience, the patient potentiates the favorable effect at all subsequent sittings by autosuggestion.

It will be found that properly relaxed patients under analgesia are in a suggestible state. Understanding this affords the dentist an additional measure of control of the situation; for example, he can suggest that all is well, that the patient is reacting extremely well. Such suggestions are commonly accepted by the patient, and a successful introduction is the end result.

THE INTRODUCTION OF ANALGESIA TO A DENTAL PRACTICE

PERSONAL EXPERIENCE BY THE DENTIST

Personal experience is the best way for the dentist to get to know analgesia and to be able to speak with assurance to his patient (Fig. 6–1). The truth of this has been amply borne out by the author's success in this regard when teaching analgesia to dental practitioners. Every member of his class is required to undergo analgesia. One may attend numerous lectures or read extensively about the sensations experienced while under analgesia, but it is only when the dentist himself has experienced these sensations that he can fully realize the experience through which he is putting his patient.

PERSONAL EXPERIENCE BY AUXILIARY PERSONNEL

For the same reason, it is important to successfully introduce analgesia to dental assistants, dental hygienists, and secretaries (Fig. 6–2). They, too, will then be able to explain it to the patient with greater assurance and sincerity, thereby making the dentist's task lighter.

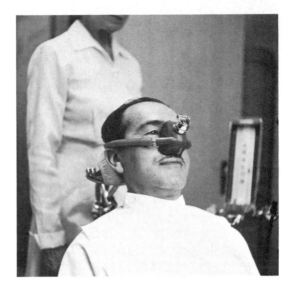

Figure 6–1 Personal experience of analgesia by the dentist.

THE CHOICE OF A SUBJECT FOR THE INITIAL TRIAL

The dentist should carefully pick his first subject for analgesia, choosing one who will afford him a good chance of success. He might start with a patient who is cooperative and relatively calm, possibly a trusting relative: the "I'll try anything once" type. It could be a patient who has had nitrous oxide–oxygen anesthesia previously and found it pleasant, or one who has such an extreme aversion to local anesthetic injection that he welcomes any substitute. The success which results from first attempts with such patients will encourage the operator and increase his self-assurance. Later, he will be able to handle the more difficult patients with greater ease and more chance of success.

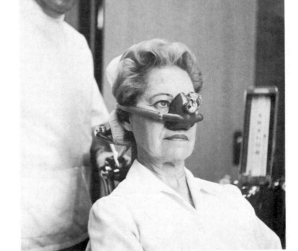

Figure 6–2 Personal experience of analgesia by auxiliary personnel.

CLASSIFICATION OF POTENTIAL ANALGESIA PATIENTS

Patients who have had no experience with analgesia and who have never heard of analgesia. This group of patients presents no particular problem. Having had no unpleasant experiences, they present a fertile field for psychological conditioning by the dentist. This is accomplished by the proper explanation of what analgesia is, why the patient is being asked to try it, and what it will accomplish.

Patients who have heard of analgesia, but have never taken it. Those falling into this group require even less conditioning than the members of the preceding group. They are usually persons who have been recommended by patients who have undergone analgesia and who have been told something about the reasons for its use, the sensations it arouses, and its benefits. In a great many instances analgesia is the very reason that these patients are applying for treatment. In a practice in which analgesia has recently been introduced, this group becomes larger and larger for, as time goes on and as more and more patients are introduced to analgesia, a greater proportion of new patients will be recommended by experienced analgesia patients. Since the new patients will already know something about the symptoms and benefits of analgesia, they will require less conditioning and explanation.

Patients with pleasant experiences with general anesthesia. The sole problem that may present itself in treating these patients is their desire to be put to sleep completely. With understanding and tact it must be explained to them that their problems can be solved successfully without complete anesthesia. It has been our finding that these patients do not fear analgesia; rather they look on it with pleasant anticipation.

Patients with unpleasant experiences with general anesthesia. It can be stated definitely that with the proper experience, analgesia will be accepted by 98 per cent of patients who enter the average dental office. Of the 2 per cent that cannot or will not take analgesia, the major proportion is composed of those who have had an unpleasant experience with general anesthesia, possibly with nausea and vomiting and a long recuperative period. It is difficult, but not impossible, to convince many of these patients that analgesia means neither general anesthesia with nitrous oxide nor the use of any other general anesthetic. With such patients it is very important to emphasize how they can control depth of analgesia by oral inhalation, and that analgesic depth *does not increase* with increased time of administration, as would occur with the administration of general anesthesia. If the use of analgesia is important to the patient's welfare, a strong attempt should be made to clear up this difference in his mind. However, if this is unsuccessful, the issue should not be forced.

Emergency patients. An emergency patient requires unique treatment. Time does not allow for the slow and deliberate approach to the use of analgesia. Ofttimes these individuals have gone sleepless for many days because of dental pain. Being overwrought and exhausted, they are quite willing to accept anything that will alleviate their pain. In this circumstance the proper approach is the so-called "short-form" introduction: the patient is told that analgesia is to be administered, that it will quickly and pleasantly rid him of his pain; then the nasal inhaler is immediately placed in position, and administration is begun. Because of the emotional state of the patient at this time, this technique is almost always successful, and not only is the patient grateful for your help but he also becomes a good analgesia patient. However, this approach is not usually successful with a fearful patient who is not in pain.

THE INTRODUCTION OF ANALGESIA TO THE PATIENT

The introduction of analgesia to a patient involves a combination of a great amount of psychology with a small amount of anesthetic gases. By the use of suggestion an attempt is made to induce an hypnotic state in which the patient will accept the procedure and the symptoms and will relax.

Suggestion is the process which results in the uncritical acceptance of an idea. The idea may be offered verbally by the logical or implied meaning of words, or it may be offered nonverbally by various means, such as gesture, facial expression, or general behavior. If, however, the idea offered is at too great a variance with a logical appraisal of the proposition, critical intellectual faculties tend to come into play and the idea is rejected. Thus we can see the importance of the choice of words, tone of voice, and general mien of the operator.

The introduction of analgesia to a patient can be divided into two phases: the education of the patient and the introductory administration.

The Education of the Patient

PRIOR PATIENTS

A patient of long standing knows his dentist, who in turn knows much about the patient: his reactions to dental treatment, his fears and phobias, his likes and dislikes. On the basis of such knowledge it is comparatively easy for the dentist to interest this patient in analgesia. The only query the operator may have to answer concerns the patient's curiosity about this "new" modality, which can readily be explained as a form of treatment that has proved to be so valuable and so successful over the years that the doctor has decided to offer its benefits to his patients. With a prior patient, the introductory administration of analgesia may be carried out at the same visit in which the subject is broached.

NEW PATIENTS: THE FIRST VISIT

Since the relationship established between the patient and the doctor is of paramount importance to the success of analgesia administration, it is wise in most instances to withhold the actual administration of the gases at the first visit of a new patient. This visit is usually spent in taking the necessary roentgenograms, the study model impressions, and the patient's history. Of course, if there is a main complaint that requires immediate attention, it should be cared for. At this first visit, as the patient and the dentist become acquainted, an excellent opportunity is afforded the dentist to project the best facets of his personality; he can show the patient how sympathetic and gentle he can be. The first gentle manipulation of the oral tissues can convince the new patient that he is being treated by someone who is aware that the sensitiveness and delicacy of these tissues demand care and a practiced hand. At this first visit, too, the dentist begins to educate his patient about analgesia.

Communication with the Patient.   If the patient is to be helped, there must be proper communication between the doctor and the patient. It should be kept in mind, however, that only a small part of this communication is transmitted through conversation; most of the significant communications are made by other means. The communications between doctor and patient can be likened to a multichannel system, each channel transmitting different messages simultaneously. Thus one set of messages is transmitted by the logical meaning of the words we use, and quite another set by the connotations of these words. Also, our expressions and gestures communicate how we feel, and our general deportment with the patient communicates a whole host of subtle meanings. If we are to understand our patient's reactions, we must be sensitive to all the various communications that take place simultaneously. We must establish *rapport*.

Basic to this establishment of rapport is the chairside manner. The patient respects the doctor within the area of his professional dealings, a relationship that is tacitly accepted by both parties. But the doctor, by his manner, attitude, and general professional behavior, can make it easier (or more difficult) for the patient to accept this relationship. The success with which rapport is established depends more on the way the doctor communicates his personal integrity than on his technical skill. It is the establishing of a successful emotional adjustment between the two concerned parties that leads the patient to place his trust and faith in a particular doctor, one who understands his problems as an individual, more than any other doctor. Once established, rapport is a therapeutic mechanism in itself, for the patient then feels that his doctor has *empathy*, that he knows how the patient feels without necessarily experiencing the same problem.

Gaining the Patient's Interest in Analgesia.   The objectives of the first visit, then, should be to gain the patient's interest in the *idea* of taking analgesia and to impart to him in simple terms a description of what analgesia is and what it can do for him. It can also be hinted that, should he be willing and if time allows, you may allow him to try it at the next visit. Of course, the next visit should be planned to allow 10 minutes for the initial introductory administration.

The following may serve to answer the patient's two basic questions about analgesia:

What is analgesia? Analgesia is induced by a mild gas which is inhaled through a simple device called a nasal inhaler. The gas is pleasant and easy to take for both children and adults. There are no unpleasant after-effects, and the patient is up and about immediately after the cessation of administration.

What does analgesia do for the dental patient?

    1. It relaxes him.

2. Fear, nervousness, and tension are eliminated.

3. It also eliminates most of the pain involved in dental treatment, and the rest is so dulled that the patient does not mind it.

4. It makes him feel warm and safe.

5. At times a feeling similar to a slight, pleasant intoxication is engendered (this analogy to be used with discretion—never to a teetotaler, nor to one who dislikes the effects of alcoholic beverages).

6. It works three ways, in that the patient finds that he is not nervous or fearful *before, during,* or *after* dental treatment.

7. When an injection is needed, the patient finds that he does not mind it at all under analgesia. Fewer injections are needed when analgesia is utilized.

8. Analgesia is like a good friend who is at hand at all times, ready to help at the moment he is needed.

9. There are no after-effects. The patient can get right out of the dental chair and immediately go about his business.

History Taking. The dental practitioner must recognize that the patient, as well as the disease and its symptoms, must be treated. Treatment requires an understanding of the patient, his general attitudes, and his psychologic values, since the whole person participates in the experiences of apprehension and pain. The first step in the control of apprehension and pain comprises the physical oral examination and the taking of a history (Fig. 6–3). The value of the information garnered from planned questioning and case study cannot be overemphasized. It is the foundation upon which the diagnosis, the approach to the patient, and recommendations for therapy are based.

Dental and medical histories, dental expectations, emotional background, occlusal neuroses, patterns of habit and activity, all are important components of history taking. This information gives a lucid picture of the patient's past and points the way to mutual satisfaction for both the patient and the dentist. When taking a history, it is mandatory that the dentist be a good listener and

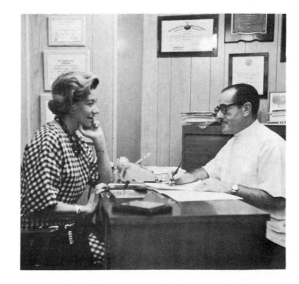

Figure 6–3 The taking of a history.

that he not hurry from one question to another. The difference in time invested by a good listener and one who hurries along may be no more than a minute, but the additional information gleaned by the former may save many, many hours and, indeed, may mark the difference between success and failure. If the history has been taken by a dental assistant, secretary or hygienist, it should be reviewed by the dentist, face-to-face with the patient. Much more significant information can be obtained by noting the *way* a patient answers: facial expressions, tone of voice, reluctance to answer, and so forth.

Fear of the needle, attitudes toward and experiences with all forms of inhalation anesthetics, reactions to surgery and tooth reduction, allergies and hypersensitivities, physical limitations or disabilities, tendencies to nausea and syncope, habits of self-medication, previous traumatic dental experiences — all may be elicited during the questioning of the patient. The information thus obtained determines the scope and extent of therapeutic recommendation and the mode of approach in gaining the patient's acceptance of relative analgesia.

The Detailed History.   In the detailed medical history the patient should be asked whether he has encountered trouble with his heart, lungs, kidneys, liver, thyroid, and so on. These organs should be enumerated so that the patient has time to think. He should also be questioned about such disorders as epilepsy, chronic cough, palpitations, chest pain, hypertension, and hemorrhage, and whether he has undergone any operations.

Medications are an excellent guide to the patient's condition. Thus medications that are forbidden the patient are a good guide to sensitivity, and those he is now taking indicate one disorder or another. For example, digitalis indicates a cardiac complication, insulin or Orinase indicates diabetes, rauwolfia may indicate high blood pressure, sedatives or tranquilizers may indicate emotional instability, and streptomycin or the amino oxidase inhibitors may indicate tuberculosis. This line of questioning is particularly helpful with the patient who is reluctant to divulge his infirmities.

The patient's past experience with dentistry, general anesthesia, and local anesthesia should also be noted for obvious reasons.

On the basis of what we discover from the patient's history we can then begin to approach him on the subject of analgesia. In order to get the patient interested in taking analgesia, it is not sufficient to speak in general terms of its benefits. It must be related to his specific needs, and the conversation must revolve on how analgesia will help solve his specific problems, which he has disclosed during the history taking. Some of these specific problems are the following:

Fear of injections or pain.

Fear of gagging during the taking of impressions or roentgenograms or when instruments are placed in the mouth.

Unpleasant sensation from the noise of the drill.

Inability to sit in the dental chair for long periods of time.

Revulsion at the sight of instruments, blood, and so forth.

Difficulty in keeping the mouth open for long periods of time.

On pages 144 to 146 are two examples of history forms from which each practitioner can choose and compose his own form.

NEW PATIENTS: THE SECOND VISIT

When the patient returns for his second visit, both he and the dentist will know each other a little better and the former will have acquired a simple working knowledge of analgesia. It now devolves upon the dentist to decide whether to continue his clinical examination and diagnosis or to administer analgesia. If irrational fear of dentistry is evident, it might be wise to introduce analgesia first. Once the doctor has successfully demonstrated the fear-eliminating properties of this procedure, a significant deterrent to acceptance of dental treatment has been abolished.

Prior Description and Prediction of All Possible Symptoms. This is of great importance because it helps immeasurably to inspire confidence and allay fear. The description of symptoms should be made in such manner as to make them appear pleasant and agreeable. Mention should be made that the patient may feel a warm, comfortable glow throughout his body, a most pleasant sensation. He may also experience a tingling in his toes or fingertips and perhaps a slight, pleasant, tingly sensation in his lips. He will feel warm and safe, light as a feather. His immediate surroundings may seem to recede so that he is hardly aware of the dental apparatus. Suggest that the entire experience will be a pleasant one.

The use of the word "may" in predicting symptoms is of great importance, since no individual ever experiences all the possible sensations under analgesia at any one sitting. This must be explained to the patient; otherwise he may become fearful and think that all is not well if he does not experience some of the symptoms the dentist has described.

Explanation of the Time Factor. Stress the fact that nothing will happen suddenly, that the onset of symptoms will be gradual and gentle. The prospective analgesia patient who thinks that symptoms should appear immediately on initiation of administration may experience unnecessary anxiety. Also, most subjects think that the longer they are under analgesia the sleepier they become, until they fall into oblivion. It must be made clear that a constant level can be maintained for hours at a time without inducing sleep.

The Fear of Falling Asleep. Some people are fearful of going into complete anesthesia. If this question is raised by the patient, and only then, assurance should be forthcoming that this cannot and will not occur.

Concern Over After-Effects. Concern over his ability to perform duties after the administration of analgesia must be dispelled by assuring the patient there will be no after-effects and that he will be completely able to pursue his activities immediately after administration.

Nasal Breathing. It must be explained that both exhalation and inhalation should take place through the nose, even though the mouth is held open. It is true that exhaling through the open mouth is easier for most people; however, an exhalation through the mouth is likely to be followed by an inhalation through the mouth. This leads to an excessive amount of oral inhaling and a consequent dilution of analgesic effect. Placing a saliva ejector in the mouth and telling the subject to practice nasal breathing with an open mouth is helpful. Also of some help is telling the patient to breathe in through the nose until he feels a cold sensation at the bridge of the nose.[8] This encourages greater concentration on nasal inhalation. Added confidence in the procedure

PRE-TREATMENT MEDICAL EVALUATION

				DATE	
NAME - LAST, FIRST, MIDDLE	MARITAL STAT.	AGE	DATE OF BIRTH MO. DAY YR.	SEX	HT. WT.
ADDRESS	PHONE	OCCUPATION			RACIAL GROUP
FAMILY PHYSICIAN - NAME, ADDRESS, PHONE NO.					

A GENERAL
1. What is your general state of health?_____
2. Are you now or have you recently been under a physician's care?_____ Reason:_____

3. Are you now taking or within the past 6 months have you taken any drugs or medications?_____
   Names:_____ Reason:_____
4. Have you ever had a serious illness or operation?_____ Describe: _____
5. Do you have any allergies?_____To what:_____
6. Have you ever had a reaction to a local anesthetic, antibiotic, or other drug?_____
   Describe:_____
7. Are you pregnant?_____Month?_____Number pregnancy? _____
8. Have you ever had hepatitis or been jaundiced?_____
9. Have you ever had venereal disease? (Gonorrhea or Syphilis) _____

B. CARDIOVASCULAR — RESPIRATORY
1. Are you able to perform your daily duties without stress or strain? _____
2. Are your activities limited for any reason?_____
3. Have you ever had any chest pains?_____
4. Have you ever had any shortness of breath?_____
5. Do you have a cough or wheeze?_____
6. Have you ever coughed up blood?_____
7. Do you ever have dizzy spells?_____
8. Can you lie flat when lying down or sleeping?_____
9. Do your ankles swell?_____When?_____
10. Have you ever been aware of a rapid heart beat or palpitations? _____
11. Have you ever had rheumatic fever?_____
12. Have you ever been told you had a heart murmur, heart trouble, or lung trouble?_____
13. Do you have frequent colds, sore throats or sinus trouble?_____
14. Have you ever had night sweats?_____When?_____

C. HEMATOPOIETIC
1. Have you ever had prolonged bleeding following a cut, tooth extraction, or other injury?_____
2. Have you ever had x-ray treatments or irradiation?_____ When?_____ Why?_____
3. Have you ever been told you were anemic?_____
4. Do you bruise easily?_____
5. Do you experience nose bleeds?_____
6. Do you have frequent infections?_____
7. Have you ever had a blood transfusion?_____Why?_____

D. NERVOUS SYSTEM
1. Have you ever had a convulsion or seizure?_____
2. Are you troubled by frequent headaches?_____
3. Are you frequently unduly apprehensive, fearful, or nervous? _____
4. Do you ever experience any pains, numbness or tingling anywhere? _____
5. Have you ever consulted a psychiatrist?_____

E. METABOLIC — ENDOCRINE
1. Have you had any recent gain or loss of weight?_____ Pounds?_____
2. Do you have a good appetite?_____
3. Does heat or warm rooms make you uncomfortable?_____
4. Do your hands sweat excessively?_____
5. Are you a diabetic?_____ How long?_____ Treatment? _____
6. Are you easily fatigued?_____

can also be obtained by explaining to the patient that he can either increase or decrease his depth of analgesia through nasal inhalation or oral inhalation, respectively.

PRECAUTIONS FOR SUCCESSFUL INTRODUCTION TO ANALGESIA

Never treat a stranger: A complete history is essential.

Do not describe analgesia as a new procedure. This is not true, since the

PRE-TREATMENT MEDICAL EVALUATION

F. GENITOURINARY
1. Do you void frequently?_____
2. Do you have to get up at night to void?_____
3. Do you have any difficulty in voiding?_____
4. Have you ever had blood in your urine?_____
5. Have you ever been told you had kidney trouble?_____

G. SOCIAL & PERSONAL
1. Is there any history of tuberculosis, diabetes, or bleeding in your family?_____
2. Do you smoke?_____ What? _____ How much?_____
3. Do you drink?_____ How much?_____
4. Are your wife and children in good health?_____

_____
_____
_____
_____

PHYSICAL EXAMINATION

BLOOD PRESSURE	PULSE RATE /MIN.	VOLUME	RHYTHM	TEMPERATURE	RESPIRATIONS /MIN.	DEPTH	CHARACTER

INDICATE WHETHER FINDINGS ARE POSITIVE (+) OR NEGATIVE (—)

SKIN -   _____JAUNDICE   _____PALLOR   _____PETECHIAE   _____ECCHYMOSIS

          _____CYANOSIS   _____RASH   _____OTHER _____

HEAD -   _____DEFORMITY   _____SWELLING   _____OTHER _____

EYES -   _____JAUNDICE   _____EXOPHTHALMOS   _____MOVEMENT

          _____REDNESS   _____OTHER _____

HANDS -   _____CLUBBING   _____PIGMENTATION   _____TREMOR   _____TEMP.

          _____OTHER _____

NECK -   _____LYMPH NODES   _____THYROID   _____VEINS   _____OTHER _____

LEGS -   _____EDEMA   _____ULCERS   _____CYANOSIS   _____OTHER _____

ANY OTHER PHYSICAL DEFECTS
_____
_____

DESCRIBE ANY ABNORMALITY OR POSITIVE FINDING
_____
_____
_____
_____
_____

modality is at least 95 years old. The thought that he is the first to try it most certainly does not instill confidence in the patient.

Do not perform dentistry at the introductory administration unless absolutely necessary. As a general rule, at this point one should not administer enough nitrous oxide to have any pain-eliminating effect. Should the patient experience pain due to a dental procedure he may lose confidence in analgesia. He has more than enough to contend with in conquering his fears of the procedure. Administering larger concentrations of nitrous oxide at this time will have no beneficial effect, because the efficacy of relative analgesia is predicated on a relaxed and fearless patient.

Patient_____ Age_____

☐ Married   ☐ Widowed   ☐ Single   ☐ Divorced

Home Address_____ Telephone No. _____

Employed By_____

Name of Spouse or Parent_____Employed By_____

Former Dentist_____Physician_____

Referred By_____

DENTAL AND MEDICAL HISTORY

THE FOLLOWING QUESTIONS WILL ENABLE US TO THOROUGHLY EVALUATE YOUR DENTAL PROBLEM. YOUR ANSWERS ARE FOR OUR RECORDS AND ARE CONSIDERED CONFIDENTIAL.

1. Are you in good health? .... Yes_____ No_____

2. Are you under the care of a physician? .... Yes_____ No_____

3. Have you had any serious illness or operation? .... Yes_____ No_____

   If so what illness or operation _____

4. Circle any of the following which you have or have had:

   Rheumatic Fever   Congenital Heart Defect   T.B.   Heart Murmur   Heart Trouble

   Stroke   High Blood Pressure   Diabetes   Hepatitis   Liver Disease   Lung Disease

   Asthma   Allergies   Epilepsy   Glaucoma   Kidney Disease   Thyroid Disease

   Anemia   Other _____

5. Are you taking any medications now? .... Yes_____ No_____

   If so what?_____For what condition?_____

6. Do you have any blood disorders or bleeding tendencies? ....Yes_____ No_____

7. Have you had any X-ray treatment for a tumor about your
   head or neck? ....Yes_____ No_____

8. Have you ever had any unusual reaction to an anesthetic
   or medicine? (i.e. Aspirin, Penicillin, Novocain).............Yes_____ No_____

   Explain _____

9. Do you wear contact lenses? ....Yes_____ No_____

10. Have you ever taken cortisone type medicines?.............Yes_____ No_____

11. Do you have any signs today of a cold or sinus condition? ......Yes_____ No_____

12. Are you pregnant (women)? ....Yes_____ No_____

13. Do you have any disease, condition, or problem not listed above? ..Yes_____ No_____

    If so, explain _____

14. Have you been hospitalized in past 5 years?_____ For what?_____

    For how long?_____

Do not administer too much nitrous oxide and do not keep the patient under too long. The sole objective of this first procedure is to obtain a pleasurable reaction, or at the very least one that will permit the patient to accept a second administration. For this purpose, only small doses of nitrous oxide are needed for a short period of time. The patient should be allowed to perceive the minimal symptoms for only 5 minutes at most. Ideally, he will then begin to sense the possibilities this instrument has for eliminating his fear.

Do not stress safety. The question of safety should never be raised by the dentist. If the patient initiates this query, only then is he emphatically assured that an extremely safe modality is being employed.

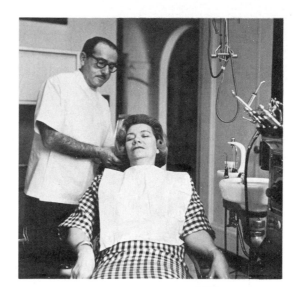

Figure 6-4 Seat the patient comfortably in the chair.

Do not converse with a third party during the introductory administration. The patient should sense that he is getting the full attention of the doctor.

The Procedure for Introductory Analgesia

For variations in procedures with various kinds of equipment, see Chapter 7, under the names of equipment.

1. Seat the patient comfortably in the chair (Fig. 6-4).

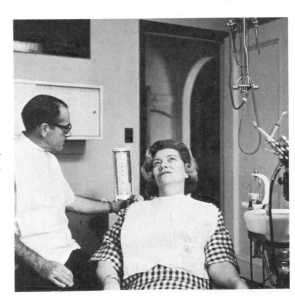

Figure 6-5 Gas machine is positioned immediately behind the patient.

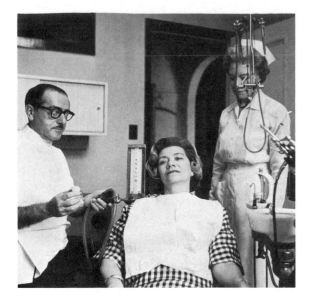

Figure 6–6   Cleansing the nasal inhaler.

    2. Bring the gas machine into position immediately behind the dental chair, where it can be reached easily by the operator (Fig. 6–5).
    3. Spray the nasal inhaler with alcohol to which a small amount of volatile oil (lavender, orange, peppermint, and so forth) has been added; dry with compressed air (Figs. 6–6 and 6–7). The oils are used because the odor of pure alcohol is obnoxious to many people.
    4. With intermittent flow machines, start the flow of 100 per cent oxygen at 1 to 2 mm. pressure with the exhaling valve set at 0 tension before position-

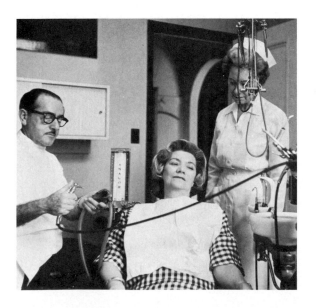

Figure 6–7   Drying the nasal inhaler with compressed air.

ing nasal inhaler. On continuous flow machines start with 8 liters per minute of oxygen. Set the air (inhaling) valve to its widest opening. Make certain that the reservoir bag is about ⅓ to ½ full. Having some gas in the reservoir bag (at this point it is oxygen) will preclude insufficient minute volume should the patient take a few deep breaths despite directions to breathe normally. It is important to bear in mind that fear causes exaggerated breathing. Position the nasal inhaler (Fig. 6–8).

Adapting the nasal inhaler to the patient's face before allowing oxygen to flow may frighten the patient. His first breath will create a sense of suffocation and he may reject the procedure at this point.

Moreover, many individuals breathe only through one nasal passageway, the other being obstructed by swollen membranes, a deviated septum, polyps, and so forth. Should the operator inadvertently position the nasal inhaler so as to occlude the one good passageway, he will then force the subject to breathe through his mouth, and no analgesic effects will result. Therefore the patient must be given permission to adjust it to his comfort and ease of inhalation.

Some patients, on the other hand, experience a feeling of claustrophobia when the inhaler is fitted. This can be overcome by pointing out the openings in the nasal inhaler through which air can enter and by mentioning the ready availability of mouth inhalation. It also helps to open the air valve on the machine to its full extent so that ease of breathing is assured. Since a subject who is breathing from a gas machine for the first time tends to breathe in an exaggerated fashion, it is important to have the reservoir bag filled so that he can draw from it without emptying it completely in one or two breaths.

5. Continue the flow of 100 per cent oxygen for at least one minute, in-

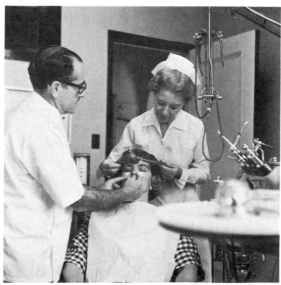

Figure 6–8 Positioning the nasal inhaler (small pieces of gauze or tissue paper prevent pressure marks on the patient's face).

structing the patient to breathe *normally,* in and out through the nose, and to adjust the nasal inhaler if necessary.

6. When exaggerated breathing ceases, start the flow of a minimal dosage of nitrous oxide — 5 per cent in intermittent flow, 1 liter in continuous flow — and reduce the flow of oxygen to 3 liters. In addition, close the air valve to the half-open position. Instruct the patient to continue normal inhalation and exhalation through the nose and to advise you of the onset of any of the symptoms which you have previously described.

7. Now assume a standing or sitting position to the right of the patient, from where changes in dosage can easily be made without moving and without the patient's being aware of the motions.

8. From time to time ask the patient, "What do you feel now?" or "How would you describe what you feel now?" He should never be asked, "How do you feel now?" This brings to mind a form of self-analysis that could be defeating. "What do you feel now?" simply calls for an enumeration of symptoms with less personal connotation. The answer to this question gives an insight into the patient's reactions and emotions. The manner in which he answers, the rapidity and choice of words signal either relaxation and acceptance or fear and anxiety. The operator's words should be chosen carefully, projecting only positive, pleasing thoughts. Everything should be conducive to a soothing, encouraging atmosphere. Well-modulated tones are used, for loud conversation or sudden loud noises will bring the subject out of his suggestible state.

9. Proceed slowly and calmly, increasing the flow of nitrous oxide very slowly by 0.5 liter increments until minimal symptoms appear. Remember that a sense of urgency on the part of the dentist is readily transmitted and is translated by the patient into a feeling of uncertainty and fear. During the entire administration the operator must be in contact with his patient, either verbally or, at times, physically by placing his hand lightly on the patient's shoulder (Fig. 6–9).

10. Once minimal symptoms have been described, stop the flow of nitrous oxide and initiate oxygenation.

The success of the introductory administration is determined by the patient's willingness to take analgesia on the next visit.

RECOGNITION AND CONTROL OF FEAR REACTIONS

The Critical Point. After the patient has inhaled the nitrous oxide for a few minutes, he begins to experience some of the sensations described to him in advance. Most patients will not mind these sensations, especially if the dentist is assuring them at the same time that the symptoms are proper and normal, just those to be expected. There are, however, an appreciable number of patients whose fear begins to take the upper hand at this very moment. These are the patients who are most fearful and who, as a consequence, have the greatest need of analgesia. Another cause of this situation is that too great a concentration of nitrous oxide is administered to a particular subject at the introductory administration.

It would be helpful for the operator to know what may be going on in the

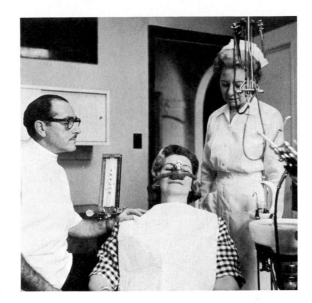

Figure 6-9 A hand on the patient's shoulder sometimes instills needed confidence.

patient's mind at the moment. Very often, it is something like this: "I have the utmost confidence in Dr. Smith. He knows what he is doing, and he has told me what to expect. And yet, how does he *really* know what is going on inside of me? How does he *really* know what I feel? Perhaps I am different. It may be that I am not reacting in the normal way. I feel odd. Something is wrong. I must tell him."

This is why it is essential for the operator—only at the introductory administration—to query his patient from time to time. For example, he might ask, "How are you doing, Mrs. Jones? What do you feel now?" If he has been

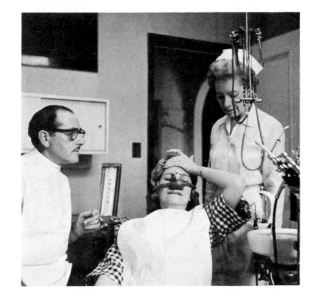

Figure 6-10 The patient experiences pressure on the head.

doing this, the patient at this critical point may describe the situation in one of several ways:

"I have a terrible pressure in my head!" (Fig. 6–10)

"I feel a great pressure in my chest!"

"My heart is pounding very rapidly and loudly!" (Fig. 6–11)

"I feel dizzy!" (This description should not automatically be evaluated as an unpleasant one. It could be "pleasantly dizzy." Find out by saying, "But you don't mind it, do you?" The answer will clarify the true situation, and suggesting that the patient does not mind the sensation may change the reaction from an unpleasant to a pleasant one.)

The concentration of nitrous oxide in the patient's bloodstream is not sufficient to cause these excessive reactions; they are the results of pure fear. Therefore the alert operator can immediately assure the patient that all is well, that the patient himself can eliminate these symptoms very easily by breathing through the mouth a few times. Explain that when he breathes through the mouth, he is breathing only atmospheric air. Show him that, for this reason, he is in control of the situation. At the same time, shut off the nitrous oxide portion of the gas flow. The flow of pure oxygen, plus reassurance by the operator, will eliminate all symptoms in a few breaths. This calms the patient and effectively demonstrates that you are in full control of the situation and that he, too, can exert control.

An interesting thing now occurs. When the same dose of nitrous oxide is reapplied, the patient seldom reacts in this way again. The fear is gone. At this point, he gives himself up to the sensations and the procedure, relaxing and allowing the gases to take over and function successfully. Although not every patient passes through this experience, the operator must be alert to its possible occurrence and ready to counteract it.

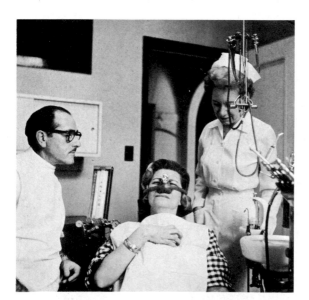

Figure 6–11 The patient feels her heart pounding very rapidly and loudly.

INITIAL AUTOSUGGESTION BY THE NERVOUS PATIENT

If after two or three inhalations through the nasal inhaler, the nervous patient immediately tells the operator that he has all the symptoms of analgesia, this should alert the dentist to the fact that he is dealing with an extremely fearful individual. This occurs most often when only oxygen is emanating from the machine, and it is due purely to autosuggestion. The patient should receive all possible encouragement and be allowed to pass through the entire gamut of symptoms on pure oxygen. In a short while he will make known the fact that he now feels no symptoms at all. At this point, and *never* before this point, the minimal flow of nitrous oxide should be started. If autosuggestion occurs immediately after the introduction of nitrous oxide, the flow of nitrous oxide should be stopped and the patient allowed to continue with pure oxygen, as just explained.

In summary, then, the introduction of relative analgesia requires a simple but well considered, psychological approach on the part of the operator. He must relax his patient and put him in a receptive mood by the proper choice of words, tone of voice, and general attitude. The degree of success is in direct proportion to the degree of relaxation obtained in the patient. This introductory procedure is carried out but once with each patient, and with a little experience it should take no more than 5 minutes.

Conversational Approach When Introducing Analgesia

At the first visit during history taking, the subject of analgesia should be broached. A typical conversation might be as follows:

Doctor: Mr. Jones, how have you had your dental work done before? Would you consider yourself a good patient?

Patient: Doctor, I think I am the worst patient in the world. My teeth are so sensitive, I can't stand the pain and noise of the drill. I even hate to have my teeth cleaned.

Doctor: Have you had any anesthetic for your dental work in the past? Were you given injections or did you take gas?

Patient: I took gas only once, Doctor, for an extraction of a wisdom tooth. I didn't mind it at all. Every time my former dentist drilled my teeth he gave me an injection. I could not have stood the pain otherwise.

Doctor: Do you mind getting an injection?

Patient: I am terribly afraid of the needle, but it is the lesser of two evils. Besides, my mouth always feels terribly numb for hours afterward, but I can stand that. It is the *thought* of being injected that terrifies me.

Doctor: Mr. Jones, we have additional ways of eliminating fear and pain. Have you heard of analgesia?

Patient: No, what is it? Is it gas?

Doctor: Yes, it is the same gas we use for putting people to sleep, *except* that for analgesia we give it in an entirely different way. It is just a mild dose of the gas. It doesn't put you to sleep.* On the contrary, you are awake at all times. You and I can carry on a conversation while you are taking it. It gives you a pleasant sensation, a relaxing sensation. It feels something like having a couple of cocktails.† You feel good under analgesia, and your fear is gone. If you are interested, perhaps we will give you a little sample of it next time.

Patient: It sounds wonderful, Doctor. I think I would like to try it.

(At the subsequent visit.)

Doctor: We have a few minutes left. I would like you to try a little of that analgesia.

Patient: If you think so, Doctor. I've been thinking about it ever since that last visit, and I must confess I'm a little bit nervous about it.

Doctor: That is perfectly all right. Everyone is a little nervous about it the first time. That's only natural. As a matter of fact, if you weren't just a wee bit nervous about it, I would think there was something wrong with you. However, there's really nothing to fear. I am going to tell you all about it, exactly what I am going to do and exactly what you may feel.‡ This first time I am going to give you very little — just enough to get you used to breathing through the nose-piece and to give you a little idea of what you feel under it.

(The doctor thereupon takes the nose-piece in his hand, and sprays it with alcohol to which a little oil of lavender, oil of roses, oil of lilac, or any other pleasant smelling volatile oil has been added. He then dries it thoroughly with air from the cut-off valve of the unit. He then starts a flow of 100 per cent oxygen with the air valve open wide.)

Doctor: Now I am going to put this over your nose and adjust it properly. However, after I've done so, if you don't think it is just right, readjust it. Make it entirely comfortable so that you can breathe easily in and out through it. Is it all right?

Patient: Yes, Doctor. It feels fine and I can breathe very easily through it.

Doctor: Good. Just continue to breathe normally, in and out through the nose-piece. That odor you smell is the alcohol with which I washed the nose-piece.§ The gas itself has little odor. In a short time you won't notice any odor at all.

(The doctor now positions his machine behind the patient, and assumes a standing or sitting position to the right of the patient).

---

*This would not be a proper concept to raise with those patients who want to go into complete anesthesia.

†Before drawing an analogy between the effects of analgesia and those produced by alcohol, make certain that the patient is not a teetotaler. He may reject analgesia on that basis.

‡'Exactly what you may feel" is an example of how we can be definite even when we use an indefinite phrase. Since no one patient will ever feel all the possible symptoms induced by analgesia administration, we must use the word "may." However, it is also important to convey to the patient that we are in full command of the situation and that we know "exactly" what will occur.

§The question of odor need not be raised, unless the patient raises it first.

Doctor: Nothing is going to happen suddenly. I'm giving you just a little bit this first time. All I want you to do is to get used to breathing through this nose-piece. Now let me tell you exactly what you may feel. You won't go to sleep or at any time be near going to sleep. You will get a little drowsy or heady at first, but after a little while this is replaced by a light, floating sensation. You will feel good, warm and comfortable. There may be a tingly sensation in your toes or fingertips and perhaps in your lips. It will be a pleasant sensation. You may also feel a warm, tingly sensation throughout your body. If you were a little child, I would call this the "magic carpet," for it gives you the sensation of flying or floating through the air on a magic carpet or in an airplane. Now, let me know when you begin to feel any of the sensations I have described.

(The doctor thereupon reaches behind the patient without moving his position and starts the flow of a minimal dosage of nitrous oxide. He then waits until the patient has breathed the mixture of nitrous oxide and oxygen for 30 to 40 seconds.)

Doctor: Do you feel anything yet?

Patient: Nothing yet.

Doctor: Fine. That's because I am giving you so little this first time. You will begin to feel it soon.

Patient: Now I am beginning to feel something. My toes and fingertips feel a little tingly.

Doctor: That's good. That's just as it should be. You are doing fine. Isn't it true, Mr. Jones, that you are much more relaxed now than you were a minute or two ago?*

Patient: That's really so, Doctor. I'm still a little bit nervous about it, but not nearly as much as before.

Doctor: Of course. Everyone is a little apprehensive the first time, but only the first time. It takes only one time to make an analgesia veteran. You cannot at this point realize the full relaxing benefits of analgesia. However, at every subsequent visit you will see how it will take away all your fear and apprehension. What do you feel now, Mr. Jones?

Patient: About the same as before, except that I am used to it now.

Doctor: Good. Are you worried about going to sleep?†

Patient: Well, perhaps just a little.

Doctor: You needn't worry about it at all, because you have full control over it.

Patient: How, Doctor?

Doctor: Very simply. It is only when you breathe through your nose that you will feel the symptoms. If at any time you want to lighten the symptoms and make yourself more wide awake, all you have to do is breathe through your mouth. When you do that, you are breathing the same air as I am. No

---

*Mr. Jones may not feel more relaxed than a minute ago, but the suggestion that he does is very often accepted and he then does feel more relaxed.

†If the patient has had no fear of going to sleep, this question could create it.

matter how much gas the machine is producing, you will feel little or no effect if you breathe through your mouth. Try it, Mr. Jones.

Patient: That's right, Doctor. It is very simple. I can control my sleepiness myself.

Doctor: Exactly. Isn't this easy?

Patient: It certainly is, Doctor.

(The doctor, having attained his objective, shuts off the flow of nitrous oxide and begins to oxygenate the patient.)

Doctor: You will now notice that all your symptoms are disappearing. That is because I have shut off the gas, and you are now breathing only pure oxygen. This makes all the headiness or fuzziness disappear in a short time. Close your mouth and breathe deeply in and out through the nose until your head is completely clear.

(The patient proceeds to breathe pure oxygen for one or two minutes, and perhaps an extra minute for this first session.)

Doctor: Is your head entirely clear?

Patient: Yes, Doctor, completely.

(The doctor removes the nose-piece and then shuts off the flow of gas from machine.)

Doctor: How did you like it, Mr. Jones? Do you think it can be of any help to you with your dental work?

Patient: I think it's wonderful but, of course, you didn't do any drilling yet. I don't know how much it will help me then.

Doctor: All in due time. I assure you, Mr. Jones, that it will be of tremendous assistance in all your dental work. I will be able to complete the work more rapidly for you, and you won't mind it. You'll see that you won't be nervous or apprehensive about making your next visit. There will be times, however, when we will have to give you an injection. But you won't mind the injection at all because you will be under analgesia at the time the injection is given. Are you willing to try this the next time for your dental work?

Patient: I certainly am, Doctor.*

THE ROLE OF THE DENTAL ASSISTANT IN AN ANALGESIA
PRACTICE †

With the continued increase in population and patient education, the demand for dental care increases. As a result, the most recent projections in-

---

*A successful introduction requires only that the patient consent to take analgesia a second time.

†By Philip E. Shipper, B.S., D.D.S.

dicate a marked increase in the patient-per-dentist ratio. One obvious way of coping with the problem is to utilize the dental auxiliary more effectively. Today, students in nearly every one of the nation's dental schools are being trained to make use of dental assistants from the very onset of their clinical training.

The significant trend toward reevaluation of the traditional roles of the dental assistant and dental hygienist suggests a broader role in the future for all ancillary personnel. As a corollary to such thinking, standards should be set up for auxiliaries in the clinical use of analgesia and the philosophy and psychology behind its successful application. Teaching programs designed for such personnel should include a thorough presentation of all aspects of the clinical applications of relative analgesia, and a description of the role that ancillary personnel should play in an analgesia practice. Such a program should embrace the philosophy, psychology, and pharmacology of relative analgesia and how this knowledge can help the dental team to build patient motivation and acceptance. Individual, personal experience with analgesia is an essential prerequisite for the auxiliary. Techniques of applying the nasal inhaler, cleansing, and sterilization; starting the flow of gases and setting the proper levels of flow at the doctor's direction; integrated training for emergency situations and supportive aid (nausea, vomiting, or fear); patient monitoring for comfort; nasal inhaler adjustments, gas level maintenance, and patient reactions; supply control, including cylinder gas level monitoring and end of day shut-off procedures; oxygenation of patient prior to end of procedures and removal of nasal inhaler, with wind-up comfort details: all of these procedures should be clearly understood by auxiliary personnel. If the value of relative analgesia is made clear to all members of the dental team, they will be in an excellent position to take advantage of the expanded duties now envisioned for them, and to function effectively within the present structure under the careful supervision of the doctor.

If office procedure normally requires that the dental assistant conduct the initial interview with a new patient, including eliciting the chief complaint and the taking of a history (both medical and dental), it is incumbent upon the interviewer to pose the proper key question, which leads directly to a discussion of the subject of analgesia. That question is: "How have you had your previous dental work done?"

The answer to this question provides the interviewer with valuable information through which the subject of analgesia can be broached. The answer could be one of several:

1. "I cannot tolerate the sound and/or the vibration of the drill."
2. "I cannot tolerate the drill without a local anesthetic."
3. "I fear the needle, but it is the lesser of two evils."
4. "I hate the numbing after-effects of the needle."
5. "I cannot keep my mouth open for any length of time."

Whatever the answers given by the patient, the statement is made that "In this office, we overcome this particular problem by the use of analgesia." This is followed by a brief simple explanation of analgesia.

So far as is known, no school provides specific training for the dental assistant in an analgesia practice. It becomes incumbent upon the dentist who practices with analgesia to provide on-the-job training to his auxiliaries, in order to fulfill the needs of the office. Each office is unique in its procedures, depending on the doctor's style of management, his preferences, and his methods of handling problems.

In some states of the United States the laws permit a wide range of duties to be performed by the dental auxiliaries, such as: (1) placement of rubber dams; (2) placement of matrix bands; (3) placement of and removal of temporary restorations; (4) insertion of cavity linings and bases; (5) placement, carving and finishing of amalgam, resin and silicate restorations; (6) placement of and removal of periodontal packs; and (7) removal of sutures.

All of these procedures would be greatly facilitated if they could be performed on the patient under analgesia.

During the routine administration of nitrous oxide and oxygen analgesia, the duties of the dental auxiliary fall under three main headings: before, during, and after the procedure.

BEFORE

1. Check the cylinders and gauges.
2. Check the machine and nasal inhaler tubing.
3. Have the patient's records ready.

DURING

1. Seat the patient comfortably.
2. Engage the patient in conversation of a pleasant nature while the doctor prepares.
3. Have necessary instruments ready.
4. Place machine in proper position.
5. Start flow of gases and position nasal inhaler.
6. Retract, aspirate, use air cut-off.
7. Adjust light.
8. Remove instruments and débris while oxygenating patient.
9. Remain with patient until fully oxygenated.

AFTER

1. Make patient comfortable—see that patient is fully recuperated.
2. Give patient any necessary instructions.
3. Record procedure.
4. Dismiss patient.
5. Prepare treatment room for next patient.

History Taking

The medical and dental history elicited from the patient at the initial interview should be thorough and detailed. Caution must be exercised lest the dental assistant, through questioning, inadvertently imply that there are hazards and problems involved in the administration of inhalation sedation with nitrous oxide. Too often a careless remark or improperly phrased question may create unwarranted fear in the mind of the patient. The proper use of semantics in our relationship with the patient is most vital in the analgesia office.

Complications during the administration of nitrous oxide and oxygen are almost nonexistent. The worst complication experienced by the patient may be nausea. This may occasionally be accompanied by vomiting. Its infrequency is authenticated by surveys conducted among dentists utilizing relative analgesia. The findings indicated an incidence of complications of 0.1%. In offices where total analgesia was administered (plane 3), the incidence was found to be much higher.

Precautionary measures necessary for any situation of this nature should include the following:

1. Emesis basin should be readily available.
2. Additional towels should be on hand.
3. A plastic apron should be used to cover patient's clothing.
4. Observe patient's color—pallor is a forewarning (except in black patients).
5. Note placement of hands—sudden positioning of hands over abdomen may possibly indicate a feeling of nausea.
6. Note if patient has given a history of habitual motion sickness.

The dental assistant should be particularly aware of any unusual comments or behavior by the patient. These unusual actions or remarks may be an early indication of the individual's fear, apprehension, and anxiety, and may occur on the telephone, in the reception room, or at the chair.

ON THE TELEPHONE

Questions posed and comments made by the patient can often give indications of anxiety, apprehension and tension. The dental assistant should be equipped to answer these questions intelligently and without hesitation, so as to reassure the patient and instill confidence, even at the time the appointment is being made.

IN THE RECEPTION ROOM

The actions, behavior and comments by the patient should be observed and noted by the dental assistant. Here again, the comments and remarks made by the knowledgeable dental assistant go a long way towards pacifying this type of individual. The extremely apprehensive patient may be escorted into the treatment room to be introduced to a veteran patient undergoing analgesia.

The observant dental assistant should quickly note any possible indication of intoxication or drug use by the patient. This may be further pursued by tactful questioning during the taking of the history at the initial interview.

AT THE CHAIR

Conversation by the dental assistant while seating and preparing the patient in the treatment room should be such as to create an atmosphere of pleasantness and cheerfulness. Avoid quick, abrupt movements and hasty, sharp remarks which tend to create a sense of urgency in the room. On the other hand, efficient and well planned actions are readily recognized and appreciated by the patient.

An effective method of conditioning a new, apprehensive patient to the use of relative analgesia:

The dental assistant, recognizing extreme apprehension, escorts the new patient into the treatment room while the doctor is still treating the veteran patient under analgesia, preferably during the terminal part of the procedure, or just as oxygenation is being instituted. The new patient is then introduced to the veteran patient. They talk with each other and the veteran, recognizing the situation instantly, is usually most prolific and helpful with words of endorsement and praise for the procedure.

After the introductory administration, and as the patient is about to leave, compliment his performance and acceptance of the analgesia procedure. It is also advisable to forecast better experiences at subsequent visits. As the patient leaves, the dental assistant might say: "You did very well with the analgesia, Mrs. Jones. You took to it beautifully. Now that you know what it's like, you will take to it much more effectively at each of the subsequent visits."

The dental assistant should ever be alert and observant of the following characteristics while the patient is under analgesia: (1) color of skin; (2) placing hands on abdomen; (3) dislodged nasal inhaler; (4) crossed legs; (5) mouth breathing; (6) unusual movements.

Color of Skin.   Nitrous oxide and oxygen in relative analgesia doses does not have any physiologic effect on the color of the skin. In very, very rare instances, a noticeable pallor may appear, indicating the onset of nausea. The patient may then be questioned as to how he feels, and the reply usually will indicate that the flow of nitrous oxide should be reduced to zero and the flow of oxygen should be increased. The patient should be informed of this. Inquire as to the food intake prior to this visit. If food was taken, then instruct the patient to refrain at the next visit. If no food was ingested, then instruct the patient to eat lightly prior to the next visit. The child patient may turn pale suddenly and regurgitate without much advance warning. Be prepared to avoid any soiling of clothes by the use of basins, plastic aprons and towels. Once relieved, the patient can usually go back to the original dosage of nitrous oxide.

Placing Hands on Abdomen.   The movement of the hands to the abdomen may be an early indication of a feeling of nausea. The patient should be asked if all is well, or the reason for the hands in that position. Any reply indicating discomfort should be followed by reducing the flow of nitrous oxide to zero. Oxygenate thoroughly for 2 or 3 minutes. After complete relief the patient can generally go back to a level just at or below that at which the discomfort originated. Here again, inquire as to food intake, and instruct the patient to do the opposite of what was done prior to this visit.

Dislodged Nasal Inhaler.   During movements of the head or manipulation of the lips and cheeks by the operator, the nose-piece may become dislodged. The patient on occasion may remark that he no longer experiences the analgesic state. Observe the position of the inhaler. It may be found that half the nares are exposed, and atmospheric air is being inhaled instead of nitrous oxide and oxygen. Readjustment of the nose-piece brings the patient back to the desired level in about 1 minute.

Crossed Legs.   Some patients in their relaxed state sit cross-legged. This position for a prolonged period of time could result in cutting off the circulation in one or both limbs. On arising from the chair, it is learned that a leg has "fallen asleep." The patient should be instructed to sit with legs outstretched.

Mouth Breathing.   Habitual mouth-breathers inadvertently forget to inhale and exhale through the nose-piece. One indication of this may be the constant fogging of the mouth mirror. It is advisable to frequently remind such a patient to breathe only through the nose. Stressing exhalation through the nose makes inhalation via the nasal passage much more likely. Greater patient cooperation may be obtained by advising him that the more frequently he breathes through his nose, the less discomfort will he feel.

Unusual Movements.   The onset of fidgety, frequent movements of the head or extremities may be an indication of pre-excitement level or plane 3 (total analgesia) level. The patient should be instructed to refrain from movement. Failure to respond to direction should indicate that the volume of nitrous oxide should be lowered. It is also advisable to check the position of the patient's head in the headrest and make any necessary adjustments.

No analgesia office should ever be without at least one dental assistant. Today, in the multichair dental practice, two, three, and even four dental assistants are considered quite feasible and useful. It is a well documented fact that "an increase of almost 64% in annual gross revenue, almost 40% in annual before-tax net income, and more than 33% in annual after-tax income demonstrates the economic feasibility of adding multiple expanded duty auxiliaries to the basic team of the solo practitioner."[13]

Special Techniques for Handling Difficult Children

FOR THE CHILD WHO WILL NOT LEAVE THE RECEPTION ROOM

Disengage the nasal inhaler from the tubing, and bring it into the reception room. Place the inhaler over your own nose, demonstrating to the child that this is what the space men use on their flights to the moon. Hand the nose-piece to the child, allowing him to place it over his own nose to demonstrate the simplicity of the procedure. This technique is successful with many children, enabling you to then escort the child into the treatment room where the complete introduction may be successfully carried through.

Another technique is to have a bulletin board on which are mounted numerous photographs of children with the nasal inhaler in position portraying the smiling or laughing face of the child. Upon showing this to the child, he is asked "Who has the happiest face, and do you think you can do better?

Let's see." With that the child is comfortably seated with the nose-piece in position, ready for photography.

THE CHILD IN THE CHAIR

The child is questioned as to his preference: "Do you like bubble gum flavor, peppermint flavor, or spearmint flavor?" Depending on the reply from the patient, a mint or other extract is sprayed on the nose-piece from an atomizer bottle and thoroughly dried with the air cut-off on the unit to comply with the child's request. From then on the procedure may be referred to as "peppermint air," or "bubble gum air."

With the child seated comfortably in the chair, the nose-piece and tubing assembly may be disengaged from the machine. The nitrous oxide control is opened to 3 or 4 liters while the child is engaged in conversation. As small talk is carried on, the open-end corrugated tubing is casually held in the vicinity of the child's nose, and the nitrous oxide is inadvertently inhaled, whereupon the patient gradually achieves a degree of analgesia and the nasal inhaler is seated in position and connected to the corrugated tubing.

One operator ingeniously bought a toy Plexiglas helmet which simulates the helmets of spacemen, and made two apertures in the helmet, into which he inserted the nitrous oxide and oxygen tubing. With the gases flowing, he puts the helmet on the child's head, explaining that this is what the spacemen wear on their trips to the moon. As the child's movements subside, indicating a light level of analgesia, the helmet is removed and replaced by the nasal inhaler, thereby continuing and possibly increasing the level of analgesia.

THE DENTAL AUXILIARY AND NITROUS OXIDE CONSCIOUS SEDATION[12]

In an analgesia practice it is essential that the dental assistant have a clear understanding of the philosophy and psychology of nitrous oxide–oxygen sedation. With this knowledge he or she can be of invaluable assistance to the dentist in building patient motivation and acceptance. In order to achieve success in this area, the primary prerequisite is that the auxiliary have personal experience with nitrous oxide-oxygen sedation. She (or he) should be thoroughly familiar with exactly what sensations may be experienced by the patient.

There are vast differences between patients. No two are alike. There are varied reactions to the analgesia experience, each of which the dental assistant should be prepared to understand and control. All of this may be attained through complete rapport with the patient, commencing with the initial telephone conversation, following through with the patient's arrival in the reception room and treatment room, and terminating with his departure until the next visit.

The rewards reaped from this approach make the workday a more pleasant experience for all. As a result of working with a relaxed and enthusiastic dentist, an atmosphere is created which permits the auxiliaries to remain relaxed and to experience less mental and physical strain. Tension and anxiety are contagious! This is evidenced by the high incidence of diseases of psychogenic origin rampant in the dental profession. This must inevitably spread to the ranks of the dental auxiliary profession. Furthermore, greater efficiency leads to better dentistry and increased productivity, and hence improved income.

Careful attention should be paid to the requirements of each state where you practice. In some areas, where it is permitted, many duties of the dental assistant are greatly facilitated by having the patient in the relative analgesia stage:

1. There is greater ease in taking x-ray pictures and in obtaining impressions on the gagging patient.

2. Discomfort in the removal of temporary fillings, cements and crowns is reduced.

3. Pain of subgingival scaling and root planing is minimized.

The dental assistant must be well versed in the techniques of proper administration.

1. Placement of nose-piece: should be comfortable but not too tight. Patient may be assured that he can adjust the inhaler to his own comfort.

2. Cleansing of nose-piece: washing with soap and water is advisable prior to immersion in antiseptic solutions which are commercially available.

3. Gas start-up: where permitted (only in certain states); otherwise must be initiated by the doctor.

4. Knowledge of possible emergency situations: fortunately a rarity, but may require turning off the flow of nitrous oxide and increasing the oxygen flow until the doctor takes over.

5. Monitoring patient by observing actions of the hands, head, and body, and noting skin-color changes.

6. Diagnosing patient reactions: by listening attentively to comments and remarks made by the patient.

7. Being concerned with patient's comfort: readjust headrest in prolonged sittings, loosen tight clothing, wipe perspiration from patient's face, remove excess saliva and water with aspirators.

8. Nose-piece adjustment: look for displacement which allows entry of excessive atmospheric air, or obstruction of nasal passages.

9. Adequate oxygenation: no patient should be dismissed from the chair without 1 to 3 minutes of 100 per cent oxygen. Patient should simultaneously be informed that he is being "cleared up" in order to avoid autosuggested analgesic after-effects.

10. Removal of nose-piece: pull forward on the nasal inhaler as the tubing clasp is released to avoid hurting the patient's face or eyes.

11. Ability to answer questions by patient: this requires a thorough knowledge of the procedure. When in doubt, refer to the doctor.

12. Record working level on patient's chart: the dosage gives the doctor a reasonable range around which to work. In addition, the auxiliary should be familiar with:

a. Turn-on and shut-off operation of the machine and wall valves.

b. Cylinder gas level monitoring.

c. Manifold switch-overs when gas is exhausted.

d. Ordering replacement of cylinders.

In lengthy procedures, when intensive and possibly painful manipulation has been completed, nitrous oxide concentration should be reduced in order to avoid an increase in the analgesic depth. At the dismissal of the patient, it is incumbent upon the dental assistant to ascertain that the machine is turned off.

"The role of the dental assistant in nitrous oxide–oxygen sedation is an important one. She is an integral part of a smooth-running practice. She actively contributes to patient comfort and peace of mind, and to the efficiency, effectiveness, and safety of the office. She is thoroughly familiar with a modality which keeps the patient, the dentist, and herself agreeable all day long—a tremendous fringe benefit."

ADDITIONAL DUTIES OF THE DENTAL ASSISTANT

1. During the administration of analgesia, the dental assistant should make her presence known in the treatment room by her physical appearance before the patient, or by an occasional verbal comment. Should she find it necessary to leave the room, the assistant should make her exit as unobtrusively as possible, so that the patient is unaware of her absence. Then she should return as rapidly as possible.

2. It is mandatory that a pleasant atmosphere be maintained at all times. Under analgesia, a patient may experience a dream, and the prevailing atmosphere may have a strong influence on the nature of the dream. Unpleasantness may generate frightening ramifications.

3. The dental assistant's personality and charisma play an important role in maintaining a cheerful, pleasant atmosphere in the office. This helps in overcoming the patient's fear and instilling a sense of confidence.

4. Machines and gauges should be carefully watched. At completion of each administration, make certain the gases have been turned off. At the end of each working day, the valve on the cylinder or central gas supply source should be closed. The level of gas remaining in the cylinder should be noted. As the level approaches zero, a new cylinder should be ordered from the supplier.

The greater the number of duties of a routine nature the auxiliary personnel can take over, the more time the dentist is permitted to spend on complex procedures. He can therefore see more patients and perform more work in a more efficient manner in the course of a normal working day.

REFERENCES

1. Breitman, F.: Psychology does half the work in nitrous oxide analgesia. Dent. Surv., 27:1081, 1951.
2. Betcher, A. M.: Preanesthetic evaluation of the ambulatory dental patient. Bull. N.Y. State Dent. Soc. of Anesthesiol. 7:4 (Dec.), 1964.
3. Langa, H.: Analgesia for modern dentistry. New York J. Dent., 27:228, 265, 1957.
4. Langa, H.: Nitrous oxide–oxygen analgesia for modern dentistry. Dent. Dig., 66:126, 173, 1960.
5. Langa, H.: Analgesia for modern pedodontics. New York Dent. J., 28:58, 1962.

6. Langa, H.: Postgraduate teaching of relative analgesia with nitrous oxide and oxygen. J.A.D.A., 67:48, 54, 1963.
7. Fox, L.: The control of pain and apprehension and use of local anesthesia in periodontics. Dent. Clin. N. America, 1961. (Reprinted in J. Am. Analgesia Soc., 4:4, 1966.)
8. Fisk, H.: Personal communication.
9. Spiro, S. R., and Jones, R. H.: Pre-treatment physical evaluation in the dental office. New York J. Dent. 32:419, 1966.
10. Henegan, J. F.: Nitrous oxide and oxygen analgesia. New York J. Dent., 11:207, 1941.
11. Shipper, P.: Personal communication, 1975.
12. Lee, B.: The dental auxiliary and nitrous oxide conscious sedation. The Dental Assistant, 42:15–17, 1973.
13. Pelton, W., et al.: Economic implications of adding two expanded duty dental assistants to a practice. J.A.D.A., 87:604, 1973.
14. Sendax, V. I.: The dental auxiliary role in relaxation analgesia. J. Am. Anal. Soc., 9:7, 1971.

TECHNIQUES OF ADMINISTRATION; POSSIBLE REACTIONS OF THE PATIENT; INDICATIONS AND CONTRAINDICATIONS

7

GENERAL METHODS OF ADMINISTRATION

The last half century has witnessed several different methods of administering analgesia. Those described below are not equally acceptable, as will be noted in the author's comments.

THE PATIENT CONTROL METHOD (HAND BULB METHOD)

In this method the patient holds a rubber bulb, and the more he squeezes it, the more nitrous oxide is available on inspiration. Possibly this method has some limited use on a very few individuals who have been thoroughly trained in the use of analgesia, but on subjects new to analgesia it is definitely contraindicated. The original reasoning behind this technique was that the patient would be less frightened and have more confidence in the procedure, for he was controlling the depth of analgesia. This assumption has proved to be faulty on two counts: In the first place, most patients are frightened at the thought of self-administration, thinking they may give themselves too much nitrous oxide, with dire results. Secondly, it is obvious that the subject will squeeze the bulb until one of two conditions ensues: he feels that he has enough depth of analgesia, or he has attained such depth that he is no longer aware of the necessity for squeezing the bulb. In either event he stops, and in a short while comes out of the analgesic state. This approach leads to a continual variation in depth, with the patient wide awake at times.

However, there is an even more important reason for condemning the patient control method. In the administration of relative analgesia, the ideal should be to induce a semihypnotic state in which the patient's thoughts will wander outside the dental treatment room. If he is given a duty to perform, such as squeezing the bulb, he will tend to stay awake in order to perform his duty properly. This creates a situation in which the operator finds it more difficult to induce in his patient the proper analgesic level, for the patient is concentrating on his task in the dental treatment room.

THE PATIENT AND OPERATOR CONTROL METHOD

This method, which is a variation on the preceding one, takes two forms. In one, the patient is permitted to give himself nitrous oxide and oxygen, but the operator varies the dosage. In the other form, the hand bulb is not a functioning part of the mechanism. It is simply there for the purpose of giving the patient something to do, to make him think he has control of the situation. This method has all the disadvantages of the patient control approach.

THE USE OF MACHINES WITHOUT OXYGEN

The use of a gas machine that does not deliver oxygen is to be strongly condemned, for oxygen permits a smoother induction of analgesia, better control of its depth, and more rapid elimination of anesthetic gases and disappearance of postadministration symptoms. Therefore nitrous oxide should never be administered with less than 20 per cent oxygen. Savings on the cost of operation are at best picayune, since oxygen is the least expensive part of the apparatus. Machines designed for nitrous oxide alone were sold for only a short time, but their use did point up the extreme safety of relative analgesia and total analgesia.

THE OPERATOR CONTROL METHOD

Unquestionably this is the method of choice. The operator controls the dosage and teaches his patient how to vary it with nasal or oral breathing. Since the patient can dilute his symptoms by inhaling through the mouth, he acquires the desired confidence without having to confine his thoughts to the immediate surroundings.

Dosage

In any discussion of dosage for the administration of relative analgesia, it is most important to realize that anesthetic drugs constitute an excellent example of an important principle in pharmacology: *there are no standard doses of anesthetic drugs for any given situation.* Dosage must be determined by the requirements of the patient, his psychological conditioning, and the dental procedure to be performed. One is not dealing here with a closed or semiclosed system; on the contrary it could be classified as a well aerated system. But it is not by choice that this situation prevails, since the procedure would be more effective and more efficient if aeration could be greatly reduced. However, clinical application has proved that a certain amount of oral inhalation will always exist, even though the patient is continually reminded to inhale and exhale solely through his nose. We are, after all, dealing with a conscious subject who must hold his mouth open during the entire administration. Moreover, proper psychology dictates that the nasal inhaler should never be pressed too tightly against the face in an attempt to totally exclude air. In any case, variations in facial anatomy preclude the possibility of perfect adaptation of the nasal inhaler, since there are a limited number of sizes.

DOSAGE AND THE NEEDS OF THE PATIENT

Because of these prevailing conditions, the total output of the gas machine will *never* reach the patient's lungs. They receive a good proportion of it, but never all of it. It becomes necessary, therefore, in evaluating the depth of analgesia to be guided by the condition of the patient—not the output of the machine. Two individuals receiving the same proportions of nitrous oxide and oxygen and the same rate of flow from the machine may react in entirely different ways: one may be in a very light plane, the other much deeper. Putting aside for the moment any consideration of variations in susceptibility to anesthetic gases, in emotional make-up, in amount of fear, and in degree of painful stimulation, there would still be wide variations at the same dosage level because of the broad range in the tendency to breathe through the mouth and because the nasal inhaler cannot be ideally adapted to all faces. One quickly learns that formal tables of dosage, even though necessary as a starting point, are to be used just as starting points from which adjustments should be made to gain the proper analgesic level in individual patients.

For the same reasons, one cannot make too precise a distinction between the dose for a child and that for an adult. Children with enlarged adenoidal tissue may often require a dose far greater than the average adult dose, because they inhale so often through the mouth. In every patient, one has first to decide how deep in analgesia the patient should be. In this, the patient can advise the operator. The flowmeters on the machine should then be adjusted to arrive at the desired level. In these adjustments the important factor is the maintaining of a mixture with a minimum of 20 per cent oxygen.

Although in the administration of general anesthesia, proper procedure calls for lightening the level of anesthesia during the later phases of an extended administration, this does not apply in the administration of relative analgesia, since the patient himself will lighten the level of analgesia from time to time by mouth breathing. Here, too, one learns to judge by the condition of the subject.

Dosages used at the introductory administration are not to be construed as guidelines for future use on the same patient. These are minimal doses designed to generate only minimal symptoms. Nevertheless, so much tension, apprehension, fear, and autosuggestion may be present at the first administration that an extreme reaction may be obtained even with this small dose. This does not automatically signify that future reactions will be similar; in fact, they are usually quite different. An individual who initially required very little nitrous oxide to evoke a reaction may require a great deal more once he has learned to relax and accept the procedure and the symptoms. The converse may also be true.

Normal Induction (One to Two Minutes). The patient is seated comfortably in the chair, the nasal inhaler is positioned, and administration is begun with the average dose. By the time the operator has washed his hands and has all instruments ready, the patient is ready for him.

Slow Induction (Two to Four Minutes). Some subjects take a little longer to relax into the state of relative analgesia. Administering a higher concentration of nitrous oxide to hasten the induction does not solve the problem, because these patients will not comfortably tolerate a greater depth of analgesia. They become unnerved and do not relax. Allowing an extra minute or two at the dosage usual for this patient is the solution.

Increased-Dose Induction (One to Two Minutes). This approach is necessary for those who cannot be made to slip into the proper state of relaxation at their average operating dose, no matter how long they are exposed to it. For example, if such a patient can be comfortably treated with 15 per cent nitrous oxide, he could be given 25 to 30 per cent nitrous oxide at the outset for one to two minutes. When he reaches the proper state, the nitrous oxide can be reduced to 15 per cent.

Anticipation of the Patient's Needs. It has been said that a good anesthesia administration is a smooth anesthesia administration. This applies equally to analgesia administration. However, a smooth analgesia administration is not always easy to maintain because of air leakage through the mouth and because of varying degrees of stimulation by instruments, water, air, and so forth. The leakage is accepted as a normal part of the procedure, even though the patient is reminded to inhale only through the nose. In spite of this reminder, if too great a dilution of gases occurs, the correction is made at the machine by increasing the volume or proportion of nitrous oxide.

When the operator is approaching a more painful or distressing part of a procedure, he should increase the depth of analgesia about one or two minutes before he reaches that point. If the patient is prone to gag and an impression is to be taken, the depth of analgesia should be increased one to two minutes before the impression material is inserted. Thus, by anticipating the patient's needs and varying the depth of analgesia accordingly, a smooth administration results. An appreciable change in depth cannot be obtained with less than a 5 per cent increase in nitrous oxide (or 1 liter on a continuous flow machine). At least one minute must be allowed for the increase to make itself evident in the patient.

OPEN AIR VALVE VERSUS CLOSED AIR VALVE

When great depth of analgesia is desired, the air valve should be closed so as to eliminate a main source of dilution. When the administration of analgesia is begun, the tissues of the body are perfused with nitrogen in equilibrium with the nitrogen content of the atmosphere. Since nitrogen is an inert gas that is 15 times more soluble than oxygen in the bloodstream, its presence in great quantity in the plasma serves to dilute the effect of nitrous oxide by slowing the rate at which it can be dissolved in the bloodstream. When air is introduced to the lungs of the patient through an open air valve, nitrogen is continually being supplied, thus maintaining a high partial pressure of nitrogen in the lung alveoli and preventing its elimination from the bloodstream. With a closed air valve the subject breathes only oxygen and nitrous oxide from the machine. Since no nitrogen is being introduced, its partial pressure in the blood plasma soon becomes greater than its alveolar partial pressure, and the gas begins to diffuse out of the bloodstream. This allows for a faster uptake of nitrous oxide by the blood, resulting in a greater nitrous oxide level, which at any given moment means a deeper level of analgesia. It is the author's definite conclusion, based on many years of clinical observation, that allowing the nitrogen to remain in the body tissues results in less interference with normal physiology—with the preservation of homeostasis. Consequently, full recuperation and return to normalcy take place more rapidly.

The closed air valve, then, is employed only when deeper levels of analgesia are desired or when dilution is so great that an average level cannot be attained with an open air valve. For example, a mouth breather or an individual with nasal block would require the closed air valve technique. Likewise, a highly emotional or fearful patient who does not respond to ordinary dosage ranges with the open air valve would also require the closed air valve approach in order to reach the proper analgesic depth. When a decision is made to close the air valve after having used a flow of 8 liters of nitrous oxide (with 3 liters of oxygen), the flow of nitrous oxide should be greatly reduced (see dosage tables).

DOSAGE IN CONTINUOUS FLOW MACHINES

In the continuous flow machines, the rates of flow of the gases are always quoted in volume per minute. The dose is determined by two factors: the proportion of nitrous oxide to oxygen and the total minute volume of gas emanating from the machine. For example, when a McKesson Analor is used to deliver 3 liters of oxygen and 5 liters of nitrous oxide, it could be said that this machine is producing a total output of 8 liters per minute, three-eighths (37.5 per cent) of this being oxygen. This does not imply that the patient's lungs are receiving 37.5 per cent oxygen and 62.5 per cent nitrous oxide, for air may enter through the air valves on nasal inhalers or through the mouth. However, since air itself has about 20 per cent oxygen, the patient is always assured of a safe minimal oxygen percentage when at least 20 per cent oxygen emanates from the gas machine.

The average adult inspires about 500 ml. of gases with each inhalation and breathes 15 to 20 times per minute. A child will take in less volume with each inhalation but will breathe more frequently. The average human being, therefore, inspires at least 7500 to 8000 ml. of gases per minute. In the absence of rebreathing, however, this minimum is not always forthcoming from a continuous flow machine, because the total volume of nitrous oxide necessary may be only 4 liters per minute. To adhere strictly to the 20 per cent oxygen factor, 1 liter of oxygen would be added. This would result in a total output of 5 liters of gases, which might create a sense of suffocation unless the patient is given access to additional air or oxygen. This is accomplished in one of three ways: opening the air valve on the nasal inhaler, increasing the volume of oxygen from the machine, or maintaining a full reservoir bag from which the patient can draw.

Proportions of Oxygen. In continuous flow machines, the maximum flow of nitrous oxide is 7 to 8 liters per minute. If oxygen is kept at 3 liters per minute, the gas machine will produce at least 20 per cent oxygen, no matter how much nitrous oxide is being used. And all levels of nitrous oxide flow below the maximum produce a higher oxygen percentage. For dosages and settings, see Table 7–1.

It should also be pointed out that almost all continuous flow machines

TABLE 7–1   Dosages and Settings for the McKesson Analor (Continuous Flow)

DEPTH OF ANALGESIA	OXYGEN SETTING	NITROUS OXIDE SETTING	POSITION OF AIR (INHALING) VALVE	POSITION OF REBREATHING (EXHALING) VALVE	DURATION OF ADMINISTRA-TION
Introductory administration	3 liters (after starting with 8 liters)	1 to 3 liters	Largest opening	Wide open	5 min.
Average levels	3 liters	3 to 5 liters	Largest opening	Wide open	Unlimited
Deeper levels Open air valve	3 liters	5 to 8 liters	Largest opening	Wide open	Limited by maintenance of open mouth
Closed air valve	3 liters	3 to 6 liters	Closed	Wide open	Limited by maintenance of open mouth

being sold today are so constructed as to preclude delivery of nitrous oxide without a minimal flow of 3 liters of oxygen per minute. Additionally, the machines cannot produce more than an 8 to 10 liters per minute flow of nitrous oxide.

Proportions of Nitrous Oxide.   The percentages of nitrous oxide can be calculated by the same simple mathematics used for calculating oxygen percentages. However, it is not important to know what proportion of nitrous oxide is being delivered, so long as a metabolic minimum of oxygen is used

TABLE 7–2   Dosages and Settings for All Other Continuous Flow Analgesia Machines

DEPTH OF ANALGESIA	OXYGEN SETTING	NITROUS OXIDE SETTING	POSITION OF AIR (INHALING) VALVE	POSITION OF REBREATHING (EXHALING) VALVE	DURATION OF ADMINISTRA-TION
Introductory administration	3 liters (after starting with 8 liters)	1 to 3 liters	Wide open at first then close to 1/2 open position	Wide open	5 min.
Average levels	3 liters	3 to 5 liters	1/2 open	Wide open	Unlimited
Deeper levels Open air valve	3 liters	5 to 8 liters	1/2 open	Wide open	Limited by maintenance of open mouth
Closed air valve	3 liters	3 to 6 liters	Closed	Wide open	Limited by maintenance of open mouth

TABLE 7–3 Dosages and Settings for the Heidbrink Model "T" Machine (Continuous Flow)

| DEPTH OF ANALGESIA | OXYGEN SETTING | NITROUS OXIDE SETTINGS | | POSITION OF AIR (INHALING) VALVE | POSITION OF REBREATHING (EXHALING) VALVE | DURATION OF ADMINISTRA- TION |
		PROPORTION	RATE OF FLOW			
Introductory adminis- tration	25%	First Λ	1 gal. per minute	¼ open after starting with wide open position	Wide open	5 min.
Average levels	25%	Between second **V** and red dot	1 gal. per minute	¼ open	Wide open	Unlimited
Deeper levels	25%	Arrow ↑ ↑ ↑	1 to 1½ gal. per minute	Closed	Wide open	Limited by main- tenance of open mouth

with it. In the administration of relative analgesia the operator works from the patient to the machine, not from the machine to the patient. That is, he decides what depth of analgesia he wishes to obtain in the patient and sets the nitrous oxide flow to produce that level, provided the level does not frighten the patient and that it permits the maintaining of an open mouth without the use of a mouth prop.

DOSAGE IN INTERMITTENT FLOW MACHINES (SEE ALSO TABLE 7–4)

In intermittent flow machines (*Euthesor, Nargraf,* and *Narmatic* machines), the proportions of the gases are known, but not the total volumetric output, since this varies with the patient's rate and depth of respiration. The force of flow can be varied and is registered in millimeters of pressure. Of course, variations in percentage of oxygen will automatically vary the nitrous oxide percentage. Thus, if one wishes to administer 15 per cent nitrous oxide, 85 per cent oxygen must be given with it. Air valves are located on the machine, if not on the nasal inhaler. On an intermittent flow machine, percentages can be read directly, but volume has to be estimated.

THE RECORDING OF DOSAGES

The new operator should keep a record of the dose administered to each patient. This does not mean that he should deliver the same dose to an individual each time. He should also recognize that gas machines can vary in their

TABLE 7–4 Dosages and Settings for the McKesson Euthesor and the Nargraf
and Narmatic Machines (Intermittent Flow)*

DEPTH OF ANALGESIA	OXYGEN (PERCENTAGE)	NITROUS OXIDE (PERCENTAGE)	MILLIMETERS PRESSURE	POSITION OF REBREATHING (EXHALING) VALVE	DURATION OF ADMINISTRA- TION
Introductory administra- tion	90 to 95	5 to 10	1 to 2	Zero tension	5 min.
Average levels	75 to 90	10 to 25	1 to 3	Zero tension	Unlimited
Deeper levels	65 to 80	20 to 35	3 to 5	Zero tension	Limited by main- tenance of open mouth

*Note: Intermittent flow machines produce so much oxygen that the open air valve is unneces-
sary.

output. Nevertheless, keeping records for the first few months will enable the
dentist to ascertain the range within which most of his patients fall with his
particular machine. In effect, he will be calibrating his machine. This procedure can eventually be discontinued.

Oxygenation of the Patient

It is imperative that 1 to 3 minutes (or more when necessary) of oxygenation be administered at the conclusion of *every analgesia administration*. It is
true that, in the past, recuperation has been allowed to take place with atmospheric air, but this is improper procedure. With oxygen, normalcy is attained
faster and more completely, for oxygenation clears the system more efficiently
and restores the abilities of the patient (to walk, drive, and so forth) in a
minimal amount of time. Good procedure dictates that oxygenation always be
used, without exception.

Rebreathing

The use of rebreathing in anesthesia administration has three objectives:
the stimulation and stabilization of respiration, the preservation of body heat
and moisture, and economy.

1. Respiration is stimulated directly by the action of carbon dioxide on
the respiratory center and indirectly by stimulation of the chemoreceptors of
the aortic sinus. Rebreathing is also a convenient and simple means of maintaining the carbon dioxide tension of the blood and thereby stabilizing the respiration.

2. Rebreathing assists greatly in the production of the optimal type of
breathing and in the preservation of body heat and moisture.

3. Rebreathing effects an economy in gas consumption, for the patient's expired nitrous oxide and carbon dioxide accumulate in the bag, tubings, or bellows. Even if no rebreathing were employed, however, acapnia would not develop, since there is always enough dead space in the lungs themselves to allow the trace of rebreathing necessary to provide the very small amount of carbon dioxide required to sustain respiration. Respiration in air occurs quite normally with a content of 0.04 per cent carbon dioxide.

The use of rebreathing assumes greater importance in the administration of anesthesia than in the administration of analgesia because, in the latter, a conscious patient is being treated, who can, of his own volition or upon direction, alter both the rate and the depth of his respiration. The anesthetized patient, being unconscious, must have his breathing conditioned by the operator. At times, analgesia patients complain of a feeling of chilliness at the end of an extended administration. Allowing them to rebreathe warm exhaled gases for a few minutes will obviate this complaint.

Carbon Dioxide and Respiration.   At one time carbon dioxide was considered to be nothing more than a harmful waste product of metabolism. It is known today, however, that it plays a very vital role in the physiology of the respiratory and circulatory systems. Some of its important functions are:

1. To maintain the acid-alkali equilibrium of the blood.

2. To facilitate gaseous interchange in the lungs and tissues (dissociation of oxyhemoglobin).

3. To control the depth of respiration.

4. To increase blood flow, blood pressure, and coagulability of the blood.

5. To increase muscle tonicity.

Effects of Increased Carbon Dioxide Tension.   An increase in carbon dioxide tension in the bloodstream causes an augmentation of both the depth and the rate of respiration: 5 per cent carbon dioxide increases the volume of ventilation four times; 10 per cent increases the volume of ventilation 10 times. Anesthetic agents alter both the reaction threshold and the sensitivity of the respiratory center to carbon dioxide in the blood.

Procedure for Rebreathing.   Rebreathing is instituted by closing the rebreathing (exhaling) valve on the nasal inhaler. To do this on the *McKesson inhaler,* increase the tension on the spring of the exhaling valve so that the valve remains completely shut or barely cracks on exhalation. On other analgesia machines, close the exhaling valve completely by turning it clockwise. Most nasal inhalers made for continuous flow analgesia machines cannot ever be closed for rebreathing. The exhaling (rebreathing) valve remains open always.

Important Considerations in Administering Analgesia

GENERAL PROCEDURES AND PRECAUTIONS

1. The gas machine should be positioned behind the patient so that the operator can manipulate the controls without changing his position. A wall-mounted machine should be used only if the operator or his assistant can reach it easily.

2. Select a nasal inhaler that is not too small for the patient's comfort and ease of respiration.

3. The patient should be *comfortably* seated.

4. The nasal inhaler should be cleansed and thoroughly dried *after* the patient is seated.

5. Before the nasal inhaler is placed on the patient's nose, a flow of 100 per cent oxygen from the machine is started. This avoids the possibility of a feeling of insufficiency at the first breath or two. The reservoir bag should not be collapsed.

6. The nasal inhaler should be positioned snugly and securely, but not tightly enough to create discomfort. See that the inhaler completely encloses both nares.

7. To prevent the formation of facial pressure marks from the nasal inhaler, insert a small piece of gauze or tissue paper under both sides of the inhaler.

8. *Proper positioning of the inhaler tubes.* The rubber tubes leading posteriorly from the nasal inhaler should be positioned for the greatest comfort of

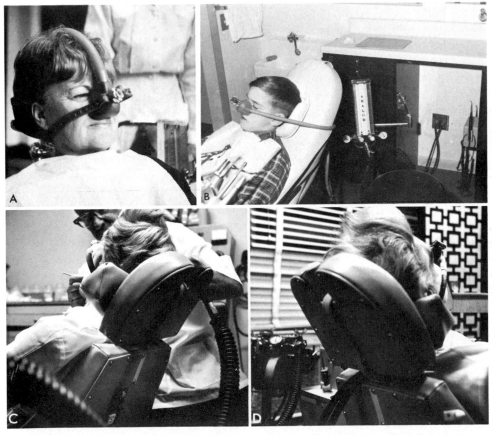

Figure 7–1 *A,* A single overhead tube for the nasal inhaler. *B,* Double lengths of tubing fit around the back of the chair. *C* and *D,* Slits in the backs of some chairs accommodate the tubing.

the patient and for proper fit of the nasal piece. Different types of dental chairs require a modification of the position of the tubes. The following are the most common variations: tubes are placed above the ears, under the ears, across the ears, or under the headrest; for high-backed chairs, a single overhead tube (Fig. 7–1A), double lengths of tubing around the chair (Fig. 7–1B), or tubing fed through a slit in the back of the chair (Fig. 7–1C and D).

9. Moderate decreases in the depth of analgesia can be obtained by opening the air valve wider or by increasing the volumetric flow of oxygen.

10. Increases in the depth of analgesia can be obtained by closing the air valve or by decreasing the proportion of oxygen (but never below 20 per cent). This takes about 2 minutes to take effect.

11. The most rapid method for increasing the depth of analgesia is through an increase in the flow of nitrous oxide (1 minute to take effect).

12. It requires at least 60 seconds for any change in dosage to become evident in the patient.

13. To compensate for excessive oral inhalation: (a) increase the pressure (in an intermittent flow machine) or increase the flow of nitrous oxide (in a continuous flow machine), (b) close the air valve if it is open, or (c) use an auxiliary oral flow tube.

14. Never leave a patient unattended when he is under analgesia.

15. Always oxygenate the patient completely.

16. When oxygenation is completed, first remove the nasal inhaler and then shut off the flow of oxygen. For the comfort of the patient, pull forward on the nasal inhaler with one hand as the other hand loosens the restraint behind his head (Fig. 7–2).

17. The patient's head should be clear before he leaves the chair, and most definitely before he leaves the office.

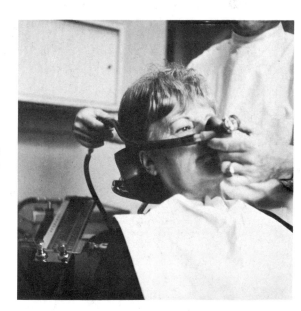

Figure 7–2 Proper technique for the removal of the nasal inhaler.

THE USE OF INSTRUMENTS DURING RELATIVE ANALGESIA

The use of relative analgesia does not necessitate the elimination or modification of any instrument that is now used for dental treatment, with the possible exception of the electric cautery (hot wire). Neither nitrous oxide nor oxygen is combustible; both, however, are good supporters of combustion, and it is conceivable that the glowing, hot cautery might flare up a little and burn neighboring tissue. All other instruments may be used. A rubber dam minimizes mouth breathing and results in a better analgesic depth (Fig. 7–3). Roentgenograms can be taken under analgesia. If the upper anterior teeth are being treated, a slight upward displacement of the nasal inhaler will permit easy access to these teeth without discomfort to the patient. The Bunsen burner may be used in its usual fashion and position (Fig. 7–4). Electrosurgery with a fully corrected current may be used.

AVOIDANCE OF A SENSE OF URGENCY OR TENSION IN THE DENTIST

It is not uncommon in the administration of general anesthesia that a sense of urgency or tension builds up in the operator. He wants to anesthetize his patient, complete the necessary dental procedures, and awaken the patient as rapidly as possible. This attitude is entirely uncalled for and, indeed, is highly undesirable during the administration of analgesia. A feeling of being rushed imparts itself to the patient, interfering with relaxation. Moreover, there is no reason to rush; most adults can withstand relative analgesia for unlimited periods. There is no reason to fear that a subject under relative analgesia will suddenly go into the excitement stage while the doctor turns his back to get an instrument. As a matter of fact, patients under relative

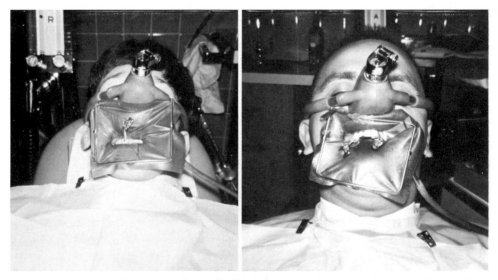

Figure 7–3 A rubber dam effectively eliminates oral inhalation. The upper border of the rubber dam can be lapped over the nasal inhaler.

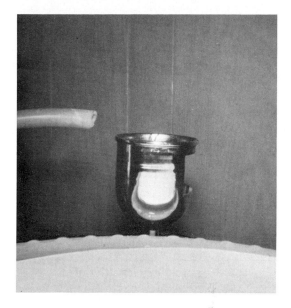

Figure 7-4 Nitrous oxide and oxygen flowing against a Bunsen burner flame; neither gas is combustible.

analgesia will *never* slip into the excitement stage. For these reasons a sense of urgency on the part of the operator during the administration of relative analgesia is entirely unwarranted. Rather it could be said that the use of relative analgesia permits the dentist to work in a much more relaxed atmosphere. The novice should bear in mind that a patient who maintains an open mouth (without mouth props) cannot be in any but the analgesic stage.

SPECIFIC PROCEDURES FOR ANALGESIA

In all of the following procedures, the preliminary steps for introductory administration are the same as those for routine administration. Therefore, in each procedure, after the instruction *Start the flow of nitrous oxide*, the operator either continues with the steps for introductory administration or proceeds to the steps for routine administration, according to his needs.

CONTINUOUS FLOW MACHINES

The McKesson Analor. *(The flow of gas is registered in liters per minute.)*
  1. Seat the patient comfortably in the chair.
  2. Open the air valve to three openings.
  3. Wash the nasal inhaler with scented alcohol. Pure alcohol may be obnoxious and nauseating, whereas pleasant odors can have beneficial psychological effects.
  4. Dry the nasal inhaler with compressed air.
  5. Start the flow of 3 liters of oxygen (8 liters for introductory administration).

6. Make certain that the reservoir bag is not collapsed, that it contains some gas. A nervous subject breathing in an exaggerated fashion may empty all available gases in the system with the first two inhalations. This may create a feeling of lack of air and cause rejection of all further administration at this point.

7. Position the nasal inhaler. Ask the patient to adjust it to his comfort (if it feels uncomfortable).

8. Start the flow of nitrous oxide.

Introductory Administration

9. Begin the administration with 1 liter of nitrous oxide. (Reduce oxygen flow to 3 liters.)

10. Instruct the patient to breathe *normally* through the nose with his mouth closed (for 2 minutes).

11. Do not hurry to increase the volume of nitrous oxide, even though the patient continues to advise you (upon questioning) that no analgesia symptoms are evident. The lack of symptoms may be due to fear and anxiety.

12. After 2 minutes without appreciable symptoms, increase the flow of nitrous oxide to 1.5 liters (or a little more).

13. As soon as minimal symptoms appear and are reported as pleasant, stop the flow of nitrous oxide and begin oxygenation with 8 liters of oxygen for 1 to 3 minutes.

14. When the patient is fully recovered, remove the nasal inhaler first and then close off the flow of oxygen.

Routine Administration

9. Set the flow of nitrous oxide immediately to the volume you estimate will be needed.

10. Allow at least 1 minute for the full effect to develop.

11. Begin the dental procedure.

12. The patient will advise you whether more nitrous oxide is needed.

13. Although the average rate of nitrous oxide flow is 3 to 5 liters, do not hesitate to advance it to 7 or 8 liters if the situation demands it.

14. If a greater depth of analgesia is desired, close the air valve.

15. On completion of the dental procedure, shut off the flow of nitrous oxide.

16. Oxygenate the patient with 8 liters of oxygen for one to two minutes.

17. Remove the nasal inhaler first, and then close off the flow of oxygen.

All Other Continuous Flow Analgesia Machines. (The flow of gas is registered in liters per minute.)

1. Where possible set the *exhaling valve* to the widest opening by turning it counterclockwise as far as it can go. The exhaling valve on these machines is the lower of the two valves on the nasal inhaler.

2. In introductory administrations, open the *air valve* to the maximum initially. When the patient's exaggerated breathing reverts to normal, close it down to ½ open position. For veteran patients, set it initially at the ½ open position.

3. Wash the nasal inhaler with scented alcohol. Pure alcohol may be obnoxious and nauseating, whereas pleasant odors can have beneficial psychological effects.

4. Dry the nasal inhaler with compressed air.

5. Start the flow of 3 liters of oxygen (8 liters for introductory administration).

6. Make certain that the reservoir bag is not collapsed; it should contain some gas. A nervous subject, breathing in an exaggerated fashion, may empty all available gases in the system with the first two inhalations. This may create a feeling of lack of air and cause rejection of all further administration at this point.

7. Position the nasal inhaler. Ask the patient to adjust it to his comfort (if it feels uncomfortable).

8. Start the flow of nitrous oxide.

Introductory Administration

9. Start with 1 liter of nitrous oxide. (Reduce oxygen flow to 3 liters.)

10. Instruct the patient to breathe *normally* through the nose with his mouth closed (for 2 minutes).

11. Do not hurry to increase the volume of nitrous oxide, even though patient continues to advise you (upon questioning) that no analgesia symptoms are evident. The lack of symptoms may be due to fear and anxiety.

12. After 2 minutes without appreciable symptoms, increase the flow of nitrous oxide to 1.5 liters (or a little more).

13. As soon as minimal symptoms appear and are reported as pleasant, stop the flow of nitrous oxide and begin oxygenation with 8 liters of oxygen for 1 to 3 minutes.

14. When the patient is fully recovered, remove the nasal inhaler and then close off the flow of oxygen.

Routine Administration

9. Set the flow of nitrous oxide immediately to the volume you estimate will be needed.

10. Allow at least 1 minute for the full effect to develop.

11. Begin the dental procedure.

12. The patient will advise you whether more nitrous oxide is needed.

13. Although the average rate of nitrous oxide flow is 3 to 5 liters, do not hesitate to advance it to 7 or 8 liters if the situation demands it.

14. If the rebreathing effect is desired, close the rebreathing valve completely by turning it clockwise, if it can be manipulated.

15. To obtain finer gradations in analgesic depth with these machines, open the air valve wider or close it completely.

16. On completion of the dental procedure, shut off the flow of nitrous oxide.

17. Oxygenate the patient with 8 liters of oxygen for 1 to 2 minutes.

18. Remove the nasal inhaler first and then close off the flow of oxygen.

The Heidbrink Model "T."   (*The flow is registered in gallons of nitrous oxide per minute.*).

1. Set the *exhaling valve* to the widest opening by turning it counterclockwise.

2. In introductory administrations, open the *air valve* to the maximum initially by turning the valve counterclockwise. When the patient's exaggerated breathing reverts to normal, close the air valve to the normal setting. This

is done by closing it completely (clockwise), and then giving it one small turn (counterclockwise) with the thumb and forefinger.

3. Set the rate of nitrous oxide flow at 1 gallon per minute.

4. Set the center lever at position "Normal" (vertical).

5. Make certain that the blow-off valve is completely closed (turn clockwise).

6. Be sure that the spigot which leads to the face mask is closed off (when the face mask is not attached).

7. Wash the nasal inhaler with scented alcohol. Pure alcohol may be obnoxious and nauseating, whereas pleasant odors can have beneficial psychological effects.

8. Dry the nasal inhaler with compressed air.

9. Start the flow of oxygen by setting the oxygen indicator at 25 per cent.

10. Make certain that the reservoir bag is not collapsed; it should contain some gas. A nervous subject breathing in an exaggerated fashion may empty all available gases in the system with the first two inhalations. This may cause a feeling of lack of air and cause rejection of all further administration at this point.

11. Position the nasal inhaler, and ask the patient to adjust it to his comfort (if it is uncomfortable).

12. Start the flow of nitrous oxide.

Introductory Administration

13. Begin the administration by setting the nitrous oxide indicator at the first ∧.

14. Instruct the patient to breathe *normally* through the nose with his mouth closed (for 2 minutes).

15. Do not hurry to increase the flow of nitrous oxide, even though the patient continues to advise you (upon questioning) that no analgesia symptoms are evident. The lack of symptoms may be due to fear and anxiety.

16. After 2 minutes without appreciable symptoms, increase the flow of nitrous oxide by moving the indicator to the second ∧ (or slightly beyond).

17. As soon as minimal symptoms appear and are reported as pleasant, stop the flow of nitrous oxide and begin oxygenation for 1 to 3 minutes. This is accomplished by turning the gallons per minute indicator to 2 or 3 gallons.

Note: As soon as oxygenation is completed, turn the gallons per minute indicator back to 1.

18. When patient is fully recovered, remove the nasal inhaler first, and then close off the flow of oxygen (by turning the oxygen indicator to position "0").

Routine Administration

13. Set the rate of nitrous oxide flow immediately to the point you estimate will be needed.

14. Allow at least 1 minute for the full effect to develop.

15. Begin the dental procedure.

16. The patient will advise you whether more nitrous oxide is needed.

17. Although the average rate of nitrous oxide flow is delivered at the setting between the second ∧ and the center dot marked "ethylene," do not hes-

itate to advance it to the arrow (on the extreme right) if the situation demands it, or increase the flow rate of nitrous oxide to 1½ gallons per minute.

18. When the rebreathing effect is desired, close the rebreathing valve by turning it completely to the right.

19. On completion of the dental procedure, turn the nitrous oxide off (to extreme left).

20. Oxygenate the patient by (a) turning the gallons per minute indicator to 2 or 3, or (b) switching the center lever to the left. This gives a direct flow of oxygen.

Note: If the gallons per minute indicator has been advanced to 2 or 3 for oxygenation, remember to turn it back to 1 at the completion of oxygenation.

21. Remove the nasal inhaler first, and then close off the flow of oxygen (turn the oxygen indicator to the extreme left).

INTERMITTENT FLOW MACHINES

The McKesson Euthesor and Nargraf and Narmatic Machines.   *(The rate of flow is registered in millimeters of pressure.)*

1. Set the exhaling valve at zero tension.

2. Wash the nasal inhaler with scented alcohol. Pleasant odors have beneficial psychological effects, whereas pure alcohol may be obnoxious and nauseating.

3. Dry the nasal inhaler with compressed air.

4. Start the flow of 100 per cent oxygen at 1 to 2 mm. pressure.

5. Position the nasal inhaler, and ask patient to adjust it to his comfort (if it is uncomfortable).

6. Start the flow of nitrous oxide.

Introductory Administration

7. Begin the administration with 5 per cent nitrous oxide. (This automatically delivers 95 per cent oxygen.)

8. Instruct the patient to breathe *normally* through the nose with his mouth closed (for 2 minutes).

9. Do not hurry to increase the proportion of nitrous oxide, even though the patient continues to advise you (upon questioning) that no analgesia symptoms are evident. The lack of symptoms may be due to fear and anxiety.

10. After 2 minutes without appreciable symptoms, increase the flow of nitrous oxide to 8 per cent (or perhaps 10 per cent).

11. As soon as minimal symptoms appear and are reported as pleasant, stop the flow of nitrous oxide by turning the wheel to the position marked "100% oxygen."

12. Oxygenate the patient for 1 to 3 minutes.

13. When the patient is fully recovered, remove the nasal inhaler, and then close off the flow of oxygen by turning the millimeter pressure indicator to position "OFF."

Routine Administration

7. Set the flow of nitrous oxide to the proportion and rate you estimate will be needed.

8. Allow at least 1 minute for the full effect to develop.

9. Begin the dental procedure.

10. The patient will advise you whether more nitrous oxide is needed.

11. Although the average rate of nitrous oxide flow is 10 to 25 per cent nitrous oxide at 1 to 3 mm. pressure, do not hesitate to advance to 25 or 35 per cent nitrous oxide if the situation demands it.

12. If the rebreathing effect is desired, increase the spring tension on the exhaling valve to 5 or 10, so that the flip valve will not lift at all or will just barely crack on exhalation.

13. If there is difficulty in breathing, increase the millimeter pressure reading to 4 or 5.

14. On completion of the dental procedure, shut off the flow of nitrous oxide by turning to the position marked "100% oxygen."

15. Oxygenate the patient for 1 to 2 minutes.

16. Remove the nasal inhaler first, and then close off the flow of oxygen by turning the millimeter pressure indicator to position "OFF."

Contingent Procedures

RESUSCITATION

In the administration of analgesia, resuscitation is almost never required; nevertheless, should it become necessary, the gas machine is an excellent and ready source of oxygen.

Resuscitation means the establishment of respiratory movements by insufflating the lung alveoli with air. Since nitrous oxide is extremely diffusible and has no affinity for the body tissues, resuscitation is readily accomplished by forcing oxygen into the lungs. When pure oxygen fills the lungs, the hemoglobin becomes saturated with oxygen, and the blood serum carries 2.2 per cent oxygen, or five times its normal amount. The blood remains in the pulmonary alveoli for only 1 second, but in two-fifths of a second the hemoglobin becomes 95 per cent saturated with oxygen; that is, it is changed from venous to arterial blood in that short interval. Oxygen is absorbed from the lungs at a little more than 1 liter per minute, a volume sufficient to saturate 20 liters of blood with oxygen. In less than 20 seconds, all the arterial blood of a patient may be saturated with oxygen.

Procedure for Resuscitation

1. Close the exhaling (rebreathing) valve. If the face mask is not being used, make certain that no gas will escape through the patient's mouth and that the nasal inhaler fits snugly.

2. Close the air (inhaling) valve, if one is present.

3. With the thumb and index finger of the right hand, press the mask or nasal inhaler to the face while the remaining fingers of the right hand elevate the chin to ensure an open airway.

4. If a direct oxygen button or lever is present, exert a steady, gradually increasing pressure on it (Fig. 7–5A).

5. When no direct oxygen lever is present, (a) open the oxygen flowmeter as wide as possible (sending the indicator beyond the calibrations of the

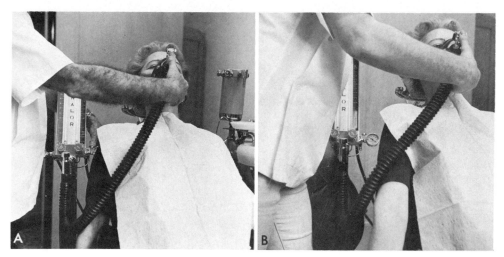

Figure 7-5   Resuscitation procedure. *A,* Left hand compresses the direct oxygen flow lever. *B,* Bag is compressed against the thigh.

flowmeter), thus inflating the reservoir bag, or (b) while an assistant holds the inhaler or mask tightly against the patient's face, compress the bag manually with both hands. If an assistant is not present, compress the bag with one hand, using the thigh for counteraction (Fig. 7–5*B*).

6. Note that the patient's chest expands, giving evidence that oxygen is entering the lungs.

7. When the patient's chest is expanded, lift the inhaler off his face to allow deflation through the elastic recoil of the lung tissue.

8. Repeat the maneuver 10 times per minute.

The use of relative analgesia in a dental office minimizes incidents in which cardiopulmonary resuscitation would be needed, and at the same time offers a ready source of oxygen. Nevertheless, it is the author's firm belief that *all* dental practitioners should know the basic principles and practices involved in life-saving procedures, in or out of the dental office.

With this thought in mind, and with the kind permission of the American Heart Association. the section on *Standards for Cardiopulmonary Resuscitation (CPR) and Emergency Cardiac Care (ECC)* has been reprinted in this text (pages 186–196).

AUXILIARY ORAL GAS SUPPLY (FIG. 7–6)

When a patient has a nasal block or is a chronic mouth breather, it is advantageous to supply nitrous oxide and oxygen through the mouth as well as through the nose. The instrument for supply to the mouth is similar to an ordinary saliva ejector and provides the same proportions of gases that are entering through the nose. (If a needle is attached to the working end, it can be used for oxygen insufflation under the free margin of the gingiva.)

Part II.—Basic Life Support*

Basic life support is an emergency first aid procedure that consists of recognizing respiratory and cardiac arrest and starting the proper application of cardiopulmonary resuscitation to maintain life until a victim recovers sufficiently to be transported or until advanced life support is available. This includes the A-B-C steps of cardiopulmonary resuscitation:

A. Airway
B. Breathing } artificial ventilation   } cardiopulmonary
                                             resuscitation
C. Circulation } artificial circulation }

These steps always should be started as quickly as possible. They are performed in the order shown above (also shown in the frontispiece and in Fig 1, Life Support Decision Tree) except in special circumstances such as: (*a*) in monitored patients or (*b*) in witnessed cardiac arrests. When cardiac arrest occurs in the monitored patient and trained personnel and defibrillators are available immediately, a precordial thump and/or advanced life support procedures should be instituted without delay. In a witnessed cardiac arrest, the A-B-C sequence should include use of a precordial thump. (See "Precordial Thump.")

There must be a maximum sense of urgency in starting basic life support. The outstanding advantage of CPR is that it permits the earliest possible treatment of respiratory arrest or cardiac arrest by properly trained persons. Optimally, only seconds should intervene between recognizing the need and starting treatment.

Indications for basic life support are:
1. Respiratory arrest and
2. Cardiac arrest. Cardiac arrest can result from:
    (a) cardiovascular collapse
        (electromechanical dissociation)
    (b) ventricular fibrillation, or
    (c) ventricular standstill (asystole).

In cases of collapsed or unconscious persons, the adequacy or absence of breathing and circulation must be determined immediately. If breathing alone is inadequate or absent, rescue breathing may be all that is necessary. If circulation is also absent, artificial circulation must be started in combination with rescue breathing. The methods of recognizing adequacy or absence of breathing or circulation and the recommended techniques for performing artificial ventilation and artificial circulation are presented below. Their proper stepwise sequence is detailed in the Life Support Decision Tree (Fig 1).

Artificial Ventilation

Opening the airway and restoring breathing are the basic steps of artificial ventilation. The steps can be performed quickly under almost any circumstance and without adjunctive equipment or help from another person. They constitute emergency first aid for airway obstruction and respiratory inadequacy or arrest.

Respiratory inadequacy may result from an obstruction of the airway or from respiratory failure. An obstructed airway is sometimes difficult to recognize until the airway is opened. At other times, a partially obstructed airway is recognized by labored breathing or excessive respiratory efforts, often involving accessory muscles of respiration, and by soft tissue retractions of the intercostal, supraclavicular, and suprasternal spaces. Respiratory failure is characterized by minimal or absent respiratory effort, failure of the chest or upper abdomen to move, and inability to detect air movement through the nose or mouth.

Airway.—The most important factor for successful resuscitation is immediate opening of the airway. This can be accomplished easily and quickly by tilting the victim's head backward as far as possible. Sometimes this simple maneuver is all that is required for breathing to resume spontaneously. To perform the head tilt, the victim must be lying on his back. The rescuer places one hand beneath the victim's neck and the other hand on his forehead. He then lifts the neck with one hand and tilts the head backward by pressure with his other hand on the forehead. This maneuver extends the neck and lifts the tongue away from the back of the throat. Anatomical obstruction of the airway caused by the tongue dropping against the back of the throat thereby is relieved. The head must be maintained in this position at all times. (See Fig 2.)

The head tilt method is effective in most cases. If head tilt is unsuccessful in opening the air passage adequately, additional forward displacement of the lower jaw—jaw thrust—may be required. This can be accomplished by a triple airway maneuver in which the rescuer places his fingers behind the angles of the

---

*The following pages (pp. 186–196) were reprinted from *Standards for Cardiopulmonary Resuscitation (CPR) and Emergency Cardiac Care (ECC).* J.A.M.A. 227 (Suppl.): 841–851, 1974. By permission of American Heart Association.

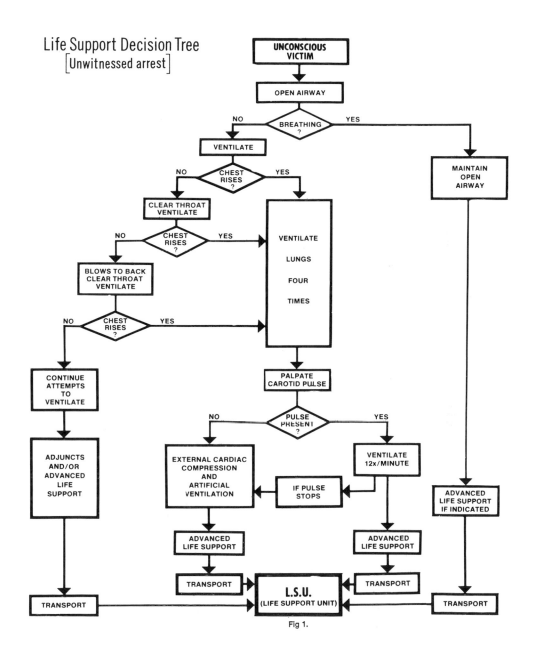

Fig 1.

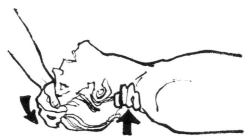

Fig 2.—Head tilt method of opening airway

victim's jaw and (1) forcefully displaces the mandible forward while (2) tilting the head backward and (3) using his thumbs to retract the lower lip to allow breathing through the mouth as well as through the nose. The jaw thrust is performed best from a position at the top of the victim's head.

However, if the victim does not resume spontaneous breathing, the rescuer must move to the victim's side to perform mouth-to-mouth or mouth-to-nose ventilation. Several variations of the jaw thrust may be used. When using jaw thrust for mouth-to-mouth ventilation, the rescuer must keep the victim's mouth open with his thumbs and seal the nose by placing his cheek against it. However, this is more difficult to teach and practice on manikins, and more difficult and tiring to perform on victims than the head tilt method. For mouth-to-nose ventilation with jaw thrust, the rescuer uses his cheek to seal the victim's mouth and does not retract the lower lip with his thumbs. Such special details of performance and the problems associated with manikin practice limit use of jaw thrust techniques to specially trained personnel.

Breathing.—If the victim does not promptly resume adequate spontaneous breathing after the airway is opened, artificial ventilation, sometimes called rescue breathing, must be started. Mouth-to-mouth breathing and mouth-to-nose breathing are both types of artificial ventilation.

To perform mouth-to-mouth ventilation, the rescuer uses his hand behind the victim's neck to maintain the head in a position of maximum backward tilt. He pinches the victim's nostrils together with the thumb and index finger of his other hand, which also continues to exert pressure on the forehead to maintain the backward head tilt. The rescuer then opens his mouth widely, takes a deep breath, makes a tight seal with his mouth around the victim's mouth and blows into the victim's mouth. He then removes his mouth and allows the victim to exhale passively, watching the victim's chest fall. This cycle is repeated *once every five seconds* as long as respiratory inadequacy persists.

Adequate ventilation is ensured on every breath by the rescuer

1. Seeing the chest rise and fall

2. Feeling in his own airway the resistance and compliance of the victim's lungs as they expand

3. Hearing and feeling the air escape during exhalation. The initial ventilatory maneuver should be *four quick, full, breaths* without allowing time for full lung deflation between breaths. (See Fig 3.)

In some cases, mouth-to-nose ventilation is more effective than mouth-to-mouth ventilation. The former is recommended when it is impossible to open the victim's mouth, when it is impossible to ventilate through his mouth, when the victim's mouth is seriously injured, when it is difficult to achieve a tight seal around his mouth, and when, for some other reason, the rescuer prefers the nasal route.

For the mouth-to-nose technique, the rescuer keeps the victim's head tilted back with one hand on the forehead and uses the other hand to lift the victim's lower jaw. This seals the lips. The rescuer then takes a deep breath, seals his lips around the victim's nose and blows in until he feels the lungs expand. The rescuer removes his mouth and the victim is allowed to exhale passively. The rescuer can see the chest fall when the victim exhales. When mouth-to-nose ventilation is used, it may be necessary to open the victim's mouth or separate his lips to allow the air to escape during exhalation because the soft palate may cause nasopharyngeal obstruction. This cycle should be repeated approximately every five seconds.

Direct mouth-to-stoma artificial ventilation should be used for persons who have had a laryngectomy. They have a permanent stoma that connects their trachea directly to the skin. It is recognized as an opening at the front of the base of the neck. Neither head tilt nor jaw thrust maneuvers are required for mouth-to-stoma resuscitation. For a patient with a temporary tracheostomy tube in his airway, it is usually necessary for the rescuer to seal the victim's mouth and nose with his hand or a tightly fitting face mask to prevent leakage of air when the rescuer blows into the tracheostomy tube. This problem can be prevented if the tracheostomy tube is provided with an inflatable cuff.

No adjuncts are required for effective rescue breathing; so artificial ventilation should never be delayed to obtain or apply adjunctive devices.

Infants and Children.—Opening the airway and performing artificial ventilation are essentially the same for children as for adults. There are some differences, however. For infants and small children, the rescuer covers both the mouth and nose of the child with his mouth and uses small breaths with less volume to inflate the lungs *once every three seconds.* The neck of an infant is so pliable that forceful backward tilting of the head may obstruct breathing passages. Therefore, the tilted position should not be exaggerated.

Accident Cases.—In accident cases, it is imperative that caution be used to avoid extension of the neck when there is a possibility of neck fracture. A fractured neck should be suspected in diving or automobile accidents when the victim has lacerations of the

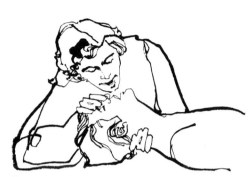

Fig 3.—Mouth-to-mouth resuscitation

face and forehead. If a fracture is suspected, all forward, backward, lateral, or turning movement should be avoided. To open the airway, a modification of the jaw thrust maneuver described above should be used. In this variation, the rescuer places his hands on either side of the victim's head so the head is maintained in a fixed, neutral position without the head extended. The index fingers should then be used to displace the mandible forward without tilting the head backward or turning it to either side (modified jaw thrust). If required, artificial ventilation usually can be provided in this position. If this is unsuccessful, the head should be tilted back very slightly and another attempt made to ventilate, using the modified jaw thrust maneuver.

Foreign Bodies.—The rescuer should not look for foreign bodies in the upper airway unless their presence is known or strongly suspected. The first effort to ventilate the lungs will determine whether an airway obstruction is present. If the first attempts to ventilate are unsuccessful despite properly opening the airway and providing an airtight seal around the mouth, an attempt should be made immediately to clear the airway with the fingers. The victim should be rolled onto his side, with the rescuer's knee placed under his shoulder. The victim's mouth then is forced open with the thumb and index crossed-finger technique. The rescuer runs his index finger or index and middle fingers down the inside of the victim's cheek toward the base of the tongue, deep into his throat. The rescuer's fingers are moved across the back of the victim's throat with a sweeping motion. Repeated attempts may be required. Where skilled, advanced life support personnel and equipment are available, direct laryngoscopy may permit the foreign body to be removed.

Larger foreign bodies frequently can be extricated by these finger maneuvers. If the rescuer is unable to dislodge the foreign body, or if it is impacted below the epiglottis, the victim should be rolled onto his side toward the rescuer, who then delivers sharp blows with the heel of his hand between the victim's shoulder blades. Further attempts at clearing the airway then should be made. If unsuccessful, there should be repeated efforts at mouth-to-mouth resuscitation, blows to the back, and probing the upper airway with the fingers. A small child having airway obstruction should be quickly picked up and inverted over the arm of the rescuer while the blows are being delivered between the child's shoulder blades.

If all of these maneuvers fail, emergency cricothyroid puncture and insertion of a 6 mm tube have been recommended for adults. However, this requires appropriate instruments and training and must be regarded as an advanced life support technique.

Gastric Distension.—Artificial ventilation frequently causes distension of the stomach. This occurs most often in children, but it is not uncommon in adults. It is most likely to occur when excessive pressures are used for inflation or if the airway is obstructed. Slight gastric distension may be disregarded. However, marked distension of the stomach may be dangerous because it promotes regurgitation, and it reduces lung volume by elevating the diaphragm. Several cases of gastric rupture resulting from overdistension have been reported. Obvious gross distension should be relieved whenever possible. In the unconscious victim, this can be accomplished without adjuncts by using one hand to exert moderate pressure over the victim's epigastrium between the umbilicus and the rib cage. To prevent aspiration of gastric contents during this maneuver, the victim's head and shoulders should be turned to one side.

Artificial Circulation
(External Cardiac Compression)

When sudden, unexpected cardiac arrest occurs, all of the A-B-C's of basic life support are required in rapid succession. This includes both artificial ventilation and artificial circulaton (external cardiac compression). Cardiac arrest is recognized by pulselessness in large arteries in an unconscious victim having a death-like appearance and absent breathing. The status of the carotid pulse should be checked as quickly as possible when cardiac arrest is suspected. In an unwitnessed cardiac arrest, the rescuer first opens the airway and quickly ventilates the lungs four times. He then maintains the head tilt with one hand on the forehead, and with the tips of the index and middle fingers of the other hand, gently locates the victim's larynx and slides his fingers laterally into the groove between the trachea and the muscles at the side of the neck where the carotid pulse can be felt. The pulse area must be felt gently, not compressed.

There are a number of reasons for recommending

palpation of the carotid pulse rather than other pulses. First, the rescuer already is at the victim's head to perform artificial ventilation and the carotid pulse is in the same area. Second, the neck area generally is accessible immediately, without removal of any clothing. Third, the carotid arteries are central and sometimes these pulses will persist when more peripheral pulses are no longer palpable. Trainees should practice palpation of the carotid pulse during classes. In hospital situations, palpation of the femoral artery is an acceptable option to use instead of the carotid artery. It is not practical to feel the carotid pulse in infants and small children. Instead, the rescuer's hand should be placed gently over the precordium to feel the apical beat.

Absence or questionable presence of the pulse is the indication for starting artificial circulation by means of external cardiac compression. External cardiac compression consists of the rhythmic application of pressure over the lower one half of the sternum, but *not over the xiphoid process*. The heart lies slightly to the left of the middle of the chest between the lower sternum and the spine. Intermittent pressure applied to the sternum compresses the heart and produces a pulsatile artificial circulation. During cardiac arrest, properly performed external cardiac compression can produce systolic blood pressure peaks of over 100 mm Hg, but the diastolic pressure is zero and the mean pressure seldom exceeds 40 mm Hg in the carotid arteries. The carotid artery blood flow resulting from external cardiac compression on a cardiac arrest victim usually is only one quarter to one third of normal.

External cardiac compression always must be accompanied by artificial ventilation. Compression of the sternum produces some ventilation, but the volumes are insufficient for adequate oxygenation of the blood. Therefore, artificial ventilation is *always* required when external cardiac compression is used.

Technique for External Cardiac Compression.—The patient always must be in the horizontal position when external cardiac compression is performed since, during cardiac arrest, there is no blood flow to the brain when the body is in the vertical position, even during properly performed external cardiac compression. It is imperative, therefore, to get the cardiac arrest victim into a horizontal position as quickly as possible in situations where he is vertical, such as in a dental chair, trapped in a vehicle, stricken on a telephone pole, while in a stadium seat, or in any similar situation. Elevation of the lower extremities, while keeping the rest of the body horizontal, may promote venous return and augment artificial circulation during external cardiac compression.

Effective external cardiac compression requires sufficient pressure to depress an adult's lower sternum a minimum of 1½ to 2 inches. For external cardiac compression to be effective, the victim must be on a firm surface. This may be the ground, floor, or a spineboard on a wheeled litter. If the victim is in bed,

a board, preferably the full width of the bed, should be placed under his back. However, chest compression must not be delayed while this support is awaited.

The rescuer positions himself close to the victim's side and places the long axis of the heel of one hand parallel to and over the long axis of the lower one half of the sternum. Great care must be exercised not to place the hand over the lower tip of the sternum (xiphoid process) that extends downward over the upper abdomen. To avoid this, the rescuer feels the tip of the xiphoid and places the heel of his hand on the lower one half of the sternum about 1 to 1½ inches away from the tip of the xiphoid and toward the victim's head. He then places the other hand on top of the first one (and may interlock the fingers), brings his shoulders directly over the victim's sternum, keeps his arms straight, and exerts pressure almost vertically downward to depress the lower sternum a minimum of 1½ to 2 inches. The compressions must be regular, smooth, and uninterrupted. Relaxation must immediately follow compression and be of equal duration. The heel of the rescuer's hand should not be removed from the chest during relaxation but pressure on the sternum should be completely released so that it returns to its normal resting position between compressions. (See Fig 4.)

Since artificial circulation always must be combined with artificial ventilaton, it is preferable to have two rescuers. One rescuer positions himself at the victim's side and performs external cardiac compression while the other one remains at the victim's head, keeping it tilted back, and continues rescue breathing. *The compression rate for two rescuers is 60 per minute.* When performed without interruption, this rate can maintain adequate blood flow and pressure and will allow cardiac refill. This rate is practical because it avoids fatigue, facilitates timing on the basis of one compression per second, and allows optimum ventilation and circulation to be achieved by quickly interposing one inflation after each five chest compressions without any pause in compressions (5:1 ratio). The rate of 60 compressions per minute allows breaths to be interposed without any pauses. Interposing the breaths without any pauses in compression is important, since any interruption in cardiac compression results in a drop in blood flow and blood pressure to zero. (See Fig 4.)

Two rescuers can perform CPR best when they are on opposite sides of the victim. They can then switch positions when necessary without any significant interruption in the 5:1 rhythm. This is accomplished by the rescuer who is performing artificial ventilation moving to the side of the victim's chest immediately after he has inflated the lungs. He places his hands in the air next to those of the other rescuer who continues to perform external cardiac compression. As soon as the other hands are properly placed, the rescuer performing chest compression removes his hands (usually after the third or fourth in the series of compressions) and the other rescuer then continues

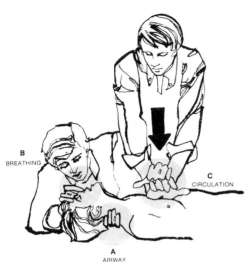

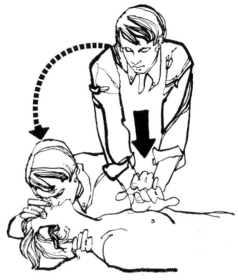

Fig 4.—Two-rescuer cardiopulmonary resuscitation
- 5 chest compressions
  - –Rate of 60/minute
  - –No pause for ventilation
- 1 lung inflation
  - –After each 5 compressions
  - –Interposed between compressions

Fig 5.—One-rescuer cardiopulmonary resuscitation
- 15 chest compressions (rate of 80/minute)
- 2 quick lung inflations

with the series of compressions. The rescuer who had been compressing then moves to the victim's head and interposes the next breath.

If the victim's trachea has been intubated, lung inflation is easier and compression rates up to 80 per minute can be used since breaths can be either interposed or superimposed following endotracheal intubation.

When there is only one rescuer, he must perform both artificial ventilation and artificial circulation using a 15:2 ratio. This consists of *two very quick lung inflations after each 15 chest compressions* (Fig 5). Because of the interruptions for lung inflation, the single rescuer must perform each series of 15 chest compressions at the faster rate of *80 compressions per minute* in order to achieve an actual compression rate of 60 per minute. The two full lung inflations must be delivered in rapid succession, within a period of five to six seconds, without allowing full exhalation between the breaths. If time for full exhalation were allowed, the additional time required would reduce the number of compressions and ventilations that could be achieved in a one-minute period.

Infants and Children.—With a few exceptions, the cardiac compression technique is similar for children. For small children, only the heel of one hand is used, and, for infants, only the tips of the index and middle fingers are used. The ventricles of infants and small children *lie higher in the chest* and the external pressure should be exerted over the midsternum. The dan-

ger of lacerating the liver is greater in children because of the pliability of the chest and the higher position of the liver under the lower sternum and xiphoid. Infants require one half to three fourths of an inch compression of the sternum; young children require three fourths to 1½ inches. The compression rate should be 80 to 100 per minute with breaths delivered as quickly as possible after each five compressions.

In infants and small children, backward tilt of the head lifts the back. A firm support beneath the back is therefore required for external cardiac compression and can be provided by the rescuer slipping one hand beneath the child's back while using the other hand to compress the chest. A folded blanket or other adjunct can also be used beneath the shoulders to provide support. For small infants, an alternate method is to encircle the chest with the hands and compress the midsternum with both thumbs.

Checking Effectiveness of CPR.—The reaction of the pupils should be checked periodically during cardiopulmonary resuscitation, since this provides the best indication of delivery of oxygenated blood to the victim's brain. Pupils that constrict when exposed to light indicate adequate oxygenation and blood flow to the brain. If the pupils remain widely dilated and do not react to light, serious brain damage is imminent or has occurred. Dilated but reactive pupils are less ominous. Normal pupillary reactions may be altered in the aged and frequently are altered, in any in-

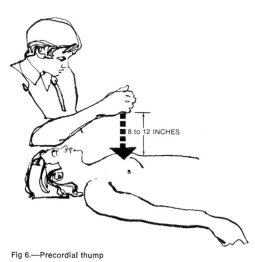

8 to 12 INCHES

Fig 6.—Precordial thump

dividual, by the administration of drugs.

The carotid pulse should be palpated periodically during CPR in order to check the effectiveness of external cardiac compression or the return of a spontaneous effective heartbeat. This should be done after the first minute of CPR and every few minutes thereafter, when additional rescuers are present and interruptions can be minimized. It should be checked particularly at the time of change of rescuers.

Precordial Thump

Continuing research and clinical experience have delineated a role for the precordial thump, but only in specific types of cardiac arrest cases. Recognizing both its limitations and usefulness, the Conference recommends the precordial thump as a basic maneuver to be used by all levels of rescuers following the detection of pulselessness in adults in these cases:

1. Witnessed cardiac arrest (basic life support)
2. Monitored patient (advanced life support)
3. Pacing known atrioventricular block (advanced life support).

The effectiveness of the precordial thump in the unmonitored patient or in an unwitnessed cardiac arrest has not been determined. Since the myocardium frequently may be anoxic in these situations a specific recommendation for precordial thump cannot be made for them. At this time the precordial thump is not recommended for use on children.

In cases where the primary cause of cardiac arrest is not hypoxia, such as in a witnessed cardiac arrest or in a monitored patient, a single precordial thump

may be effective in restarting circulation and may reverse certain dysrhythmias if performed within the first minute after arrest. In those situations, an initial thump on the midsternum using the fist may be the first maneuver performed following the determination of pulselessness.

Such a blow generates a small electrical stimulus in a heart that is reactive. The thump may be effective in restoring a beat in cases of ventricular asystole due to block, and in reversing ventricular tachycardia, or ventricular fibrillation of recent onset. When necessary it may be possible to use the fist as a pacemaker in some cases of heart block. When a series of chest thumps are used for this purpose, the pulse should be palpated before each thump.

The precordial thump is not useful for anoxic asystole and cannot be depended upon to convert an established ventricular fibrillation, nor is it useful for electromechanical dissociation associated with exsanguination. It should not be used for a ventricular tachycardia that is providing adequate circulation.

The precordial thump should be used to provide a stimulus to a potentially reactive heart. However, it is not a substitute for effective external cardiac compression.

There are also hazards associated with the precordial thump. In cases of an anoxic heart that is still beating, the low voltage stimulus may induce ventricular fibrillation. In addition, persons who do not restrict themselves to the recommended single blow may delay starting effective CPR.

In delivering the precordial thump, these rules should be followed:

1. Deliver a sharp, quick single blow over the midportion of the sternum, hitting with the bottom, fleshy portion of the fist struck from 8 to 12 inches over the chest. (See Fig 6.)
2. Deliver the thump within the first minute after cardiac arrest.
3. If there is no immediate response, begin basic life support at once.

The precordial thump is integrated into the basic pattern of CPR differently, depending upon the circumstances surrounding the cardiac arrest. The techniques for using the thump in cases of witnessed arrest or an arrest of a monitored patient are given below.

Technique for Witnessed Cardiac Arrest

1. Tilt the head to open the airway and simultaneously palpate the carotid pulse.
2. If the pulse is absent, give a precordial thump.
3. If the victim is not breathing, give four quick, full lung inflations.
4. If pulse and breathing are not immediately restored, begin one-rescuer or two-rescuer CPR.

Technique for Monitored Patient (For use with patients who have sudden ventricular fibrillation [VF], asystole, or ventricular tachycardia [VT] without pulse.)

1. Give a single precordial thump.

2. Quickly check the monitor for cardiac rhythm and simultaneously check carotid pulse.

3. If there is ventricular fibrillation or ventricular tachycardia without a pulse, countershock as soon as possible.

4. If the pulse is absent, tilt the head, give four quick, full lung inflations.

5. Check the carotid pulse again.

6. If the pulse is absent, begin one-rescuer or two-rescuer CPR.

It must be emphasized strongly that no time should be lost in waiting to assess the results of the precordial thump or by delivering repeated precordial thumps.

Pitfalls in Performance of CPR

When CPR is performed improperly or inadequately, artificial ventilation and artificial circulation may be ineffective in providing basic life support. Enumerated below are important points to remember in performing external cardiac compression and artificial ventilation.

1. Do not interrupt CPR for more than five seconds for any reason, except in the following circumstances.

(a) Under emergency conditions, endotracheal intubation usually cannot be accomplished in five seconds. However, it is an advanced life support measure and should be performed only by those who are well trained and well practiced in the technique and *only* after the victim has been properly positioned and all preparations made. Even under these circumstances, interruptions in CPR for endotracheal intubation should never exceed 15 seconds.

(b) When moving a victim up or down a stairway, it is difficult to continue effective CPR. Under these circumstances, it is best to perform effective CPR at the head or foot of the stairs, then interrupt CPR at a given signal and move quickly to the next level where effective CPR is resumed. Such interruptions usually should not exceed 15 seconds.

2. Do not move the patient to a more convenient site until he has been stabilized and is ready for transportation or until arrangements have been made for uninterrupted CPR during movement.

3. Never compress the xiphoid process at the tip of the sternum. The xiphoid extends downward over the abdomen. Pressure on it may cause laceration of the liver, which can lead to severe internal bleeding.

4. Between compressions, the heel of the hand must completely release its pressure but should remain in constant contact with the chest wall over the lower one half of the sternum.

5. The rescuer's fingers should not rest on the victim's ribs during compression. Interlocking the fingers of the two hands may help avoid this. Pressure with fingers on the ribs or lateral pressure increases the possibility of rib fractures and costochondral separation.

6. Sudden or jerking movements should be avoided when compressing the chest. The compression should be smooth, regular and uninterrupted (50% of the cycle should be compression and 50% should be relaxation). Quick jabs increase the possibility of injury and produce quick jets of flow; they do not enhance stroke volume or mean flow and pressure.

7. Do not maintain continuous pressure on the abdomen to decompress the stomach while performing external cardiac compression. This may trap the liver and could cause it to rupture.

8. The shoulders of the rescuer should be directly over the victim's sternum. The elbows should be straight. Pressure is applied vertically downward on the lower sternum. This provides a maximally effective thrust, minimal fatigue for the rescuer, and reduced hazard of complications for the victim. When the victim is on the ground or floor, the rescuer can kneel or stand at his side. When he is on a bed or high-wheeled litter, the rescuer must be on a step or chair or kneeling on the bed or litter. With a low-wheeled litter, the rescuer can stand at the victim's side. Problems arise with the use of low-wheeled litters in ambulances. Special arrangements must be made for proper positioning of the rescuer based on the design of the ambulance.

9. The lower sternum of an adult must be depressed 1½ to 2 inches by external cardiac compression. Lesser amounts of compression are ineffectual since even properly performed cardiac compression provides only about one quarter to one third of the normal blood flow.

10. While complications may result from improperly performed external cardiac compression and precordial thumps, even properly performed external cardiac compression may cause rib fractures in some patients. Other complications that may occur with properly performed CPR include fracture of the sternum, costochondral separation, pneumothorax, hemothorax, lung contusions, lacerations of the liver, and fat emboli. These complications can be minimized by careful attention to details of performance. It must be remembered, however, that during cardiac arrest, effective cardiopulmonary resuscitation is required even if it results in complications, since the alternative to effective CPR is death.

Special Resuscitation Situations

Drowning.—Extensive research has delineated the events and mechanisms of drowning and the detailed physiological variations between fresh water and sea water submersion. However, basic life support resuscitation procedures following drowning are the same as basic life support principles presented above, and CPR should be performed as quickly as possible. There are a few special considerations, given below:

1. When attempting to rescue a drowning victim, the rescuer should get to him as quickly as possible, preferably with some conveyance, such as a boat or surfboard. If a conveyance is not available, a flotation

device should be carried by the rescuer. The rescuer always must exercise care not to endanger himself while trying to aid a drowning person.

2. External cardiac compression should never be attempted in the water because it is impossible to perform it there effectively.

3. Mouth-to-mouth or mouth-to-nose ventilation may be performed in the water, although it is difficult and often impossible in deep water unless the rescuer has some type of flotation device to support the victim's head.

4. Artificial ventilation always should be started as soon as possible, even before the victim is moved out of the water, into a boat or onto a surfboard. As soon as the rescuer can stand in shallow water he should begin artificial ventilation.

5. In cases of suspected neck injury, the victim must be floated onto a back support before being removed from the water. If artificial respiration is required, the routine head tilt or jaw thrust maneuvers should not be used. Artificial ventilation should be accomplished with the head maintained in a neutral position and using a modified jaw thrust maneuver (as described under "Accident Cases.")

6. When removed from the water, the victim should have standard artificial ventilation or cardiopulmonary resuscitation performed according to the standards previously described.

7. Drowning victims swallow large volumes of water and their stomachs usually become distended. This impairs ventilation and circulation and should be alleviated as soon as possible. To relieve the distension, the victim may be turned on his side and his upper abdomen compressed or he may be turned over quickly into the prone position and lifted with the rescuer's hands under the stomach to force water out. This is referred to as "breaking" the victim.

8. There should be no delay in moving the victim to a life support unit where advanced life support capabilities are available. Every submersion victim, even one who requires only minimal resuscitation, should be transferred to a medical facility for follow-up care.

Electric Shock.—Electric shock may induce a variety of phenomena ranging from the benign to the lethal. The outcome depends largely upon the amplitude and duration of contact with the current. Other than burns of varying severity and injuries due to falls, the possible emergency events to be recognized include:

1. Tetany of the musculature of breathing, which is usually confined to the duration of the shock but may produce secondary cardiac arrest if the tetanizing shock is of a prolonged duration.

2. Prolonged paralysis of respiration, which may result from a massive convulsive phenomenon and may last for minutes after the shock current has terminated.

3. Ventricular fibrillation or other serious cardiac arrhythmias (such as runs of premature ventricular contractions or ventricular tachycardia that may prog-

ress to ventricular fibrillation) produced by low voltage currents (110 to 220 v) sustained for several seconds.

The prognosis for victims of electric shocks is not predictable easily since the amplitude and duration of the charge usually are not known. Failure of either respiration or circulation is likely to result.

After safely clearing a victim from an energized object, the rescuer should determine his cardiopulmonary status immediately. If spontaneous respiration or circulation is absent, the technique of cardiopulmonary resuscitation outlined in this statement should be initiated.

In cases where electric shock occurs on a public utility pole, a precordial thump should be delivered and mouth-to-mouth ventilation started at once. The victim must *then* be lowered to the ground as quickly as possible. CPR is only effective when performed on a victim in the horizontal position.

Beginning and Terminating Basic Life Support

CPR is most effective when started immediately after cardiac arrest. If cardiac arrest has persisted for more than ten minutes, cardiopulmonary resuscitation is unlikely to restore the victim to his pre-arrest central nervous system status. If there is any question of the exact duration of the arrest, the victim should be given the benefit of the doubt and resuscitation started.

Basic life support is not indicated for a victim who is known to be in the terminal stages of an incurable condition. When resuscitation is indicated and started in the absence of a physician, it should be continued until one of the following occurs:

1. Effective spontaneous circulation and ventilation have been restored.

2. Resuscitation efforts have been transferred to another responsible person who continues basic life support.

3. A physician assumes responsibility.

4. The victim is transferred to properly trained and designated professional medical or allied health personnel charged with responsibilities for emergency medical services.

5. The rescuer is exhausted and unable to continue resuscitation.

The decision to stop resuscitative efforts is a medical one. (See sections on "Advanced Life Support" and "Medicolegal Considerations.")

Training and Certification in Basic Life Support

Artificial Ventilation Only.—Every effort should be made to teach artificial ventilation to all members of the general public. Training the entire population should be accomplished through American National Red Cross courses, as well as through schools, YMCA's, clubs, local groups, and medical, paramedical and rescue organizations. All school children should be required to have annual training in artificial ventilation beginning in the fifth grade, and a major national effort should be mounted to achieve this objective in the shortest possible time.

The Conference further recommends that training should be provided by courses conducted by trained and certified instructors according to the technique described above and in accordance with the training standards of the American Heart Association. For optimum results, training should include such media as lectures, demonstrations, posters, slides, and movies. Actual practice on training manikins is required to assure efficiency of performance. Acceptable manikins must simulate obstruction of the airway when the head is not tilted back maximally, allow mouth-to-mouth and mouth-to-nose ventilation, and simulate rise of the chest when the lungs are inflated. Training should be to a level of demonstrated proficiency in mouth-to-mouth and mouth-to-nose resuscitation on adult manikins and mouth-to-mouth-and-nose resuscitation on infant manikins.

Basic Life Support.—CPR is an emergency procedure that requires special training both to recognize cardiopulmonary arrest and to perform artificial ventilation and artificial circulation. In order to ensure the widest possible benefits of its application, programs should be started to train the general public in basic life support according to the recommended American Heart Association standards. Initially, groups with the greatest need such as policemen, firemen, rescue workers, lifeguards, high-risk industry workers, and families of cardiac patients may receive preference, but the goal should be to train the general public, starting with school children at the eighth grade level.

Basic life support training of the public should be under the auspices of the American National Red Cross, the YMCA, and comparable volunteer and public service agencies concerned with saving lives. Training programs must adhere to the standards of the American Heart Association. These agencies should participate in training CPR instructors to teach basic life support and in certifying allied health personnel and nonmedical groups, public specialty groups, school children, and other segments of the population according to the training and performance standards of the American Heart Association as recommended by the National Research Council.

In addition to lectures, demonstrations, and films, actual practice and demonstration of proficiency in both the ventilatory and the circulatory components of cardiopulmonary resuscitation are required on training manikins. CPR cannot be taught or practiced on conscious or unconscious human subjects.

Manikins used in CPR training programs must provide (a) airway obstruction when the neck is flexed, (b) effective chest movement as a result of proper lung ventilation via mouth or nose, and (c) adequate movement of the sternum as a result of properly applied external cardiac compression against resistance. In addition, it is desirable for training devices to provide a simulated carotid pulse and an objective means (lights, gauges, strip chart) by which the student or instructor can determine adequacy of lung inflation and chest compression and mistakes in hand position. Palpation of the actual carotid pulse should also be practiced on other trainees.

To simplify instruction in basic life support, initial training should cover the recommended A-B-C sequence used for an unwitnessed cardiac arrest. When the trainee understands and can perform this effectively, further instruction should include use of precordial thump for witnessed cardiac arrest and for monitored patients.

Certification in CPR.—The purpose of certification is, as far as possible, to maintain adherence to uniform national standards established or recognized by the American Heart Association. Certification will be accomplished through the use of national cognitive (written or oral) and performance examinations. Receipt of certification will be contingent on satisfactory completion of such examinations and will indicate that the person certified was found to be qualified at the time of examination to perform and/or teach those, and only those, emergency techniques indicated by the certifying individual or agency. The process of training, certification, and recertification is intended to develop and maintain a mechanism for emergency cardiac care and resuscitation that is both broadly available and uniformly effective, in a manner most consistent with the public interest and safety. Certification does not imply that the American Heart Association or any designated certifying individual or agency either warrants or assumes responsibility for the performance of individuals subsequent to their certification.

An initial course leading to certification in CPR should be for small groups and should include didactic presentations and sufficient supervised, intensive manikin practice for every student to become proficient in detecting breathlessness and pulselessness and in performing the sequential steps of rescue breathing and external cardiac compression. Both one-rescuer and two-rescuer CPR should be practiced.

Periodic recertification or refresher courses that include retesting on manikins are required for all personnel, including instructors. The exact frequency for such recertification may need to be regulated on the basis of the professional skill and experience of particular groups. At present, suggested requirements for nonmedical groups are recertification one year from the initial course and then at least every three years thereafter, or more frequently where indicated.

CPR Instructors.—CPR instructors should be highly motivated individuals who represent special or organized groups in the community in which they will provide CPR training, have a background in or the capability for teaching, have an interest in or a role in the delivery of CPR, have completed an initial CPR course, and have successfully completed the CPR instructor's course according to American Heart Association standards and have a valid instructor's certificate.

Certification of instructors will indicate that the

recipient has passed the examination for instructor certification as defined elsewhere in this statement, and it will authorize the holder to conduct CPR courses according to standards of the American Heart Association. Certification of instructors is not intended to imply that the American Heart Association or any other certifying agency warrants or assumes responsibility for the performance of individuals trained by such certified instructors.

Certification of instructors is valid for a specified time and must be renewed periodically. If instructors are actively engaged in CPR instruction or performance and are familiar with new techniques, they may be recertified after review by local certifying authorities. If they are not actively engaged in training, they should attend a recertification course as detailed above.

Conference Recommendations.—The Conference recommends that CPR training be given to all eighth grade pupils and that it be repeated each year through high school. Additional pilot studies are required to determine the effectiveness of newer training methods.

The Conference mandates that CPR courses be required as part of the curriculum of all medical, dental, nursing, osteopathic, respiratory therapy, and other allied health schools. In order to implement this, the Association of American Medical Colleges should be made aware of this requirement so that all schools include instruction in basic life support and require a demonstration of proficiency in performance of this technique as part of their curricula.

The Conference recommends that every hospital with acute care facilities must assign to a specific committee the responsibilities for providing CPR teams on a 24-hour-per-day basis and that they be capable of performing CPR and all aspects of emergency life support. The CPR or emergency life support team should consist of nurses, technicians, respiratory therapists, house staff, and on-call attending staff. Wherever possible, the CPR hospital committee should be composed of, at least, a surgeon, a cardiologist, an anesthesiologist, an in-service nurse, and an administrator. The committee should be responsible for providing a written plan of action (protocol), CPR training and practice sessions, and a record of CPR occurrences available for periodic audit and review.

The Conference recommends that all nurses and physicians, including house staff, should be competent in all phases of CPR. To accomplish this, it is recommended that all hospitals require that, for annual staff reappointment, all physicians must either:

1. Demonstrate proficiency in basic life support through participation in actual resuscitation efforts or in teaching CPR to others, or

2. Agree to attend an approved training or retraining course offered by the hospital or their local heart association.

All hospital medical and nursing emergency department personnel must be trained and certified in basic and advanced life support, and all allied health personnel must be trained in basic life support.

The Conference further recommends that all hospitals and all state boards of health, divisions of hospital licensing, change their rules to conform to the above requirements and that they be included in the standards for hospital accreditation by the Joint Commission on Accreditation of Hospitals and as a stated policy of the American Hospital Association.

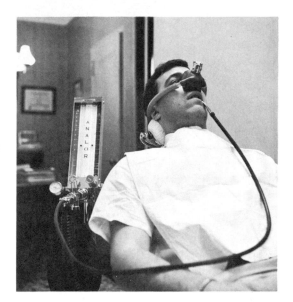

Figure 7–6 Auxiliary oral gas supply.

NASAL TUBES (FIG. 7–7)

Nasal tubes are not nearly as efficient in maintaining analgesic depth as a nasal inhaler, nor are they as comfortable to the patient. They are, however, serviceable for extreme cases of claustrophobia and in endodontic treatment of the lower anteriors when a lingual approach is necessary. The usual nasal inhaler might interfere with proper entry into the canal in these cases. With nasal tubes, higher flows of gases are necessary because of uncontrollable dilution of the gases with air. Additionally, irritation of the mucous membranes may occur whenever gases are projected directly against them, unless they have been previously moistened by passing them through water.

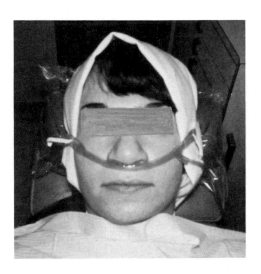

Figure 7–7 Nasal cannula.

MUSIC AND ANALGESIA (FIG. 7–8)

The use of music with analgesia seems to help some patients and to annoy others. Among those dentists who have made use of the combination, opinion seems to be about evenly divided as to its efficacy. The author has used quiet background music in the office with no definitive results. In contrast, those who have tried earphones or a stethoscope-like instrument feel that analgesia administration is enhanced by music, especially if white sound is also employed.

PREMEDICATION

The fear of pain and all the reactions related to apprehension may be modified by the use of drugs which are termed hypnotics and sedatives. In selected patients, sedation may be of great value in reducing tension and raising the pain reaction threshold. In direct contradistinction to analgesics, the hypnotics and sedatives have little if any effect on pain when it is already present, but they are used primarily because of their value in modifying untoward reactions to the potentials of a procedure, or what is commonly termed the mood of the patient.

When treating a subject as complex as a human being, any and every rule must have its exceptions. Nevertheless for most occasions the use of relative analgesia has eliminated the necessity for employing a host of other drugs now used in the practice of dentistry. In a sense, the dentist himself acts as the initial premedicant. By the projection of the best facets of his personality, by his kindliness and calming effects on his patient, he almost always succeeds in obtaining a successful introduction to relative analgesia. Once the patient has realized the calming and relaxing effect of the procedure, the experience itself acts as effective premedication in subsequent visits.

However, when kindliness, cajolery, flattery, bribery, and all other avenues of approach have been used without success — and yet the patient still wants to be treated and to take relative analgesia, but cannot overcome his fears — then premedication should be used to overcome this initial hurdle. The

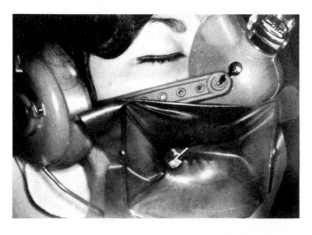

Figure 7–8 Music and analgesia.

sole purpose of the premedication should be to obtain the patient's acceptance of the nasal inhaler and the procedure. When premedication is indicated, it is usually required only at the first (rarely the second) administration. As one gains experience in introducing analgesia, he will find that his patients' need for premedication decreases.

The operator should keep in mind that, with premedication, he may no longer have a fully aware, ambulatory patient. The indiscriminate use of premedication is therefore to be avoided, for it makes relative analgesia a less practical instrument and poses other problems as well.

Iatrogenic Disorders.[5]   A problem of rapidly increasing significance for the dentist is *iatrogenesis*. Iatrogenic disorders are those disorders arising from the activities of physicians or dentists. In this discussion, we will deal only with complications resulting from properly administered therapy.

In dentistry there are three broad categories of useful chemotherapeutic agents that sometimes elicit unanticipated disease while solving a specific dental or oral problem. They are the antibiotics, corticosteroids, and tranquilizers.

Today antibiotics are the most widely prescribed therapeutic agents. No one questions their effectiveness in overcoming acute bacterial disease. Certainly, we as dentists know that their use has effectively controlled many hitherto dangerous and disfiguring oral infections. No brief is being held here for elimination of the use of antibiotics. However, it is important that the dentist be alerted to their possible side effects: hypersensitivity, illness from drug-induced toxicity, and infections by antibiotic-resistant strains after the normal flora have been suppressed. These effects follow previous exposures and the build-up of antibodies.

Corticosteroids, which are frequently used for the relief of painful temporomandibular joint syndromes, provide another example of the iatrogenic process. In cases of rheumatoid arthritis with painful limitation of motion, these steroids may, after effectively relieving the pain, inflict severe trauma to the involved joint, leading to degenerative changes.

In like manner, many dentists have been led to embrace the *routine* use of tranquilizing agents as preoperative sedatives in extensive restorative procedures and for every fearful dental patient. The literature abounds with reports of habituation, withdrawal symptoms, and skin eruptions after the use of these agents. Caution in the use of preoperative sedation is certainly warranted.

Precautions for Patients on Drug Therapy[41]

Introduction.   A considerable responsibility is imposed on the dentist treating patients taking one or more therapeutic agents for medical disorders. The agent, as well as the disease, may constitute a treatment problem and necessitate modification of treatment. The onslaught of new drugs being released (with their lists of contraindications and side effects occasionally representing the greater part of the information supplied by the manufacturer) compounds the factors which must be considered by the dentist prior to treatment of the patient.

Therapeutic agents with all their benefits on occasion produce undesirable side effects. Pickering, Cranston, and Pears[18] point out that therapeutics can, on occasion, make the patient miserable, and state: "Depressed by rauwolfia, made constipated, giddy, and impotent by ganglion blockers, the patient can soon be very ill indeed." Other iatrogenic possibilities are emerging: lupus erythematoid states, ulcers and asthma, nasal congestion and diarrhea, fever and liver damage, manic excitement, and terrorizing dreams, to name a few. To these have been added the induced risk of partaking of wine and cheese, avoidance of nose drops, and adverse reactions from anesthesia and premedication.[19]

Problems Involved. Concomitant administration of drugs for combined medical and dental treatment, in light of the growing number of sophisticated therapeutic agents, increases the likelihood of unanticipated drug reactions. Iatrogenic disease, secondary to medical (and dental) treatment, is of increasing concern and may be noted by the growing number of texts dealing with drug therapy. One text dealing with the problem of drug-induced disease[20] lists over 2500 references in discussing "diseases of medical progress." If the medical status of the patient is to be altered as little as possible during dental treatment, the dentist must be aware of the implications of the patient's disease and the pharmacology of the drugs being employed. Since both the disease being treated by the physician and the drugs being employed may present problems in treatment, the following procedures are recommended:

1. A good history of the patient's physical condition, as well as present medical treatment, drugs being taken, and allergies or sensitivities, should be noted.

2. If not known to the dentist, drugs currently being taken by the patient should be investigated with particular reference to contraindications and side effects. One of the standard references should be available in the practitioner's office for this purpose.

3. If any doubt exists relating to the history obtained or drugs currently being employed, elective procedures should be deferred until consultation has been obtained with the patient's physician.[21]

4. A complete understanding with the patient's physician regarding the treatment being employed by each, and rational caution on the part of the dental practitioner.

Finally, the dentist must question himself: Will the drug I am employing do more harm than good? Will this drug alter the effects of the drug or drugs already being taken by the patient? This should result in increased safety for the patient, and a reduction in administration of drugs of unproved value and unknown side effects.

General Pharmacological Considerations. Within reasonable limits it seems prudent to attempt to maintain the patient on the drug being used for treatment of his general medical condition.[22] Withdrawal should never be undertaken without express consent of the patient and the physician involved.

Few absolute contraindications exist regarding drugs employed in the dental office for patients on other current therapy; however, many relative contraindications exist and must be recognized prior to initiating medication by the dentist.

It should be kept in mind that drugs never create new cellular functions, they merely modify existing functions. This alteration of function may occur as the result of stimulation or depression of cellular function, initiation of a cellular response, or act of a mechanical, physical, or chemical nature. Generally speaking, drugs tend to act either as depressants or stimulants.[23]

Drugs employed together may cause enhancement or antagonism. Enhancement may reflect potentiation in which an exaggeration of response is produced. Addition (an effect greater than either active agent) and synergism (more than double the effect of either active drug alone) also contribute to enhancement. Antagonism effects a reduction of response. Specific antagonism may occur by "blocking action" (at the receptor sites). Antagonism may also occur by the production of effects which negate each other, by drug combinations forming inert compounds, or by creation of a compound with lessened activity.[23]

The patient's drug therapy may easily be modified unknowingly by the administration of drugs by the dentist. These modifications may block the action of drugs being employed or seriously increase the number and severity of side effects. Any drug, no matter how seemingly innocuous, can have serious consequences for some patients.[21] Examples of these consequences may be seen in barbiturate administration to patients with porphyria or the administration of belladonna derivatives (usually atropine) to the patient with glaucoma.[23] Steiner[24] has eloquently stated: "Geriatric patients and others may depend on delicately balanced programs of chemotherapy, and have every right to expect that their precarious existence will not be jeopardized by careless or ignorant administration of agents which disturb this balance or are incompatible with drugs already in use."

It is evident, then, that both the general medical condition of the patient, as well as the drugs being employed for treatment, may constitute a problem in dental treatment. The benefit of consultation between the physician and dentist concerned should be considered for any patient requiring drug therapy for a medical condition.

Agents and Diseases Requiring Precaution: Cardiovascular Considerations. As our geriatric population increases, vascular disease increases, thus increasing the numbers of patients with cardiovascular disease who will be seen in the dental office. This is one area where "adapting the procedure to the patient rather than the patient to the procedure" should be kept in mind. These patients have a decreased ability to withstand and recover from stress. Experience has shown that they respond well if properly handled; cooperation with the patient's physician again is the key to proper management. Commonly used drugs in cardiovascular disease include the diuretics, antihypertensive agents, nitroglycerine, rauwolfia type compounds, guanethidine, and the ganglionic blocking agents. Anticoagulants, as well as antiarrhythmic drugs and monamine oxidase inhibitors, may also be employed.

The diuretic group of drugs are represented by the carbonic anhydrase inhibitors (Diamox, Daranide, Cardrase, Neptazane), the mercurial diuretics (Neohydrin, Mercuhydrin, Diucardyn, Thiomerin, Mercuzanthin, Dicurin, Salygan), and the thiazide and thiazide-like diuretics (Diuril, Hydro-Diuril, Esidrix, Na-Clex, Saluron, and so forth). Some of the side effects inherent in this group of drugs of interest to the dental profession include possible paresthesia, orthostatic hypotension, drowsiness, nausea, and vomiting.[19] Oral symptoms may appear in treatment with the mercurials and must be differentiated from gingivostomatitis and the blood dyscrasias.[21]

Antihypertensive drugs include phenoxybenzamine (Dibenzyline), the ganglionic blocking agents (Ansolysen, Ostensin, Inversine), guanethidine (Ismelin), hydralazine (Apresoline), methyldopa (Aldomet), rauwolfia and rauwolfia-like compounds (Reserpine, Rauwiloid, Singoserp, Moderil, Harmonyl, Raudixin), and veratum and its derivatives (Veriloid, Unitensen, Provell, Veralba, Protalba). This group of drugs may manifest the following clinical symptoms: postural hypotension, nausea, restlessness, mydriasis, anhydrosis, lethargy, and bradycardia. Inversine has been reported to cause glossitis in some patients, secondary to xerostomia.[25] Guanethidine has been reported to cause parotid swelling.[19] Rauwolfia and its derivatives have been reported to cause severe hypotension with general anesthesia,[23] and extreme caution should be exercised when anesthetizing these patients.[26]

Nitroglycerine is a commonly used drug for anginal symptoms. Patients using this drug will almost invariably have a supply with them. If an attack occurs during dental treatment, treatment should be stopped and additional nitroglycerine given. The vasodilatation associated with nitroglycerine is not selective; hypotension and syncope may occur.[21]

The monoamine oxidase inhibitors, such as isocarboxazid (Marplan), phenelzine (Nardil), pargyline (Eutonyl), tranylcypromine (Parnate), and nialamide (Niamid), are occasionally prescribed for anginal pain and may produce significant hypotension. These drugs appear to be falling into disuse for angina but continue in use as "psychic energizers" and in the treatment of hypertension. They appear to interfere with the release and cause an accumulation of tissue catecholamines. Ephedrine and amphetamine are reported to cause severe hypertension by releasing the previously stored catecholamines.[19] In addition to hypotensive and hypertensive episodes, effects of dental interest include xerostomia, muscle twitching, nervousness, and drug enhancement. Severe enhancement may occur from the administration of narcotics, general anesthesia, barbiturates, tranquilizers and antihistamines, and from alcoholic intake.[25] These drugs should obviously be given with extreme caution, if at all.

Anticoagulant therapy when employed in cardiovascular diseases may be represented by one of the following: bishydroxycoumarin (Dicumarol), warfarin sodium (Coumadin), ethyl biscoumacetate (Tromexan), acenocoumarol (Sintrom), and the indandione derivatives (Danilone, Hedulin, Indon, Dipaxin, Miradon). These drugs, if being taken by the patient, should indicate need for caution if surgical procedures are anticipated. Nausea and vomiting, as well as bleeding tendencies, may appear in patients taking anticoagulants.[19] Spontaneous gingival bleeding may occur.[27]

Patients with heart failure may be on any one of a long list of antiarrhythmic agents, including the cardiac glycosides (digitalis and digitalis-like drugs: Lanoxin, Digoxin, Davoxin, Digitaline, Acylanid, Crystodigin, to name only a few). These agents have dental implications in that they may cause nausea and vomiting,[19] and care should be exercised to avoid stimulating the vomiting reflex and to prevent aspiration of vomitus, should such occur.[21]

Other antiarrhythmic agents are represented by the quinidines (Quinaglute, Hydromox, Quinicardine, Cardioquin, Quinera) as well as quinidine hydrochloride. The procainamides may also be utilized (Parcaine, Pronestyl). Side effects include anorexia, nausea, dizziness, fever, and hypoprothrombinemia.[19] A precipitous fall in blood pressure may follow slight provocation. Leukopenia and granulocytopenia may follow the use of procainamides, and ulcerative lesions of the mucous membranes may be associated with agranulocytosis.[21] A cross sensitivity between the procainamides and local anesthetics may exist.[19]

Additional precautions to be considered for patients with cardiovascular disease include omitting or using with caution atropine and methantheline (Banthine), which may cause tachycardia. Premedication of cardiovascular patients is advisable to reduce apprehension. The short-acting barbiturates are probably the drugs of choice, although tranquilizers are occasionally used. Careful titration according to the needs and cardiac status of the patient is a necessity. Hypotension varying in degree from severe episodes to postural or orthostatic hypotension may be precipitated when sedatives are given to these patients. This is particularly true if the patient is being treated with drugs such as the ganglionic blocking agents, hydralazine, guanethidine, methyldopa, phenothiazines, or the rauwolfia drugs. These agents will also prolong the action of analgesics, sedatives, and tranquilizers.[28] The dosage of any analgesic, sedative, or tranquilizer must therefore be carefully and cautiously given to any cardiovascular patient being treated with any of the agents mentioned. Orthostatic hypotension is a common side effect of many of the cardiovascular agents. Suitable "stabilizing" time should be allowed between changes of body position, particularly from a prone to an upright position. It is wise to have these patients stand by the dental chair for a period of time after arising.

Other considerations in the treatment of patients with cardiovascular disease include prophylactic antibiotic therapy (preferably penicillin) for patients with a history of rheumatic or congenital heart disease. The dentist should be familiar with and follow the suggested prophylactic treatment plan suggested by the American Heart Association. Vasoconstrictor reactions should be avoided by carefully aspirating to prevent intravascular injection, and omitting vasoconstrictors for gingival retraction or hemostasis.[28]

For those patients on anticoagulant therapy, experience has shown that the dangers of withdrawing the patient from the anticoagulant are probably greater than the hemorrhage which may ensue from maintaining the patient within a therapeutic range of anticoagulation. Several studies have indicated the feasibility of oral surgery on the fully anticoagulated patient.[29-31] This again is a matter of mutual understanding between the patient, the physician, and the dentist. Hemorrhage from oral procedures can usually be brought under control using local measures, such as prolonged pressure to the bleeding area, ice bags, and gelatin sponges placed in extraction sites.[32] Anticoagulant dosage adjustment by the physician may be necessary. If faced with a hemorrhagic episode, the dentist should never, short of a life-saving emergency, administer any vitamin K preparation, since sudden thrombosis or embolism may occur.[33]

Tranquilizers and Sedatives. These agents have a wide range of application in altering emotional states. Some have been used as antiarrhythmics and antiemetics, as well as for premedication. The tranquilizers suppress anxiety and tension and alter behavioral patterns without producing a profound hypnotic effect. Meprobamate, hydroxyzine, and benactyzine are widely used for anxiety states, while reserpine and the phenothiazines appear more effective in the treatment of neurosis and psychic agitation.[33] The various drugs are far too numerous to list. The drug groups, with examples, include the rauwolfia drugs (previously mentioned), the phenothiazines (Thorazine, Trilafon, Phenergan, Compazine), the meprobamates and related preparations (Miltown, Equanil, Ultran), the diphenylmethanes (Atarax, Vistaril), and sedative-hypnotics (Doriden, Placidyl), as well as the barbiturates. Miscellaneous agents include chlordiazepoxide (Librium) and diazepam (Vallium). The bromides and chloral hydrate are sometimes included in this group. Side effects include drowsiness, nausea, vomiting, hypotension, extrapyramidal syndromes, and convulsions.[19] Hypotension in the phenothiazine group should not be treated with epinephrine, as an epinephrine reversal occurs and dangerous hypotension may ensue. Levarterenol or phenylephrine are considered the vasopressors of choice.[34] A reduction in leukocytes with a tendency to infection and a granulocytosis has been reported for the phenothiazine group. Mucosal lesions have been noted in patients taking meprobamate.[21] These drugs are potentiators of depressant drugs and concomitant use may pose problems. The extrapyramidal reactions are of particular interest to the dentist, since the effects on the muscles of mastication, the tongue, and the face may be the only manifestations.[35] This produces bizarre discordant movements of the face and jaws, and tetanus may be simulated. Slurred speech may be the earliest sign.[36] These reactions do not appear to be dose related. Although the sedatives and narcotics have been used as antidotes, diphenhydramine (Benadryl) appears to be the drug of choice.[20]

Central Nervous System Stimulants. These drugs are employed in diet control and in stimulating physical and mental activity. This group includes the amphetamines (Benzedrine, Raphetamine, Dexedrine, Norodin, Syndox, and others), epinephrine and norepinephrine, ergotamine, imipramine (Tofranil), amitriptyline (Elavil), piperidine derivatives (Meratran, Ritalin), xanthine derivatives (aminophylline, Tedral, Isuprel, caffeine, and so forth). The previously mentioned monoamine oxidase inhibitors are occasionally employed.[19] Side effects of interest to us include hypertension, angina, agitation, and rapid pulse. These patients may require greater amounts of premedication and postoperative sedation; however, if they are on one of the monoamine oxidase inhibitors, narcotics should be avoided.[21]

The Diabetic and Diabetic Drugs. Drugs commonly employed for the treatment of diabetic patients include chlorpropamide (Diabinese), insulin (Iletin, Lente, NPH Iletin, Protamine Zinc, and others), phenformin (DBI), and tolbutamide (Orinase). Nausea and vomiting are side effects common to all the antidiabetic drugs, and a "brassy" taste has been attributed to phenformin therapy. Approximately 40 per cent of diabetic patients seen will be taking insulin preparations; the remainder will be on oral hypoglycemics or diet modification alone. The "juvenile" ("growth onset," "ketotic," "insulin dependent") diabetics will always be on insulin. The "mature" or "adult-onset" ("stable" or "nonketotic") diabetics may at times be on insulin, but diet restriction alone or oral hypoglycemics are more commonly effective.[19] Aspirin is a mild hypoglycemic agent and may reinforce the other agents.[20]

The uncontrolled diabetic should be subjected to oral surgery procedures as a matter of emergency only. Consultation with the patient's physician is imperative, and elective procedures should be undertaken only on the controlled diabetic.[21] Infection intensifies the disease,[37] and antibiotic coverage should be considered. Associated disease, such as arteriosclerosis, hypertension, periodontal disease, and increased caries rates in the uncontrolled diabetic, should be kept in mind. Surgical appointments should be timed according to the antidiabetic agent being taken; corticosteroids should be avoided.[23] The dentist should be familiar with the signs, symptoms, and emergency treatment of diabetic acidosis and insulin shock.

Thyroid Disease and Medications. Drugs commonly used to treat hypothyroidism include thyroid extracts, sodium levothyroxine (Synthroid), and liothyronine (Cytomel). Myxedema coma is rare but carries a high mortality rate, as does its counterpart, thyroid crisis.[19] Side effects of drug therapy are mainly a result of overdosage and include tachycardia, excitability, tremors, sweating, and vomiting.[25]

Hyperthyroid agents commonly employed are radioactive iodine, propylthiouracil, methimazole (Tapazole), methylthiouracil (Methiacil, Muracil, Thimacil), and potassium perchlorate.[19] Side effects of dental interest include agranulocytosis and infections of the mouth, secondary to thiourea.[23] Parotitis has been reported.[21] Also of dental interest is the characteristic exophthalmos associated with the disease, and thyroid crisis. The hyperthyroid patient must be under absolute medical control and adequately premedicated prior to dental treatment, since undue stress may precipitate a crisis.

Corticosteroids and Corticotrophins. Over 150 of these preparations are available in the United States. They have a wide range of use, including in rheumatoid arthritis, allergic states, and pemphigus.[21] Since their original use to reduce the inflammation and pain of rheumatoid arthritis they have been used in practically every known disease state. These agents suppress natural body responses, including inflammation, and may mask serious disease. They should not be used on patients with diabetes, tuberculosis (active or healed), peptic ulcers, emotional disturbances, and certain infections.[20] Since they are so commonly employed, many patients will be seen who are, or have been, on steroid therapy. These patients, and particularly those with Addison's disease, may have hypofunctional adrenals. They must be under a physician's care and have adequate steroid reinforcement prior to any surgical procedure.[32]

Side effects common to these agents are many. Some effects of dental interest include: osteoporosis with fracture tendencies, spread of systemic bacterial, fungal, and viral infections, and prolonged healing time.[20]

Agents for Treatment of Allergy. Agents employed in the treatment of allergies include the xanthines, vasoconstrictors, iodides, steroids, and antihistamines.

The antihistamine preparations are many—approximately 160 are available. Examples include: diphenhydramine (Benadryl), tripelennamine (Pyribenzamine), chlorpheniramine (Chlor-Trimeton, Teldrin), and brompheniramine (Dimetane). Allergies comprise a group of disorders with many manifestations, the symptoms of which may range from mild itching to severe anaphylaxis. Side effects of treatment include drowsiness, blurred vision, diplopia, nausea, vomiting, and hypotension.[19] Xerostomia has been noted,[21] as well as delirium, narcolepsy, shock-like states, fever, syncope, and dermatitis following the administration of normal doses.[20] Patients on iodides may experience orofacial edema, parotitis, and burning sensations of the throat and gingiva.[21] The xanthine derivatives and vasoconstrictors may give rise to nervousness and tachycardia, and patients taking these medications may require increased doses of sedatives, if such are used in dental treatment. This is not true, however, for patients on antihistamines, as the antihistamines may potentiate depressant drugs.

Patients with allergic histories should be carefully evaluated for possible reactions to antibiotics, analgesics, local anesthetics, and any other drug which the dentist may contemplate using.[21]

Anticonvulsants. These agents are employed in the treatment of the epilepsies. Many are in use, chiefly diphenylhydantoin (Dilantin), mephanytoin (Mesantoin), ethotoin (Peganone), primidone (Mysoline), and others. Adjunctal medications may be employed using the various stimulants, barbiturates, and tranquilizers. The most common side effect of dental interest is gingival hyperplasia.[20] Primidone has been reported to provoke gingival pain.[21] All may be associated with ataxia and drowsiness. These agents are all employed on a long-term basis, and the medication should not be discontinued. The patient's physician should be consulted prior to treatment; premedication may be desirable to prevent any seizures which might occur under stress of treatment.[21]

Central Nervous System Depressants. These include a wide range of drugs, chiefly the barbiturates and tranquilizers, which have already been mentioned. They may be employed for a variety of diseases, including Parkinsonism, epilepsy, gastric ulcers, hyperthyroidism, menopausal symptoms, and motion sickness.[19] The therapeutic agent being used frequently causes significant sedation; if additional depressant agents are employed, they should be given with caution.

Antibiotics and Antibacterial Agents. Antibiotics are probably the most widely used and abused of all the therapeutic agents. Drug toxicity, hypersensitivity (including anaphylaxis), and production of resistant organisms are the major undesirable effects. A survey by the Food and Drug Administration of 1070 serious reactions in 1957 includes the following: 809 were anaphylaxis reactions, 107 were superinfections, 70 were skin reactions, 46 were blood dyscrasias, and 38 were angioneurotic edema reactions with cerebral or respiratory involvement. Penicillin was most often involved in anaphylaxis; chloramphenicol was the agent most frequently associated with blood dyscrasias.[20]

It has been estimated that 5 to 6 per cent of all individuals are sensitive to penicillin,[38] and all antibiotics may produce hypersensitivity. For this reason it is imperative that patients be questioned regarding allergic and sensitivity states prior to treatment.

Side effects of antibiotic treatment are extensive. Effects of dental interest, in addition to those already mentioned, are: stomatitis, glossitis, black hairy tongue, chelitis, sore throat, dysphagia, xerostomia.[20] Neonatal deposition of tetracycline, causing pigmentation of deciduous teeth, has been reported, as has enamel hypoplasia and loosening and discoloration of the nails.[39]

Of the antibacterial compounds, the sulfonamides have been implicated in anemias, agranulocytosis, thrombocytopenia, and Stevens-Johnson syndrome (erythema multiforme).[40]

Miscellaneous. Atropine and atropine-like drugs block the cholinesterase inhibitors, such as neostigmine (Prostigmin), pyridostigmine (Mestinon), and ambenonium (Mytelase), which myasthenia gravis patients may be taking. These patients may have oropharyngeal involvement, and care should be taken when performing intraoral procedures to prevent posterior displacement of objects.[19, 23] Lingual or pharyngeal weakness may cause sudden obstruction of the upper airway.

Atropine, the nitrates, and probably the steroids should not be given to patients with glaucoma, and premedication may be indicated.[23]

Patients on antineoplastic agents such as aminopterin, mercaptopurine (Purinethal), and busulfan (Myleran) may develop necrotic lesions of the gingiva. Patients with Hodgkin's disease have been reported to bleed excessively postoperatively.[21]

Spontaneous bleeding has been reported secondary to the use of streptokinase-streptodornase (Varidase).[20]

Patients with liver disease who manifest jaundice may have clotting difficulties due to hypoprothrombinemia.[23] Drugs should be given to these patients with caution, as they detoxify drugs poorly.[19]

Although few in number, patients with primaquine-sensitive erythrocytes should not be given any of the following drugs commonly prescribed by the dentist, as hemolytic anemia may result:[19] acetanilid, phenacetin, acetylsalicylic acid, and sulfanilamide.

Summary. In addition to the desired effect, almost any drug will produce toxic effects, as well as side effects. These varying therapeutic manifestations, together with treatment problems related to the disease for which the drug is being taken, must be considered by the dentist. Some of these diseases and their related drugs have been discussed to refresh the practitioner's memory; representative trade names have been included, since it is these that are usually given by the patient when a history is taken.

By possessing current information, by taking an adequate history, and by appropriate consultation with the patient's physician, the dentist will be in a position to weigh the calculated risks against the potential benefits of treatment.

Purposes and Effects of Premedication.[2]   Premedication is used to alleviate anxiety, fear, and apprehension; to produce amnesia; and to lower the metabolic rate.

In decreasing general body metabolism, premedication lowers the demand of the tissues for oxygen and raises the threshold of irritability to decreased concentrations of both carbon dioxide and oxygen.

The lessening or abolition of fears and apprehensions is produced in part by the action of premedications on endocrine gland activity. In addition, by reducing the activity of the cerebral cortex, premedication diminishes the discharge of epinephrine ordinarily stimulated by fear.

Today many different types of chemicals are available for this purpose. In choosing the agent to be used in a given patient, the most important factor to consider is his metabolic activity. In general, the greater the metabolic activity, the greater the tolerance to the depressant drug. Some factors that influence the rate of metabolic activity are:

Age. A mature, active individual will tolerate larger doses than infants or old people. Young's formula for children's dosage is:

$$\frac{age}{age + 12} \times \text{average dose}$$

Physical Status. A healthy, strong, active patient will tolerate larger doses than one who is suffering from a debilitating illness or chronic infection.

Emotional State. Fear, anger, irritability, and worry call for larger doses than pleasant, cooperative, or lethargic behavior.

Bodily Comfort. The presence of pain requires a larger dose.

Endocrine Activity. Hyperthyroidism, in which there is greater tolerance, calls for larger doses and, conversely, hypothyroidism calls for smaller doses.

Some Available Drugs. Many depressant drugs are used; here, however, only some of the more common types are listed.

Belladonna Derivatives. In some cardiovascular conditions, these drugs are contraindicated. Included are *atropine* and *scopolamine*. The latter has amnestic properties owing to its action in primary depression of the higher centers; it also creates great psychic depression with a lesser degree of physical depression.

Sedatives, Hypnotics, and Soporifics. The agents of this group most commonly used are the intermediate and short-acting barbiturates: pentobarbital (Nembutal elixir for children), secobarbital (Seconal), and amobarbital (Amytal), and the ataractic drugs (phenaglycodol and meprobamate).

The Choice of a Premedicant.[14] In determining where, when, and how a drug may be used, potency, curve of action, characteristics of absorption, and elimination all play a decisive role. One must often decide whether it should be used at all, despite desirable pharmacologic actions.

The potency of a drug, which is the amount by weight necessary to produce a pharmacologic effect, is of obvious practical importance, since it determines the amount necessary to produce a therapeutic response. In some instances, however, the potency of drugs as expressed in the literature is actually misleading. For example, there are barbiturates for which the average hypnotic dose is appreciably smaller than the usual barbiturate dosage. Such barbiturates have been advertised as being safer than others, of which more has to be used for similar effect. The implication here is that the smaller dose is less likely to cause difficulties. On the other hand, less potent barbiturates which require more drug per hypnotic dose than usual have been advertised as being preferable because a larger than usual amount is required for toxic effects. The implication here is that difficulties are not so likely to be encountered because a larger amount is necessary to cause toxicity.

Obviously both arguments cannot be correct. However, what is of even greater importance is that both are wrong. The relative difference in therapeutic ratio is more important than relative potency. The therapeutic ratio is the physical amount of a drug which will produce a pharmacodynamic effect in relation to the amount of the same drug which will produce untoward effects under the same circumstances. The therapeutic ratio is the relationship between therapeutic and toxic potency.

Dosage depends upon potency, toxicity, urgency of the condition, and the influence of the patient's condition in reacting to or eliminating the drug. The dose which may be used implies a consideration of the amount necessary to produce a useful therapeutic effect in the face of the danger of producing untoward effects. The average dose is a term which would ordinarily mean an arithmetic average of all doses given. It is, however, the dose given to the average patient. It usually signifies the safe dose with which to start the medication and is calculated to induce a relatively low incidence of untoward effects.

The attitude of the practitioner as well as that of the patient is important in shaping responses to treatment. Both hope that the medication will be effective. The use of suggestion when presenting the prescription to the patient will very often do much more good than just handing it to him without comment. For example, when prescribing a drug for preoperative sedation, it helps immeasurably for the dentist to say, "If you take this medicine as I suggest, you should experience very little or no difficulty at all."

The placebo is another important factor in prescribing medication. It has a definitive place in the practice of the healing arts, and cannot be too easily discounted as a means of helping many patients.

Ideally, we are searching for a sedative that will produce calmness without anxiety. Ideal sedatives should adequately reduce preoperative psychic tension without concomitant depression of respiration and circulation. If possible, they should permit the patient to come to the office alone, and leave without being accompanied by another person.

The use of the following prescriptions will generally result in a much more cooperative patient if taken as prescribed. The patient need not be accompanied by anyone.

Rx: Dilone
    M. tab. No. XV
    Sig. tab. 1 one hour before dental appointment

Hexobarbital	50 mg.
Acetylsalicylic acid	224 mg.
Phenacetin	160 mg.
Caffeine	32 mg.

Rx: Miltown
    M. tab. No. X
    Sig. tab. 1 one hour before dental appointment
        Meprobamate   400 mg.
Rx: Equagesic
    M. tab. No. XV
    Sig. tab. 1 at bedtime and tab. 1 one hour before dental appointment
        Meprobamate   150 mg.
        Ethoheptazine citrate   75 mg.
        Acetylsalicylic acid   250 mg.
Rx: Phenaphen
    M. caps. No. XV
    Sig. caps. 1 at bedtime and caps. 1 one hour before dental appointment
        Phenacetin   194.0   mg.
        Acetylsalicylic acid   162.0   mg.
        Phenobarbital   16.2   mg.
        Hyoscyamine sulfate   .031 mg.

THE TRAINING OF THE PATIENT

Elimination of the fear of analgesia and of the procedure and apparatus involved takes but one careful introductory administration. To ensure success, the patient should be trained in certain simple but important procedures.

The Patient as Guide to the Operator

ADJUSTMENT OF THE NASAL INHALER BY THE PATIENT

A certain amount of air leakage is accepted in analgesia administration; however, gross leakage is undesirable because the analgesic effect will be minimal. For this reason, the adjustment of the nasal inhaler assumes great importance. Since an analgesia patient is a conscious subject and since the dentist should at all times strive to obtain maximum comfort for his patient, it is highly undesirable to position the nasal inhaler too tightly against his face. Then, too, holding the nasal piece against the patient's face is not good procedure psychologically.

Many people have one nasal passage occluded, owing to swollen membranes, deviated septa, or nasal polyps. If the operator positions the inhaler on a patient new to analgesia but does not give him permission to adjust it to his comfort and to afford the greatest ease of respiration, the patient will rarely feel free to do it himself (Fig. 7–9). In this circumstance, the patient's one good passageway may be occluded and he will have difficulty in breathing. As a result, a good deal of oral inhalation ensues, and poor analgesia results. Nasal obstruction can be minimized by the use of Neo-Synephrine or Afrin nose drops prior to the administration of analgesia. This shrinks the nasal mucosa and opens the nasal airway.

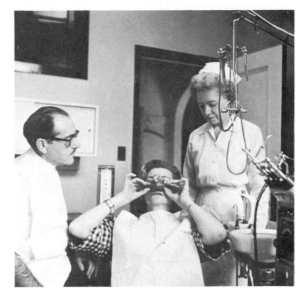

Figure 7–9 The patient adjusts the nasal inhaler.

The patient should understand that he is to tell the dentist whether he needs more or less analgesia. If he feels discomfort, the onus must be put on him for not having advised the doctor of his needs.

Claustrophobia and the Nasal Inhaler (Fig. 7–10). The fear of claustrophobia can be overcome by pointing out to the patient that:

1. His nose is not completely shut off from air, because (a) the valves in the nasal inhaler are holes through which air can enter freely and (b) air enters between the nasal inhaler and his face.

2. He can always breathe through his mouth if he so desires.

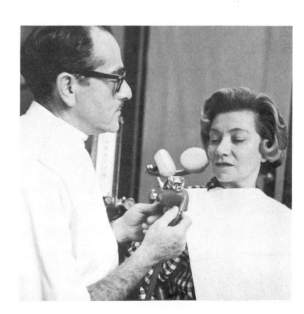

Figure 7–10 Overcoming claustrophobia.

Nasal Respiration

In the stage of relative analgesia, the patient maintains an open mouth. For most individuals in this posture, exhalation through the mouth is easier than through the nose. However, when one exhales through the mouth, the next inhalation will most likely occur through the mouth. Consequently the patient should be trained to inhale and exhale only through the nose, and the importance of this should be emphasized. If the patient finds he is suddenly wide awake after having been in a good analgesic state for some time, it must be impressed on him that he should immediately revert to nasal respiration, that he awoke because he inhaled excessively through the mouth and not because the doctor "shut off the machine," as is most often thought.

Mouth-breathing in the absence of nasal obstruction is very often a result of nervousness and apprehension.[13] It occurs reflexly in order to help improve the ventilation of the lungs. At rest, a person normally breathes through the nose, and yet seldom does one observe a person under tension take a deep *nasal* inspiration. Of course, the first step toward the encouragement of nasal respiration is the relaxation of the patient. In addition, it is helpful to suggest that the patient "blow the gas away through the nose" or "breathe in through the nose deeply until a cold sensation or cold spot is felt at the bridge of the nose."[7]

These suggestions aid in establishing nasal inspiration and expiration. Allow the patient to practice nasal respiration with a saliva ejector placed in the open mouth (Fig. 7–11).

The Patient in Control

If suddenly the depth of analgesia is not sufficient to obtund the pain of some part of a dental procedure, the patient is trained to take deep breaths

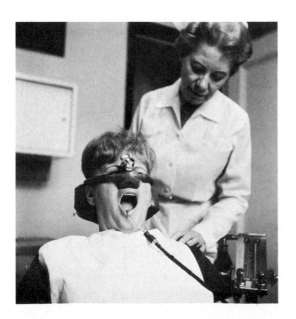

Figure 7–11 The patient practices nasal respiration with mouth open.

through the nose *immediately*. This has a certain value from a psychological viewpoint, although not from a physiological one, since the instantaneous nasal breathing of the patient cannot result in a sudden marked increase in the concentration of nitrous oxide in the bloodstream. The *act* of breathing and of concentrating on it does, however, have value. The principle of distraction enters into this effect. It helps also to increase the patient's confidence in his ability to control the situation.

POSSIBLE REACTIONS OF THE PATIENT UNDER RELATIVE ANALGESIA

Nitrous oxide has psychological as well as physiological effects in analgesic concentrations, a fact which must always be kept in mind when evaluating a patient's reaction. If the physical reaction of the subject were to be the sole criterion, an incorrect evaluation would very often result. Since under relative analgesia the thinking processes are stimulated and the feelings and emotions are altered, the individual new to analgesia may be somewhat fearful of losing contact with his surroundings, partially or fully. Perhaps he has not built up enough confidence in the procedure to permit him to relax fully, to give himself up to the symptoms, to accept them passively, and to allow these novel sensations to flow through him without resistance. This partial acceptance produces certain signs and symptoms.

Then there are the signs observed in individuals who *do* accept the procedure and the symptoms willingly and eagerly and who even add autosuggestion in order to intensify the effects. Lastly, there are the physical reactions of patients who are approaching the deeper phases of the maintained analgesic stage.

The maintenance of an open mouth and a relaxed mandible by the patient, without the use of mouth props, is a foolproof sign that the patient is in the analgesic range. Even taking into consideration the fact that individuals may vary greatly in their sensitivity to nitrous oxide, it can be stated as a fact that the dental practitioner who uses relative analgesia will never observe the true excitement stage.

Repeated Closing of the Mouth.   Under this circumstance, the subject is still in the maintained analgesic stage and is usually perfectly relaxed, but performing dentistry is difficult. An oral direction to "open" is not always necessary; slight pressure on the lower lip may suffice (Fig. 7–12). If closing continues, decrease the concentration of nitrous oxide until the patient opens his mouth on direction.

Rigid Mandible.   In relative analgesia the mandible is loose and relaxed. Patients who otherwise find it difficult to open their mouths wide and to keep them open for any length of time find that they can do so more easily under relative analgesia. If the mandible becomes set and rigid, the patient is approaching the state of total analgesia. To correct this, decrease the concentration of nitrous oxide.

Diaphoresis.   Nitrous oxide has a vasomotor excitation effect which dilates the surface blood vessels and stimulates the sweat glands. A small part

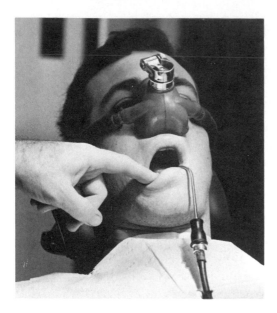

Figure 7–12 An oral direction to "open" is not always necessary; use slight pressure on the lower lip.

of the excretion of nitrous oxide also takes place through intact skin and the sweat glands. In diaphoresis, beads of perspiration become visible on the forehead. This effect is visible in 2 to 3 per cent of treated patients. It has no clinical significance.

Nausea and Vomiting.   It is a high tribute to the safety and effectiveness of relative analgesia that the most untoward effect of its administration is nausea or vomiting. This is certainly not a serious result, nor is it frequent enough to be considered a problem. It occurs in less than 1 per cent of the total number of administrations.

Causes and Signs of Vomiting.   When vomiting does occur, it is usually caused by (a) a full stomach from recently ingested foods or liquids, (b) the central effect of the drug on the medulla, which stimulates the vomiting center, or (c) hypoxia, which, regardless of the cause, is usually followed by vomiting. The vomiting center is depressed in stage 3, plane 1.

Nausea and vomiting may occur more often in children 10 years of age or younger during an administration of more than 30 minutes. Yet this does not make necessary the automatic limitation of administration time for children. Experience with the child should dictate the procedure. If the child is prone to nausea and has so advised the doctor, he should observe the patient carefully during the first administration. Children under six years of age will usually not give advance warning by facial pallor, but they may show some signs: they may place a hand on the abdomen, or there may be less movement than previously of the body, lips, cheeks, and tongue. Once nausea is suspected, the flow of nitrous oxide is reduced to zero and oxygenation is begun. An emesis bowl and protective covering for the patient's clothes should be in readiness. If emesis has occurred, and the patient is willing to continue treatment, the operator may continue.

With adults, advance warning signs of nausea usually appear, taking the form of a grayish, greenish pallor of the forehead and nose. Here, too, the emesis bowl and protective covering should be the concern of the operator.

Prevention of Vomiting. Whether the patient is a child or adult, if nausea or emesis occurs once and there is no history of proclivity toward this condition, it is unnecessary to give directions relative to eating or not eating before analgesia administration. However, if it occurs more than once it would be wise for the doctor to determine what the patient consumed immediately before treatment. With young children the story is usually one of overeating before the dental visit. Advise abstaining from food for two to three hours before each visit. In the case of adults, nausea can occur just as often when no food has been taken for three or four hours previous to administration as when eating took place immediately before. Directions should be given accordingly. If the nauseated patient has had no food for about three hours before the visit, advise a light meal several hours before his next visit. If he has eaten, advise no food for three hours before analgesia administration. The dentist must realize, however, that it would be mistaken procedure to lay down eating rules routinely for all patients. This would be constructing an unnecessary barrier to the routine use of relative analgesia. Quite often verbal suggestion against nausea is helpful. Antinauseant drugs may also be prescribed.

Nausea may occur more often in hot, humid weather. The solution is, of course, an air-conditioned treatment room. If nausea occurs several times in succession in different patients within a short span of hours or days, one should suspect that he has reached the bottom of the nitrous oxide cylinder. The impurity that will most often cause nausea is moisture. Discard the cylinder.

Expectoration. Expectorating, rinsing, and taking small drinks of water during dental treatment are phenomena well known to all dental practitioners. It is also common knowledge that they can be, and often are, great time wasters. Typical is the child (or adult) who leans over the bowl and wants to drink, expectorate, or rinse every time the dentist removes his hands from the mouth. Very often this constitutes a defense mechanism. The patient knows that when he is leaning over the bowl, the dentist cannot work on his teeth. He goes to the bowl often and stays there a long time.

Under relative analgesia, expectoration and rinsing are almost entirely eliminated. In the first place, an analgesia patient is less aware of an excessive amount of fluid in the mouth, for the gagging reflex is depressed. Secondly, he is not fearful and has no conscious need for such defense mechanisms. Then, too, the evacuators commonly used today prevent the accumulation of an excessive amount of fluid or debris in the mouth. Debris can also be removed very easily with a square of gauze or a piece of tissue paper.

Infrequently, however, the patient must be allowed to expectorate. At this point, it should be borne in mind that, because he is not in full control of his movements, he may bump his head or face. The following procedure should be followed:

1. Place one hand on the forehead of the patient.

2. With the other hand, hold the tubings immediately behind the patient's head.

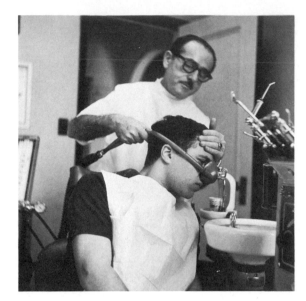

Figure 7–13 Controlling the patient during expectoration.

3. With both hands now in position, guide the patient's head to the bowl and then back to the headrest (Fig. 7–13).

A Hard, Angry Look in the Eyes. The eyes of the patient under relative analgesia have a calm, relaxed, faraway look (Fig. 7–14A). If the expression changes to a hard, angry look, it means that the individual is too deep in relative analgesia (Fig. 7–14B). Decrease the concentration of nitrous oxide.

Sitting Forward or Rigid Posture. Should the patient sit forward or

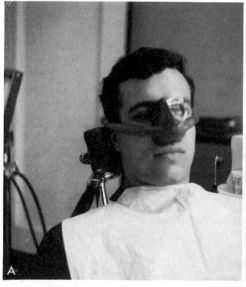
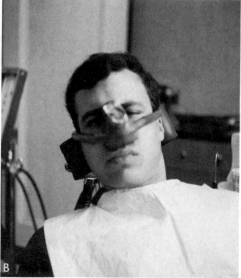

Figure 7–14 A, Typical relaxed, far-away look of a patient under analgesia. B, Hard, angry stare indicates excessive analgesic depth.

become rigid, it is evidence of fear of becoming unconscious (Fig. 7–15). The subject wants to do something about it. He "travels" or becomes tense. Decrease the concentration of nitrous oxide.

Wincing and Withdrawal Signs.   Wincing and withdrawal signs are invariably taken to be evidence of reactions to pain. This is not always true. When wincing or withdrawal occurs, ask the patient if he feels pain. If he answers, he is too wide awake and *is* being hurt. (Increase the concentration of nitrous oxide.) If he cannot hear the question and does not answer, he is approaching the deeper phases of the maintained analgesic stage and will soon close his mouth, if he has not already done so. (Decrease the concentration of nitrous oxide.)

Reluctance to Awaken.   The individual who reacts ideally to analgesia is in a semihypnotic state. He is often a person who is more open to suggestion and who can practice autosuggestion. He likes the feeling of being in a state of euphoria to such a degree that many times he keeps himself there even though he is being oxygenated. He may hear the dentist speaking but wishes that he would not bother him. He wants to "hang on" to his good feeling. When this occurs, a possible solution is suggesting to the patient, "When I tap you on the shoulder you will be wide awake."

Desire to Record Thoughts.   A great amount of cerebration takes place under relative analgesia. The patient's thoughts may focus on philosophy and religion, and he may attempt to solve the world's problems. These thoughts seem to be of such depth and importance that the thinker wants to record them for posterity and consequently asks for paper and pencil. Unfortunately, he does not remember them when he comes out of the analgesic state. Attempts to record such thoughts in writing usually fail because the act of writing wakes the patient out of the proper depth of analgesia and interferes with his thoughts.

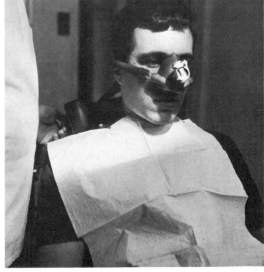

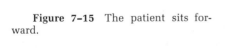

Figure 7–15 The patient sits forward.

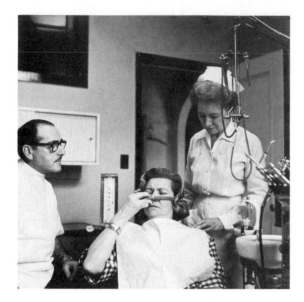

Figure 7-16 Tearing off the nasal inhaler.

Tearing Off the Nasal Inhaler (Fig. 7-16). When this happens the patient has become frightened by the initial sensations of relative analgesia, even though they have been described to him in advance. To prevent this result, see discussion of *The Critical Point* on page 150.

The Talkative Patient. The act of speaking results in overstimulation and excessive oral breathing and therefore makes it difficult and time-consuming for the patient to reach the proper depth of analgesia. It is frequently a sign of nervousness. Calm the patient and tell him to close his lips and breathe deeply through the nose; at the same time, increase the proportion of nitrous oxide.

Expressive Hand Movements. The hands of the patient under relative analgesia for the first or second time constitute a rich source of information:

Hands gripping the arm rests: The patient is tense, fearful, anticipating pain (Fig. 7-17A). When the gripping action of the fingers relaxes, the patient is a little more relaxed (Fig. 7-17B).

Hands in lap: If the hands are tightly clenched at first, the patient is tense (Fig. 7-18A). If later, they lie loosely in the lap, tension is decreased (Fig. 7-18B).

Hands fall off lap or armrests (Fig. 7-19): This action can signify one of two conditions: (a) a voluntary expression of a euphoric, "high" feeling, or (b) the reaching of a deep analgesic level, with the law of gravity taking over. Neither result is cause for concern. If the operator wishes to discriminate between the two, he may ask his patient a question (any question). If he answers, he is experiencing the euphoric, "high" feeling. If no answer is forthcoming, he is in a deeper analgesic level and is not aware of the position of his hands and arms. Continue the level of administration as long as his mouth is open.

Subjective Tension and Increased Muscular Tone.[12] There is a close reciprocal relationship between the state of physical relaxation or tension of

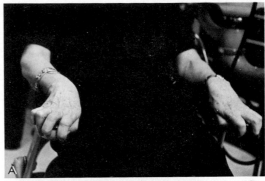

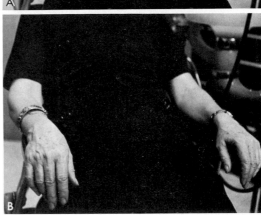

Figure 7–17 *A*, Hands gripping armrests; the patient is tense. *B*, When hands relax, the patient is also mentally relaxed.

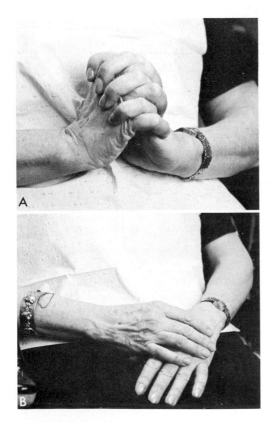

Figure 7–18 *A*, Tightly clenched hands denote mental tension. *B*, When hands relax, the patient is more relaxed mentally.

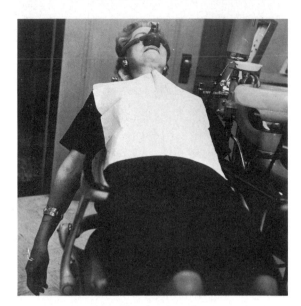

Figure 7–19   Hands fall off lap or armrests.

the muscles and the subjective state of relaxation or tension of the mind. Anxious patients show a general increase in muscular tone, which at times may be sufficiently severe that it produces pain. If such a patient can be brought to relax his muscles, there will be a corresponding loss of mental tension—in other words, a reduction of anxiety. Muscular relaxation seems also to reduce reactivity to pain and other stimuli.

Salivation.   Nervous tension, the experiencing of pain, or the anticipation of pain is sometimes the cause of excessive salivation, especially in children. This can exist to such a degree that it interferes with both the procedure and the quality of the end result. Relative analgesia, by relaxing, distracting, disorienting, and eliminating pain, obviates this.

Emotional Reactions.   Infrequently, tears stream from the eyes of the patient under relative analgesia. The novice might immediately guess that this sorrowful state is one of the disadvantages of analgesia administration. Nothing could be further from the truth. It is true that the tears are the result of the subject's thoughts wandering to some sad event, such as the recent death of a loved one and, unquestionably, pleasant thoughts would be more desirable. However, the important fact to bear in mind is that the patient's thoughts *did* wander from the immediate surroundings, away from the dental treatment room and from the dentistry being performed on him. To the dentist who uses relative analgesia, it is an unending source of gratification to be able to treat a patient who has had a lifelong history of fear of the dental experience while he is so relaxed that he does not even think about the dentistry being performed.

It must be remembered that these reactions occur only when the subject is new to analgesia. Once the patient's mind and body have become accustomed to the sensations—once the patient realizes the benefits of taking analgesia—he begins to relax, and with the help of the operator he learns to control unpleasant thoughts, and they disappear.

Eyeglasses and Contact Lenses.   After proper oxygenation, the patient is asked whether he is fully recuperated and clear-headed before he is allowed to leave the chair. Individuals who wear thick lenses will need them before they can decide properly. Contact lenses should be removed if the nasal inhaler will press too tightly against them.

Postanalgesia Headache, Dizziness, Sleepiness, or Nausea.   Although very infrequent, the complaint of headache, dizziness, sleepiness, or nausea for several hours after administration must be dealt with properly. Any one of these symptoms may occur after the initial introductory administration, in which case it is usually a reaction to the emotional experience and to the novelty of the effects of nitrous oxide on the body. However, there may be other reasons. For example, there may be retention of nitrous oxide. In this regard it has been found that nitrous oxide is not demonstrable in the bloodstream 4 minutes after anesthesia administration. By far the greatest volume of this gas is excreted through the lungs; however, a small amount is eliminated through the sweat glands, the skin, and the bladder and as bowel gas.[3] It is this latter portion that may remain for a longer period of time in the body. It has also been suggested that some cases of postanalgesia symptoms may arise from a concomitant viral infection which the patient is developing.

Again, it must be stressed that a patient should be well ventilated with 100 per cent oxygen after every analgesia administration. Fink demonstrated that, following the administration of nitrous oxide–oxygen anesthesia, arterial oxygen saturation may fall 5 to 10 per cent, often reaching levels below 90 per cent.[6] This type of hypoxia arises because the rapid outward diffusion of nitrous oxide lowers the alveolar partial pressure of oxygen when the patient breathes room air after the nasal inhaler is removed. In other words, the inhaled atmospheric oxygen (20 per cent) is diluted by the exhaled nitrous oxide, causing temporary hypoxia despite the fact that the patient is breathing room air containing sufficient oxygen. This diffusion hypoxia may account for some postanalgesia symptoms on rare occasions.

The changed emotional status, relaxation, and some residual nitrous oxide may also be causative factors in the production of postanalgesia headiness, dizziness, sleepiness, or nausea. If these symptoms occur in a patient who has taken relative analgesia several times, it usually means that this subject is more sensitive to the effects of nitrous oxide and will react very well with lesser concentrations. However, sufficient oxygenation during and after administration is the most important preventive measure.

SUMMARY OF REACTIONS AS DESCRIBED BY PATIENTS AND THE OPERATOR

1. Breaking into a cold sweat; nightmares.
2. Dreaming of the end of world.
3. Frightening daydreams, "weird" feeling.
4. Recall of anesthesia experiences, the operating room, the delivery room.
5. Complaint of a pain in the back of the skull. The patient may have ex-

erted excessive pressure against the headrest. (Change the position of his head in relation to the headrest.)

6. Fear of losing control emotionally and physically. (Assure the patient that this cannot happen.)

7. Hallucinations. In one instance, an extremely tense woman saw many people crowding around her, most of whom she had not seen in 30 years.

8. Fear of "fainting." (Assure the patient that this cannot occur.)

9. Very depressing thoughts. (Suggest pleasant topics at the next administration.)

10. Expressions such as "I hate it." This phrase was used by a patient at the beginning of every administration. Upon the doctor's suggestion that he do without it, the answer was invariably "Oh, No!" The sensations of analgesia are disliked, but the thought of doing without it is even more distressing and the patient accepts analgesia as the lesser of two evils.

11. Hearing the same phrases of music over and over again.

12. Thoughts such as "The doctor thinks I am not in full control, but I certainly am."

13. Laughter, giggling (rare).

14. Snoring (but cooperative).

15. Attitudes such as "I hear the doctor giving me a direction, but I just can't be bothered answering him."

16. An imagined communication with God. In this connection it is extremely interesting to note what the great philosopher William James says about his religious experiences under nitrous oxide:

> Nitrous oxide, when sufficiently diluted with air, stimulates the mystical consciousness in an extraordinary degree. Depth beyond depth of truth seems revealed to the inhaler. This truth fades out, however, or escapes, at the moment of coming to; and if any words remain over in which it seemed to clothe itself, they prove to be the veriest nonsense. Nevertheless, the sense of a profound meaning having been there persists; and I know more than one person who is persuaded that in the nitrous oxide trance we have a genuine metaphysical revelation.
>
> Some years ago I myself made some observations on the aspect of nitrous oxide intoxication, and reported them in print. One conclusion was forced upon my mind at that time, and my impression of its truth has ever since remained unshaken. It is that our normal waking consciousness, rational consciousness as we call it, is but one special type of consciousness, whilst all about it, parted from it by the filmiest of screens, there lie potential forms of consciousness entirely different. We may go through life without suspecting their existence; but apply the requisite stimulus, and at a touch they are there in all their completeness, definite types of mentality which probably somewhere have their field of application and adaptation. No account of the universe in its totality can be final which leaves these other forms of consciousness quite disregarded. How to regard them is the question—for they are so discontinuous with ordinary consciousness. Yet they may determine attitudes though they cannot furnish formulas, and open a region though they fail to give a map. At any rate, they forbid a premature closing of our accounts with reality. Looking back on my own experiences, they all converge towards a kind of insight to which I cannot help ascribing some metaphysical significance.*

---

*William James wrote this in 1902 in his book *The Varieties of Religious Experience.*

INDICATIONS AND CONTRAINDICATIONS FOR THE USE
OF RELATIVE ANALGESIA

Clinical experience has amply demonstrated the high margin of safety obtained with the use of nitrous oxide accompanied by sufficient oxygen. This statement was made with respect to the use of nitrous oxide–oxygen as a general anesthetic. When used as analgesia, either relative or total, it has never caused morbidity or mortality. However, the fact that a drug will not cause death does not automatically mean that it is always proper, safe, or wise to employ it. Fortunately there are very few contraindications to the use of nitrous oxide as relative analgesia. As used in the dental office, it does not seem to enter into any chemical union with the tissues of the body and its action is readily reversible.

Indications for Relative Analgesia

1. The patient is fearful of the dental experience.
2. The patient refuses both local anesthesia and general anesthesia.
3. The patient's physician has prohibited the use of a vasoconstrictor, and good local anesthesia cannot be obtained.
4. The patient gives a history of anaphylactic shock reaction to local anesthesia.
5. The patient gags readily.
6. The patient cannot tolerate long sittings for dental treatment.
7. *Age.* People of all ages can safely take relative analgesia. At the younger end of the scale, so long as the subject is old enough to sit in the dental chair and receive treatment he can be given relative analgesia. Likewise, old age is no deterrent. Older people, as a rule, take to the administration of relative analgesia very easily and react well with a higher concentration of oxygen and a lower concentration of nitrous oxide (Fig. 7–20).
8. *Cardiac conditions.* If an individual suffering from any form of cardiac disease is ambulatory, his condition is either wholly or partially compensated for. Therefore he can safely be given relative analgesia. Cardiac patients are usually tense individuals who do not look forward to dental treatment with equanimity. Creating tension, worry, and pain in such a subject is definitely contraindicated. With the use of relative analgesia the patient is relaxed and is at all times receiving a safe minimal percentage of oxygen. If no question is raised by the patient with a cardiac condition regarding the administration of analgesia, no precaution on the part of the dentist is necessary. However, should the patient question the advisability of using analgesia, it becomes mandatory that the physician be consulted. It devolves upon the dentist to explain the necessity for using analgesia and to differentiate between it and general anesthesia. From a medicolegal point of view, the physician's concurrence should be forthcoming before administration of analgesia in such a situation is attempted.

Should the physician not agree to analgesia and at the same time request that his patient not be given epinephrine, the dentist is presented with an all too familiar problem. One way to deal with this is to study the arithmetic of

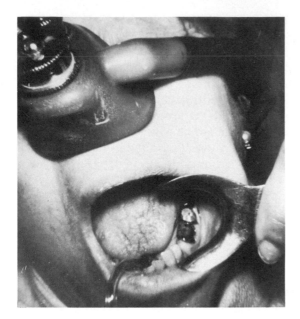

Figure 7–20   Age is no contraindication to the use of relative analgesia, as can be seen in this preparation for full coverage on lower left first molar of a 79 year old woman.

dosages and then to use your knowledge diplomatically and intelligently.[4] The problem is that the average physician, unschooled in the science of anesthesiology and unaware that a solution as potent as 1:1000 of epinephrine is unnecessary for local anesthesia, assumes that all epinephrine solutions are similar to the 1:1000 solution in the vial he carries around for emergency use. He therefore feels that 1 ml. of every solution of epinephrine contains 1 mg. of the potent drug.

Actually various doses have been advocated for use with patients with a history of coronary occlusion and other heart diseases. Some authorities say 0.2 mg.; others, 0.4 mg. For the sake of argument, let us agree on an arbitrary maximum dosage of 0.1 mg. for a patient with a recent history of coronary occlusion and let us also agree that this maximum dose should be injected very slowly and extravascularly. Then, 1 ml. of a 1:1000 solution is 10 times the maximum. Obviously, a solution of such potency should never be used with a cardiac patient. But what happens when a solution of 1:100,000 of epinephrine is injected? Through simple mathematics, we determine that 1 ml. of such a solution contains 0.01 mg. or one tenth of the maximum allowable dose. Assuming that the solution is injected slowly and extravascularly, a dentist using a local anesthetic solution containing 1:100,000 epinephrine could safely inject 10 ml. of the solution—assuming also that such a large amount of the accompanying local anesthetic would not hurt the patient.

This problem is a common one, but the difficulty of having to treat a patient without epinephrine, when you know that you need epinephrine to establish adequate and profound anesthesia and to cut down on bleeding, should be easily resolvable. Simply explain to the physician the mathematics involved, that you use a solution of local anesthetic that contains minute amounts of epinephrine and that, if you use a local anesthetic without epinephrine, you are quite likely to cause some pain. Pain, in turn, causes a flow of endogenous epinephrine which usually far surpasses the amount of epinephrine in a dental anesthetic ampule.

Epinephrine, therefore, in the concentrations we are accustomed to using, is a safe drug. As a matter of fact, contrary to the belief held by some, it is usually indicated in patients with a history of cardiac pathology, rather than contraindicated.

9. *Asthma*. An asthmatic patient breathes more easily from a gas machine. At times the gases come into his lungs under greater than atmospheric pressure, and he receives a plentiful supply of oxygen.

10. *Diabetes*. This condition is not a contraindication, since nitrous oxide does not seem to enter into any chemical union with the tissues of the body when used as relative analgesia in the dental office.

11. *Hypertension and hypotension*. Neither of these conditions constitutes a contraindication to the use of relative analgesia. During the maintained analgesic state, there is no alteration in blood pressure. Moreover, the patient suffering from hypertension is most commonly a nervous, tense individual whose blood pressure would rise when faced with the prospect of undergoing painful dentistry. The proper introduction and use of relative analgesia would negate this increase in blood pressure.

12. *Epilepsy*. The use of nitrous oxide and oxygen as relative analgesia minimizes the possibility of a seizure during dental treatment.

13. *Cerebral palsy*. With the use of relative analgesia it has become possible to perform dentistry on patients whose condition heretofore precluded any treatment whatsoever. (See Chapter 11.)

14. *Mental retardation*. Tender loving care plus relative analgesia is indicated. Treat the patient at his age level. (Chapter 11.)

15. *Neuroses*. Patients with any one of the so-called ordinary neuroses make excellent analgesia patients. They ardently desire the euphoric sensation and enhance it with autosuggestion. This applies also to individuals undergoing psychoanalysis.

16. *Pregnancy*. Nitrous oxide–oxygen analgesia has been used for many years during labor with no harm to mother or child. Indeed, it is believed that the concept of analgesia for dentistry was introduced to the United States by a French obstetrician. In pregnancy, nitrous oxide should be given with equal parts of oxygen. This mixture will produce adequate analgesia. The relative amount of nitrous oxide should never be exceeded. Wylie and Churchill-Davidson, in their discussion of placental transmission of drugs, state that:

> *No foetal depression* has been demonstrated following the use of nitrous oxide and oxygen mixtures. Some impediment to the passage of nitrous oxide across the placenta exists, as the concentration in the foetal circulation rarely rises above 50 per cent of that in the mother's circulation. Sufficient nitrous oxide to produce foetal depression does not occur.[15]

After initial analgesia is obtained, the nitrous oxide level may often be reduced to 15 per cent. The low concentrations of nitrous oxide with an always sufficient concentration of oxygen preclude any untoward results. However, should the patient question the wisdom of analgesia administration during pregnancy, the physician must be consulted. If he thinks it inadvisable to use analgesia at this time (no matter what the reason) it should not be administered. It is advisable to consult with the physician in all cases.

17. *Hemophilia.* Fewer injections needed; therefore, there is less chance of hemorrhage.

18. *Emphysema.* The relaxed patient and a plentiful supply of oxygen allow for ease of respiration.

19. *Treating the sickle-cell anemia dental patient.*[16] *Sickle-cell anemia, although not peculiar to black people, is endemic in that population.* It is a disease of children and young people, and shortens life span considerably. *Awareness of this disease in dental patients is vital;* thus the dentist, upon taking a medical history, should ascertain if the patient previously has been tested for the disease. If not, especially in the case of young black children, he should do a screening test prior to treatment. A test smear can be taken in the office. *If the patient has sickle-cell anemia, significant changes in treatment planning and procedures are indicated:* (1) long and extensive dental procedures must be avoided; (2) local anesthetic use should be minimized; if used, 2% lidocaine is recommended; (3) if general anesthetics are considered, anoxic episodes must be avoided; oxygen–nitrous oxide and fluothane are reasonable choices; (4) antibiotic therapy should be administered before and after surgical procedures to reduce sickling potential; (5) hemoglobin levels should be restored to 70 to 80% of normal before surgery; (6) preoperative sedation causes a decrease in respiration, and aspirin reduces blood pH; both conditions can precipitate a "crisis"; and (7) treatment must not be done during a "crisis."

Contraindications for Relative Analgesia

1. *The common cold.* Acute rhinitis makes breathing through the nose difficult, and the resultant excessive mouth breathing leads to poor, ineffective analgesia. Furthermore, since the gases from the machine are sometimes pushed into the respiratory system under greater than atmospheric pressure, there is a remote possibility of pushing nasal or pharyngeal infection farther into the respiratory system.

2. *Tuberculosis and other acute pulmonary conditions.* Nitrous oxide is one of the least irritating inhalation anesthetics. For this reason it has been the anesthetic of choice for tuberculosis and other pulmonary conditions when an inhalation anesthetic *must* be used. For the performance of dentistry it is not essential to use an inhalation anesthetic, since there are other media. Although nitrous oxide is an exceedingly mild and nonirritating gas, it is more irritating than not using gas at all. When a history of pulmonary disease is given, it should be discussed with the patient's physician.

3. *Patients undergoing psychiatric treatment.* Subjects undergoing any form of shock therapy (insulin, electric, or Metrazol) or those under psychiatric care for any severe emotional illness, should be given relative analgesia only after consultation with the psychiatrist. It is true that a change in emotional status is effected in most individuals with the use of relative analgesia

and that this change is usually for the better. However, a patient whose emotional state is rather precarious might be upset by any change. Consult the psychiatrist before administering analgesia. By no means should these patients automatically be considered as ineligible for analgesia administration. Most are good analgesia patients when approached with tender, loving care. In this connection it is informative and interesting to learn the opinions of over 100 clinical psychiatrists.[17]

NITROUS OXIDE PSYCHOSEDATION IN THE DENTAL TREATMENT OF PATIENTS WITH PSYCHIATRIC DISORDERS: A SURVEY OF PSYCHIATRISTS' OPINIONS[17]

Introduction.   Literature dealing with the dental treatment of the psychiatric patient or of patients with psychiatric histories has been conspicuous by its absence. This factor has contributed to the widespread reluctance on the part of the dentist to treat a potentially large category of patients. For example, in sections on contraindications to various dental treatments appearing in most dental texts, "psychiatric patients" are almost always included. Such exclusions occur, it would seem, on the basis of repetition of previous contraindications, without the authority of any scientifically sound literature or data.

It is particularly interesting that dentists tend to ignore, as threatening, dental problems of these patients because of the large body of contemporary literature which promulgates an image of the psychiatric patient as one whose behavior is irrational, taxing,[44] uncooperative, and possibly life-threatening to the dentist.

Because of the paucity of information currently available on this subject and as part of a continuing project at our laboratories on nitrous oxide–oxygen psychosedation, the present study was undertaken to determine the state of psychiatric opinion on the suitability of psychiatric patients for nitrous oxide–oxygen sedation in conjunction with dental treatment.

Materials and Methods.   One hundred and forty-five certified clinical psychiatrists were randomly selected from the 1972–1973 Directory of Medical Specialists.[42] These persons were mailed questionnaires (with self-addressed return envelopes) describing the use of nitrous oxide–oxygen sedative techniques in the treatment of the apprehensive dental patient. The questionnaire included the following questions:

   1. Before treating a patient with a history of psychiatric problems, should the dentist seek a consultation from the therapist?

   2. What specific psychiatric patients would you feel should not have nitrous oxide sedation with dental treatment?

   3. What guidelines would you offer the dentist in general in treating patients with psychiatric histories?

Results and Discussion.   Of the 145 questionnaires mailed, 114 were returned for a percentage response of 78.6 per cent. Four others were returned because the addresses of the subjects were unknown or incorrect.

Need to Seek Consultation.   In reply to the question whether the dentist should seek consultation before administering nitrous oxide to a patient with a psychiatric history, the responses were essentially equally divided. Fifty-two per cent (52.6 per cent) indicated the dentist should seek consultation with the therapist and 47.4 per cent indicated that a consultation was unnecessary. Those respondents who believed a consultation was appropriate stated that it was desirable to do so from a medicolegal standpoint. In addition, these same respondents claimed that most psychiatric patients currently in treatment would probably be ingesting various psychotropic drugs and information regarding the nature of the medication would be of use to the dentist.

Interestingly, psychiatrists who reported a consultation as unnecessary viewed the eliciting of this information from the patient as an "invasion of privacy." Perhaps more important were their reasons for this somewhat strong position. These therapists pointed out that most psychiatric patients routinely exhibit behaviors that are little or no different from that of non-psychiatric patients. They expressed the view that labeling a patient as a "psychiatric" patient would result in the dentist's seeing in a specific patient behaviors that are inherent in stereotypes rather than in actuality. That this does indeed occur has been documented in the literature.[45] The result, these respondents felt, would be to reduce unnecessarily the dental treatment potentially available to these patients.

Contraindications to Nitrous Oxide–Oxygen Sedation. In reply to the question about what psychiatric categories of patients were contraindicated for nitrous oxide sedation, 39.4 per cent claimed there were none based on the classification per se. In other words if the patient wanted this modality in conjunction with dental treatment, there were no contraindications to it. However, some 60.6 per cent felt there were definite categories for whom it would be prudent to exercise caution in its use. The most frequently cited categories included the paranoid patient, fragile schizophrenics, and acute psychotics. These categories of patients logically require caution in treatment because of their desperate attempts to maintain control of themselves and their ideations. Because of some of the dissociative symptoms (floating feelings, and so forth) which may be experienced by the patient undergoing nitrous oxide–oxygen psychosedation, acute psychotic episodes theoretically could be precipitated or potentiated.

Guidelines for Treating Patients With Psychiatric Histories. In response to this question, a large percentage (72.8 per cent) of the psychiatrists reported that the patient should be treated for medical and dental problems as necessary. With a close relationship with the patient's therapist, any psychiatric sequelae could be dealt with after dental treatment. The respondents also indicated that the dentist should prepare the patient for treatment by explaining in sufficient detail the various aspects of the proposed treatment procedure. They believed that concerted preparation of the patient would minimize potential difficulties and facilitate his cooperation. The importance of preparing the patient has repeatedly received support in the literature.[43]

Case Report. The following rather typical consultation is included in the present report because it illustrates many of the findings obtained in the above survey results. The patient was initially seen for a dental appointment where it was determined that she had received psychiatric treatment for a prolonged period. At the initial appointment she was noticeably anxious about the kind of treatment she would receive. Because of her exacerbated anxiety and some impressions of impaired thought processes, it was deemed advisable to seek a consultation from her therapist.

Therapist's Report.   This 36 year old married female was regularly involved in therapy at Mental Hygiene Service on a weekly to monthly basis during the period May 1971 to April 1973. At various times during this period, she received the following medications: Stelazine, 5 mg. t.i.d., and Cogentin, 1 mg. b.i.d.; Naldal and Mellaid, 25 to 50 mg. q.i.d. At her request she discontinued therapy and medication in June 1973 and has not received treatment or reevaluation since that time. Reports have indicated she has been functioning adequately without medication.

A report of the present mental status examination is as follows. Patient presently demonstrates mildly increased and anxious motor behavior. She relates with appropriately articulate and normal speech. She is oriented to person, time, and place. Memory and recall are intact. The patient presents an adequate attention span with moderately restricted judgment, especially concerning the antecedent dental procedures. Mood is enthusiastic and mildly elevated, with affect mildly to moderately elevated and appropriate. Thought processes are organized, rational, and goal directed. Associations are intact, although decidedly unsophisticated concerning the dental care previously attempted. The content of thoughts is characterized by indecisiveness but no evidence of delusions, paranoid ideation, and so forth. Perception is free of hallucinatory phenomena, insight is restricted but appropriate, attitude is passive-dependent, mildly suspicious. The patient reports no significant physiological complaints, and reports no drug or alcohol abuse.

Impressions and Recommendations.   According to her reports and information on consultation request, the patient appears to have demonstrated an acute exacerbation of neurotic anxiety reaction with mild to moderate paranoid thought content. She presently is free of psychotic processes in mood, thought, or behavior. She understands the importance of the prescribed dental treatment and is motivated to undergo nitrous oxide–oxygen sedation due to present anxiety. Thus, the following recommendations are made:

1. The dental appointment should be rescheduled as soon as possible.

2. A thorough explanation of procedures should be provided before treatment is administered to patient.

3. The stabilizing influence of patient's husband's presence during treatment should be considered.

4. The Mental Hygiene Clinic should be consulted should further complications develop following treatment.

Summary and Conclusions.   The results of a survey of psychiatrists' opinions on the use of nitrous oxide–oxygen as a sedative adjunct in the treatment of patients with histories of psychiatric treatment have been presented. The findings indicate:

1. Consultation with the patient's therapist was considered important by the majority of respondents. Consultation would provide the dentist with potentially useful information concerning medications which

the patient might be ingesting. In addition, communication is open between the dentist and the psychotherapist should any complications develop.

2. Emphasis was placed on treating the patient's medical and dental problems. Any untoward psychiatric sequelae could be dealt with by the therapist afterwards.

3. The majority of respondents pointed out the necessity of preparing the patient, and of explaining in some detail the stages of the procedure.

REFERENCES

1. American Medical Association: Fundamentals of Anesthesia. Philadelphia, W. B. Saunders Co., 1954.
2. Clement, F. W.: Nitrous Oxide–Oxygen Anesthesia. Philadelphia, Lea & Febiger, 1951.
3. Eastwood, D. W. (Ed.): Clinical Anesthesia. Clinical Use of Nitrous Oxide. Philadelphia, F. A. Davis Co., 1964.
4. Editorial: J. Amer. Dent. Soc. Anesthesiol., 12:91, 1965.
5. Editorial: Dentistry's stake in iatrogenics. N.Y. State Dent. J., 306, 1965.
6. Fink, B. R.: Diffusion anoxia. Anesthesiology, 16:511, 1955.
7. Fisk, H. M.: Personal communication.
8. Langa, H.: Analgesia for modern dentistry. New York J. Dent., 27:228–265, 1957.
9. Langa, H.: Nitrous oxide–oxygen analgesia for modern dentistry. Dent. Dig., 66:126, 173, 1960.
10. Langa, H.: Postgraduate teaching of relative analgesia with nitrous oxide and oxygen. J. Amer. Dent. Assoc., 67:28, 1963.
11. James, W.: The Varieties of Religious Experience. New York, Modern Library.
12. Meares, A.: The Management of the Anxious Patient. Philadelphia, W. B. Saunders Co., 1963.
13. Shane, S.: Handbook of Balanced Anesthesia. Baltimore, Lowry & Volz, 1958.
14. Sniderman, M.: Rx for dentists — prescribe. The Fortnightly Review of the Chicago Dental Society, August 15, 1963, p. 15.
15. Wylie, W. D., and Churchill-Davidson, H. C.: A Practice of Anaesthesia. 2nd ed. Chicago, Year Book Publishers, Inc., 1966.
16. Quart. National Dental Association, 31:72, 1973.
17. Ayer, W. A., and Getter, L.: Nitrous oxide psychosedation in the dental treatment of patients with psychiatric disorders: A survey of psychiatrists' opinions. Anesthesia Progress, 22:17–19, 1975.
18. Pickering, G. W., Cranston, W. I., and Pears, M. A.: The Treatment of Hypertension. Springfield, Ill., Charles C Thomas, 1961.
19. Modell, W.: Drugs of Choice 1966–1967. St. Louis, Mo., The C. V. Mosby Co., 1966.
20. Moser, R. H.: Diseases of Medical Progress. 2nd ed. Springfield, Ill., Charles C Thomas Co., 1964.
21. Treatment considerations of dental patients receiving medical care. In Accepted Dental Remedies. Chicago, American Dental Association, 1966.
22. Tarsitano, J. J.: Never treat a stranger. J.A.D.A., 73:856–862, 1966.
23. Kutscher, A. H., Zegarelli, E. V., and Hyman, G. A.: Pharmacotherapeutics of Oral Disease. New York, McGraw-Hill, 1964.
24. Steiner, R. B.: Drug intoxication. Dental Clin. N. America, pp. 727–754, Nov. 1964.
25. Physicians' Desk Reference to Pharmaceutical Specialties and Biologicals. 20th ed. Oradell, New Jersey, Medical Economics, Inc., 1966.
26. Munson, W. M., and Jenicek, J. A.: Effect of anesthetic agents on patients receiving reserpine therapy. Anesthesiology, 23:741–746, 1962.
27. Williams, J. L.: A case of acute gingivitis apparently caused by administration of dicumarol. J. Periodont., 21:95, 1950.
28. Management of dental problems in patients with cardiovascular disease: Council on Dental Therapeutics, Am. Dent. Assoc. and Am. Heart Assoc., Joint Report. J.A.D.A. 68:333–342, March, 1964.
29. Shira, R. B., Hall, R. J., and Guernsey, L. H.: Minor oral surgery during prolonged anticoagulant therapy. J. Oral Surg., Anes. Hosp. D. Serv., 20:93–99, 1962.
30. Behrman, S. J., and Wright, I. S.: Dental surgery during continuous anticoagulant therapy. J.A.M.A., 175:483–488, 1961.

31. Frank, B. W., Dickhaus, D. W., and Claus, E. C.: Dental extractions in the presence of continued anticoagulant therapy. Ann. Intern. Med., *59*:911–913, 1963.

32. Irby, W. B., and Baldwin, K. H.: Emergencies and Urgent Complications in Dentistry. St. Louis, Mo., C. V. Mosby Co., 1965.

33. Riddick, F. A.: Long term anticoagulant therapy in an outpatient department; techniques and complications. J. Chron. Dis., *12*:622, 1960.

34. Martin, E. W. (Ed.): Remington's Pharmaceutical Sciences. 13th ed. Easton, Pa., Mack Publishing Co., 1965, p. 1167.

35. Ayd, F. J., Jr.: A survey of drug induced extrapyramidal reactions. J.A.M.A., *175*:1054–1060, 1961.

36. Scine, I. A., and Tallant, E. J.: Tetanus-like reactions to prochlorperazine (Compazine). J.A.M.A., *171*:1813, 1959.

37. Cecil, R. L., and Loeb, R. F.: A Textbook of Medicine, 10th Ed. Philadelphia, W. B. Saunders Co., 1959.

38. Johnson, A.: Hypersensitivity to penicillin. Med. J. Australia, *2*:432–433, 1962.

39. Orentreich, N., Harber, L., and Tromovitch, T. A.: Photosensitivity and photo-onycholysis due to demethylchlortetracycline. Arch. Derm., *83*:730–737, 1961.

40. Weinstein, L., Madoff, M. C., and Samet, C. M.: The sulfonamides. New Eng. J. Med., *263*: 952–957, 1960.

41. Waldrep, A. C.: Precautions for patients on drug therapy. South Carolina Dental J., *27*:21–27, 1969.

42. Directory of Medical Specialists, 15th Edition, Vol. 2. Marquis Who's Who. Chicago, 1972.

43. MacKenzie, R. D.: Psychodynamics of pain. J. Oral Med., *23*:75–84, 1968.

44. Scheman, P.: Pharmacology of sedatives and amnesics. *In* Amnesic Analgesia Techniques in Dentistry. Edited by S. R. Spiro. Springfield, Ill., Charles C Thomas, 1972.

45. Szasz, T. S.: The Myth of Mental Illness: Foundations of a Theory of Personal Conduct. New York, Harper, 1961.

CLINICAL APPLICATIONS OF RELATIVE ANALGESIA IN THE PRACTICE OF DENTISTRY

8

> The practice of pain- and fear-control is a major factor in building peace of mind in the dentist and in his patients. For dentistry to be socially acceptable it is not enough that it be technically competent: it must be humanely presented.[11]

The philosophy of dental practice and the needs and demands of dental patients have changed considerably in the last 25 years. And these, in turn, have stimulated the development and acceptance of modalities that formerly were not too well understood. With the development of methods to lengthen the duration of the dental sitting, a variety of procedures may now be accomplished at one sitting. At the same time, the dentist has found that, in order to utilize each visit effectively on a continuing basis, he must provide a means not only of obtunding pain but also of eliminating fear and apprehension.

Dentists almost always deal with ambulatory patients. Consequently, general anesthetic agents are used infrequently and then only by a limited number of dentists, for such agents cause problems unrelated to dental complaints. Likewise, heavy and prolonged premedication brings collateral problems. With local anesthetics, although they can effectively block the passage of painful stimuli, the dentist must still cope with the problem of overriding anxiety and fear. In contrast, with the use of nitrous oxide and oxygen as relative analgesia, the dentist has at his disposal an instrument which is safe, easily mastered, and effective in its application to all phases of dental practice.

RELATIVE ANALGESIA AND LOCAL ANESTHESIA

Dental practitioners have a tendency to categorize procedures as "major" and "minor." On the one hand, the preparation of a quadrant for full coverage and the removal of an impacted tooth are considered to be major procedures. On the other, an oral prophylaxis, blowing air into a cavity, and applying medicaments are considered to be minor procedures. Most dentists offer the patient local anesthesia for cavity preparation. How many routinely give local

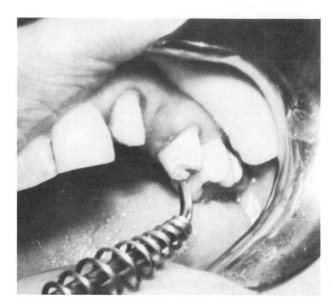

Figure 8–1 Blowing air into sensitive dentine: a minor procedure with major effect.

anesthesia to their patients at subsequent visits for fitting a fixed bridge, blowing air into sensitive dentine (Fig. 8–1), applying irritating and painful medicaments, and cementation of a restoration is open to question. In each of these procedures, resulting pain is of major importance to the patient. Similarly, the preparation of hypersensitive cervical cavities is often painful even with the use of local anesthesia.

In many of these instances, relative analgesia obtunds pain to an even greater degree than does local anesthesia. The reason for this is, as the dentist knows full well, that tooth reduction is by no means the sole cause of pain and discomfort. He knows, too, that the elimination of pain stimuli to the central nervous system is not the complete answer to all the reactions that are the cause of wasted operating time. In relative analgesia, not only are pain and fear eliminated, but also the contraction of the orbicularis oris (Fig. 8–2) and the movements of the tongue, the cheeks, the head, and the body are all controlled.

The dentist also finds that a high percentage of procedures in routine operative dentistry (90 per cent) can be done without local anesthesia and that, when local anesthesia is discarded, his work is not limited to one quadrant of the mouth. He is thus able to accomplish much more work at one short sitting. Moreover, if multiple crown or jacket preparations are to be done, the patient will be less aware of the lapse of time and the noise and vibration of the instruments will be greatly dulled. All this makes for a less nervous, less harried, and more cooperative patient, and such a patient is less averse to undergoing dentistry of a similar nature in the future. Finally, if local anesthesia must be used, the patient will not mind the injection when he is under relative analgesia.

The question often arises, When can relative analgesia be used alone? or When does the situation call for the combination of local anesthesia and rela-

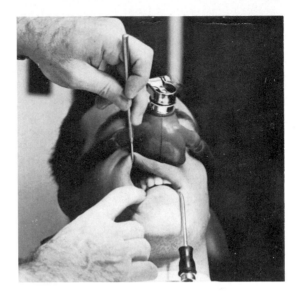

Figure 8–2 The orbicularis oris does not "fight back" in relative analgesia.

tive analgesia? Each procedure has to be judged by the patient's needs, for, in the final analysis, the patient's comfort and freedom from pain and apprehension must be our criteria. Let him be the judge. However, when a patient under relative analgesia evinces pain or discomfort, there should be no hesitation to increase the flow of nitrous oxide (as long as the mouth is maintained in an open position) before deciding to use local anesthesia. Then, if complete comfort is obtained only by an analgesic depth that causes repeated closure of the mouth or generation of fear, local anesthesia is necessary.

When an injection of local anesthetic solution is utilized with the patient under analgesia, the dental practitioner will find that his injection results in *complete* anesthesia more *frequently* and more *rapidly* for the following reasons:

1. More accurate injection technique can be employed because the sedated, relaxed patient offers no interference by tensing of muscles or by moving the head.

2. Metabolic rate and rate of blood flow are not increased due to fear and apprehension, so that the anesthetic solution is not carried away from the desired site too rapidly.

3. Translating pressure, sound and vibratory sensations into pain sensation does not take place under analgesia.

ORAL RECONSTRUCTION

Extensive mouth reconstruction has become an increasingly significant subject in contemporary dentistry.[22] In correlating the complex disciplines necessary for successful oral rehabilitation, concern must be directed toward the intrinsic feelings of the patient who may be asked to undergo a series of treatments describable at best as unnerving. Major care requires time and minute attention to details, no matter how skillful the operator. The patient in turn should be able to weather these demanding sessions.

An immediate and pressing goal for the dentist in oral reconstruction is the transformation of a harrowing extended course of treatment into a relatively benign experience. If the advantages of modern dental procedures are not to be negated by psychological attrition, greater concern for the patient's psyche is demanded. Otherwise, the patient may find the cure worse than the disease.

The use of relative analgesia for oral reconstruction combines the advantages of active patient cooperation with the quiet detachment of a general anesthetic, and yet it has none of the disadvantages and dangers of the latter modality. The advantages of analgesia in a total treatment plan for complex procedures are even greater than those in simpler procedures, because analgesia is singularly suited to meet the multiple problems encountered. These problems affect both the dentist and the patient, for the dentist works under a greater relative strain with increased responsibilities, and the patient must endure repeated lengthy sessions.

The very concept of analgesia, properly explained to the patient, can be a crucial factor in gaining acceptance and creating sufficient motivation for full mouth rehabilitation. In instances in which there have been contraindications to local and general anesthesia, extensive procedures have been carried out with relative analgesia alone. Even when local anesthesia must be included, it is a valuable asset to be able to limit the number of local injections, thus reducing the incidence of drooping of the face and the numb after-sensations to a much more tolerable level. Almost complete elimination of local anesthesia is routine for such trying procedures as crown and bridge impressions and try-ins, and temporary and permanent cementations. Of course, when an injection is used to supplement analgesia, the typical needle shock trauma is eliminated. Multiplied over many sessions, these advantages add up to much higher patient morale.

Patients who are in need of extensive oral therapy have often neglected their oral condition because of fear and anxiety. They often present a typical syndrome of gagging, bruxism, salivation, and highly motile tongue and lip reflexes. They are ideal patients for relative analgesia. Many such patients have severe functional and constitutional problems that complicate dental rehabilitation, for example:

1. The patient who is allergic to local anesthetics, barbiturates, and other drugs.

2. The patient with severe temporomandibular joint problems associated with malocclusion, stress, muscle spasm, bruxism, and hypermotility.

3. The psychically disturbed patient.

4. The patient on whom it is impossible to obtain centric relation under typical office conditions owing to stress, tension, or spasm.

5. The patient who insists on speaking, rinsing, moving, swallowing, coughing, gagging, and watching.

6. The patient who requires local anesthesia for impressions, cementations, fitting of restorations, and periodontal treatment.

All such patients can be helped to a better final result with the use of relative analgesia. From the patient's point of view, the technical success of major dental therapy often depends on a continuing, favorable dentist-patient relationship. In analgesia, with the patient gently cushioned in a state of euphoria and comfort, a difficult case can be seen through to a conclusion that is mutually satisfying to both the patient and the doctor, without the usual emotional resentment and backlash from a long, grueling ordeal. The stage is thus set for the crucial follow-up maintenance care so necessary for the continued success of the work already accomplished. The use of relative analgesia not only helps make the original rehabilitation possible, but encourages the patient to return at the proper intervals.

OPERATIVE DENTISTRY

Relative analgesia is indicated in each of the following procedures:

Cavity Preparation for All Types of Filling Materials (Fig. 8–3). Ninety per cent of all cavity preparations can be done under relative analgesia without the addition of local anesthetics. This statement is based on the reaction of patients to the procedure both during and after treatment. With this procedure, not only may many teeth be prepared at one sitting, but teeth in all four quadrants may be treated at one sitting (Fig. 8–4). Even the pain and discomfort resulting from the preparation of hypersensitive cervical cavities is ofttimes eliminated more completely when relative analgesia is used, as opposed to local anesthesia. Moreover, should an injection be needed, the pain and fear of that procedure is controlled when the patient is under analgesia.

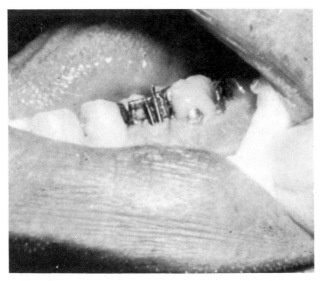

Figure 8–3 Under relative analgesia, the more detailed techniques such as threaded pin reinforcements for silver amalgam restorations can be accomplished deliberately.

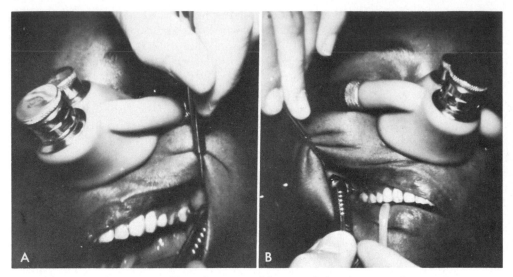

Figure 8–4 Preparation of buccal cavities of the upper left and upper right second molars at the same sitting (no local anesthesia).

Inserting Matrix Bands and Gingival Wedges (Fig. 8–5). These procedures are certainly minor from the dentist's point of view, and yet they sometimes generate a disproportionate reaction in the patient, especially the child-patient. It is wise therefore to complete all the necessary steps before the cessation of analgesia administration.

Blowing Air Into Cavities. It is common knowledge that blowing air against sensitive dentine, even air at the proper temperature, is painful to the

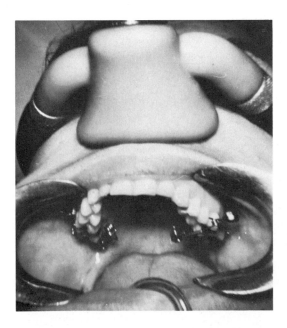

Figure 8–5 Matrices inserted in both maxillary quadrants.

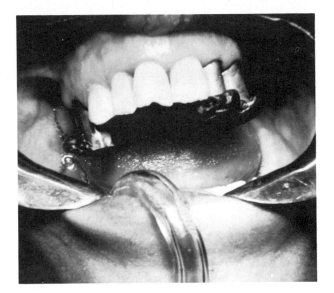

Figure 8–6 Copper band impressions are accomplished without the use of local anesthesia.

patient. Analgesia is effective in eliminating the pain of this procedure—a minor one to the dentist, a major one to the patient.

Taking Band Impressions (Fig. 8–6). At any given analgesic level, the pain resulting from the manipulation of soft tissue is experienced at a lower threshold than the pain resulting from the treatment of hard tissue. To anticipate the patient's needs and to ensure his freedom from pain and discomfort, deepen the analgesic level about 1 to 2 minutes before fitting the bands and taking the impression.

Removing Provisional Splints or Bridges (Fig. 8–7). Force must be exerted in order to loosen a restoration, and sensitive dentine is exposed in the

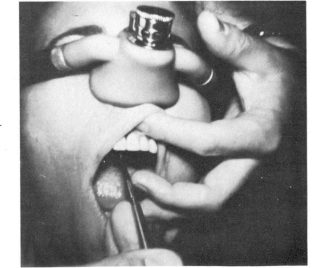

Figure 8–7 Removing a restoration.

process. The tense, apprehensive patient contracts his lips and cheeks, thus making the removal more difficult for both the patient and the operator. Many provisional acrylic bridges and splints are broken because of such interference by the patient. Debridement of the prepared teeth may also create a problem. The subject under analgesia is insensitive to the force exerted and to temperature changes.

Inlays, Crowns, and Pin Splints (Fig. 8–8). Pain and discomfort are involved in the preparations for gold inlays, gold crowns, porcelain or acrylic jacket crowns, and pin splints, as well as in seating the restorations, tapping them into place, and removing them. Under relative analgesia, the patient remains calm and free of pain.

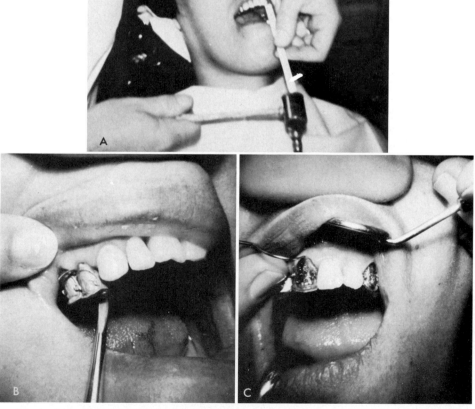

Figure 8–8 Using relative analgesia to minimize the trauma of (A) seating of the castings; (B) tapping off crowns after fitting; (C) checking subgingival margins, a minor procedure which can be highly disturbing to an apprehensive patient.

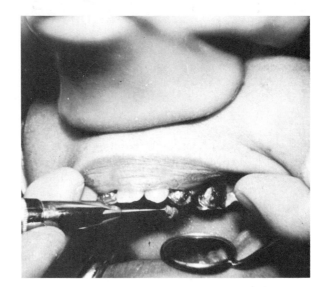

Figure 8–9 Adjusting occlusal relationships (under a light plane of analgesia, so that the patient can guide the operator).

Adjusting the Occlusal Relationship of an Inlay or Crown (Fig. 8–9).
Pain and discomfort may be created by thermal changes or by the translation of vibratory and sound sensations into pain sensations by a nervous, tense patient. This is eliminated by analgesia.

Sterilization and Cementation (Fig. 8–10). These "minor" procedures can generate much pain even when all possible precautions are taken. The use of relative analgesia is invaluable here, for when local anesthetics are used, it is sometimes difficult to explain several hours of numbness after a 5 or 10 minute procedure.

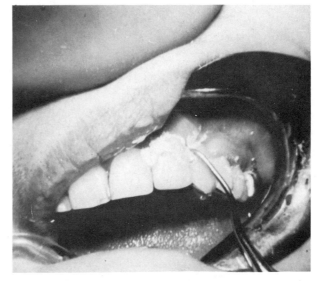

Figure 8–10 Eliminating the pain of cementation by means of analgesia.

PERIODONTICS

It is in the variety of its applications to the practice of periodontics that analgesia excels. In this respect, there is no adequate substitute for it. Whether it be the general practitioner giving an oral prophylaxis or the periodontist executing deep scaling, curettage, or surgical procedures, analgesia helps the doctor and the patient immeasurably. Familiar to all is the patient who cries, "I would rather have a tooth pulled or drilled than have my teeth cleaned!" This cry can be eliminated by analgesia. And it is important to remember that, although there is a degree of central nervous system depression associated with relative analgesia, it is well tolerated by patients in the extremes of age, those with cardiovascular disease, and the debilitated.

PERIODONTAL PROCEDURES WITH RELATIVE ANALGESIA

Scaling and Curettage (Fig. 8–11).　Scaling consists of the removal of calculus. Since these accretions are firmly attached to the tooth and are adjacent to soft tissues, the latter must be displaced and force must be exerted to engage the calculus by the instrument utilized for the removal of this substance. When hypersensitivity of the cervical and root surfaces exists, scaling or curettage can be an extremely painful experience, so painful, in fact, that it is difficult for the operator to perform adequately and even more difficult for the patient to submit to treatment. Much operating time is therefore lost, and the patient does not look foward to the visit. Consequently, many do not complete all the necessary treatments. The use of relative analgesia in periodontal procedures permits the operator to work better and faster, with no discomfort to the patient.

Occlusal Adjustment of the Natural Dentition.　This procedure, even if

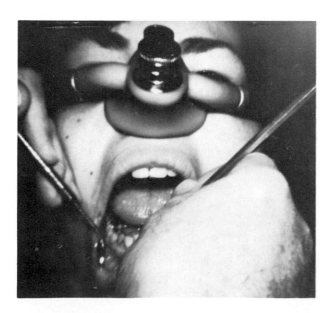

Figure 8–11 Subgingival curettage: the use of analgesia permits a greater number of areas to be treated at one sitting.

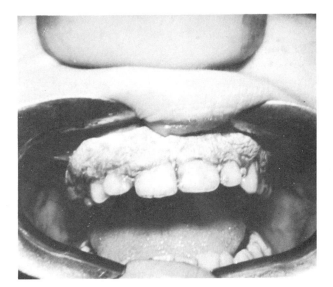

Figure 8-12 The insertion and removal of periodontal packs following gingivoplasty can be done painlessly.

there is extensive pericementitis, will be of little concern to the patient under analgesia.

Changing Packs After Periodontal Surgery (Fig. 8-12). The use of analgesia reduces the uncomfortable sensations that may accompany the removal of the surgical dressing and the exposure of the raw wound surfaces. The replacement of new dressings is also carried out with a minimum of discomfort.

Eliminating Premature Contact Points. This can be done with great dispatch under analgesia because the relaxed patient with a relaxed mandible performs properly.

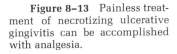

Figure 8-13 Painless treatment of necrotizing ulcerative gingivitis can be accomplished with analgesia.

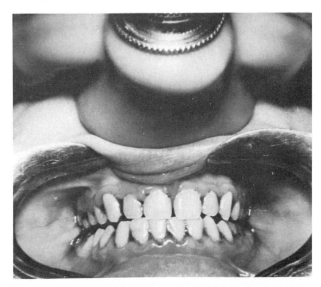

Emergency Treatment of Necrotizing Ulcerative Gingivitis (Fig. 8–13). With the administration of analgesia, this procedure can be performed painlessly and rapidly.

Initial Periodontal Examination (Fig. 8–14). Pocket probing and the like are also done painlessly when analgesia is administered.

Ultrasonic Instruments. These instruments can be employed with no discomfort to the patient under analgesia.

SURGICAL PROCEDURES WITH ANALGESIA AND LOCAL ANESTHESIA

The administration of relative analgesia precedes the injection of the local anesthetic solution. As Fox has stated:

> In periodontal procedures where there is trauma from surgical technique causing laceration of tissues, there is need for a prolonged anesthetic or even solutions that subsequently become analgesic. . . . The type of local anesthetic drugs as well as the volume of the solution injected should be determined by the nature and extent of the procedure. Wherever possible, [and as indicated] prolonged postoperative paresthesia [should be avoided].
>
> The surgery of the marginal and attached gingival areas of the periodontal tissues, which include the interdental papillae, can be cared for in terms of the local anesthetic needs by the papillary injection. The local anesthetic solution is injected into the interdental papillae from the buccal aspect. The site of the injection is at the junction of the marginal and attached gingiva.
>
> Where mucogingival surgery and vestibular procedures are demanded, supplementary injections of the local anesthetic solution are inserted by infiltration technique into the mucobuccal fold areas of either the upper or the lower jaw. Palatal and lingual infiltration injections are given where necessary and indicated.[10]

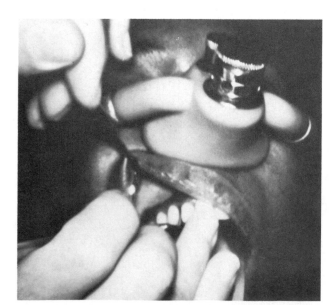

Figure 8–14 Probing a periodontal pocket—a minor procedure which may assume major proportions to the patient—is made painless by relative analgesia.

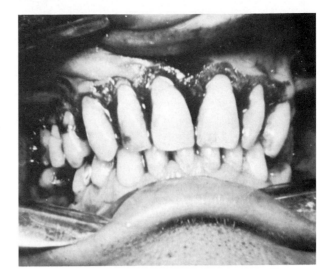

Figure 8–15 Gingivectomy-gingivoplasty (with analgesia and local anesthesia).

However, *the entire treatment is carried out under relative analgesia* (Figs. 8–15 and 8–16).

THE CONTROL OF GAGGING

Gagging is a reflex action produced by the transmission of afferent impulses to a nerve center and their outflow, thence as efferent impulses independent of volition. The afferent impulses provoking the reflex of gagging may result from tactile, visual, acoustic, olfactory, or psychic stimuli.

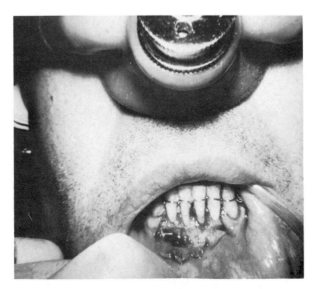

Figure 8–16 Flap operation with analgesia supplemented with local anesthesia.

IMPRESSION TAKING

Familiar is the individual who gags at the sight of an impression tray coming toward him. Even more familiar is the gagger who cannot bear the impression material to come in contact with his palate especially, as often occurs, when it runs down his soft palate. Many agents, drugs, and topical anesthetics are recommended to make that first impression successful. None, however, are necessary if relative analgesia is used.

Gagging often presents a serious problem in treating children. This problem can be solved easily with the use of relative analgesia. Although it does not totally eliminate gagging in extreme cases, it depresses the gag reflex sufficiently that a good impression is obtained at the first attempt in *all* cases (Figs. 8–17 and 8–18).

ROENTGENOGRAPHY (FIG. 8–19)

The patient with a hypersensitive palate or the nervous patient may gag during the taking of roentgenograms. This is an example of a so-called minor procedure which may assume major proportions to the subject and consume much valuable time. If gagging is discovered to be a problem (during history taking), it would be wise to delay the taking of roentgenograms until the patient has been properly introduced to relative analgesia.

The upper molar areas are usually the most difficult to x-ray, although in many patients the lower molar areas present a problem. Some nasal inhalers have tubings containing metal wiring, which would appear in the picture. Others are made entirely of plastic and rubber, which would not interfere with the result. To ensure success and save much valuable operating time, the following procedures should be followed:

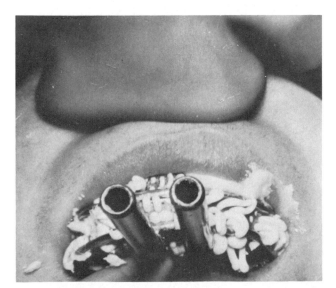

Figure 8–17 Alginate impression under analgesia (gagging controlled).

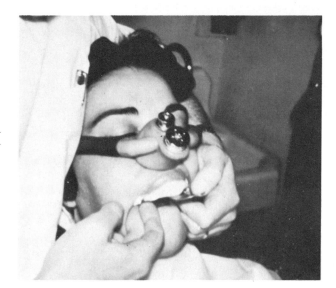

Figure 8–18 Plaster impression under analgesia (gagging controlled).

Apparatus Containing Metal

1. Place the subject into the proper analgesic depth (depending on the severity of gagging).

2. Remove the nasal inhaler; do not oxygenate.

3. Expose the molar and bicuspid films.

4. If the patient begins to gag before all the problem films are exposed, it will be necessary to administer analgesia again and to repeat the preceding steps.

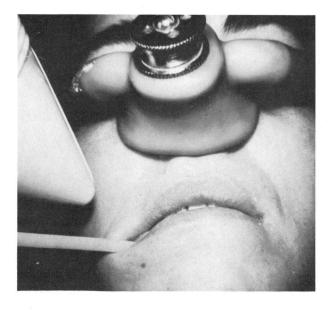

Figure 8–19 Analgesia and the control of gagging during the taking of roentgenograms.

5. Expose the anteriors (which rarely are a problem) and raise the nasal inhaler to the forehead of the patient.

6. Oxygenate the patient.

Apparatus Without Metal

1. Place the subject into the proper analgesic depth and maintain him there during the exposure of all films except the upper anteriors.

2. Raise the nasal inhaler to the forehead and expose the upper anterior films.

3. Oxygenate the patient.

Note: The Tongue Technique. Many patients who gag when asked to hold the film with their finger, or when a film holder is used, will be able to keep the film in proper position with their tongue, without gagging. This technique is applicable only to maxillary films.

ORTHODONTICS

Relative analgesia is used in orthodontic procedure to control salivation and during the following:

1. Impression taking. See the section on impression taking and the control of gagging.

2. Fitting and cementing bands; adjusting orthodontic wires.

3. Intra-oral adjustments.

4. Determining the centric relation.

ORAL SURGERY

Analgesia performs with telling effect in surgical procedures. The *reduction of awareness,* including the dulling of the sounds of the instruments,

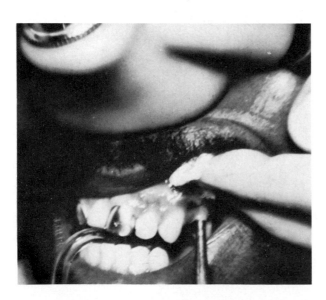

Figure 8–20 Use of the elevator: under analgesia the sound of the instrument is not misinterpreted as pain.

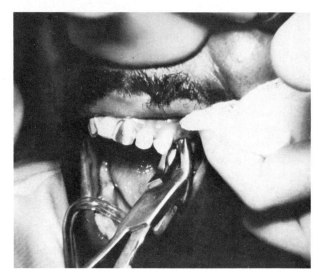

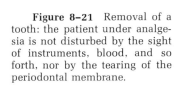

Figure 8-21 Removal of a tooth: the patient under analgesia is not disturbed by the sight of instruments, blood, and so forth, nor by the tearing of the periodontal membrane.

makes the entire procedure much less of a trial to the patient (Figs. 8–20 to 8–22).

Analgesia and Local Anesthesia. Analgesia is used synergistically with local anesthesia: the patient is first put into the analgesic state and then the injection is made (Fig. 8–23). The level of analgesia is maintained throughout the entire surgical procedure. Complete elimination of pain is more likely to result when local anesthesia and analgesia are employed together.

Radically Involved Teeth. Teeth that are extremely loose can be removed with analgesia alone.

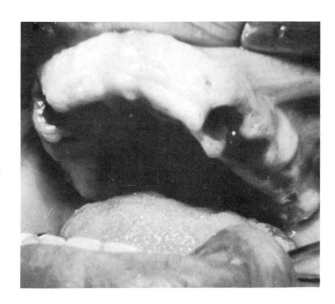

Figure 8-22 Alveolectomy of the left and right tuberosity areas. If two sessions are required, the patient who has been given analgesia will not fear the second procedure.

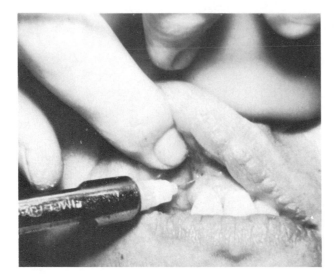

Figure 8–23 Elimination of the fear and pain of injection by means of analgesia.

Lengthy Surgical Procedures (Figs. 8–24 and 8–25). Since a patient under analgesia is unaware of the lapse of time, he does not become apprehensive and uncooperative during lengthy surgical procedures. The operator is thus less harried and can perform more efficiently and with greater dispatch. At the end of the procedure, no matter how much time it has taken, the patient does not feel "all in." Neither does the operator.

Analgesia as Conditioning for General Anesthesia. A patient who has been trained in the use of analgesia makes an excellent anesthesia patient: he is accustomed to breathing through the nasal inhaler; he knows what his preliminary symptoms will be; and, accepting them readily, he slides smoothly into the proper stage of anesthesia.

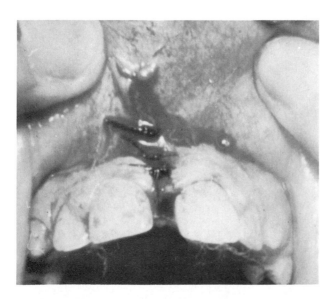

Figure 8–24 A frenectomy done with analgesia and local anesthesia. The orbicularis oris does not contract to interfere with the placing of sutures, and the nasal inhaler does not hinder the dentist performing the surgical procedure.

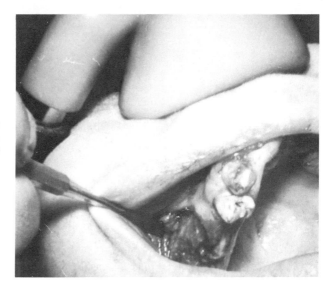

Figure 8-25 Alveolectomy of the right tuberosity area. Under analgesia, the patient is unaware of the lapse of time.

Postoperative Sequelae. After one has used analgesia for a considerable period of time, he is forcibly struck by the paucity of postoperative sequelae. This does not mean that in every case there is a complete absence of postoperative symptoms. However, every dentist who employs analgesia for surgical procedures agrees that, because patients under analgesia are relaxed and are not apprehensive before or during surgery, they are less likely to develop adverse postoperative sequelae.

Treating Abscesses. Analgesia is used to great advantage in the incision and drainage of abscesses and in postoperative irrigations and the removal of sutures (Figs. 8-26 and 8-27).

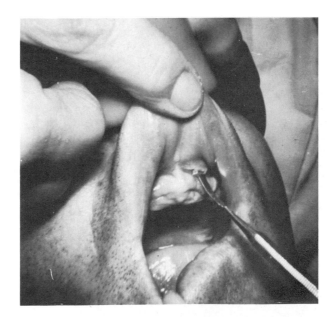

Figure 8-26 The incision and draining of an abscess with analgesia alone.

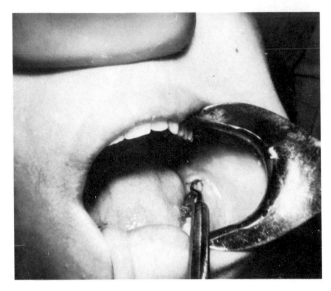

Figure 8-27 Curettage: establishing drainage for a pericoronal infection with the patient under analgesia (no local anesthesia is necessary).

ENDODONTICS[29]

In no field of dentistry is there greater patient apprehension than in the practice of endodontics. Fear of having a "nerve removed" is almost universal. In the view of endodontists who have made extensive use of relative analgesia, nothing is of greater efficacy in obtaining better patient acceptance of treatment.

PREMEDICATION

Rarely is it necessary to use sedatives or tranquilizers when relative analgesia is utilized, especially when the referred patient has undergone the experience of the sedative and analgesic effects of nitrous oxide. Those who have never experienced analgesia present a somewhat different but not difficult problem. In endodontic practice, patients are usually seen for no more than two to four visits. However, many patients arrive at the office with pain, fear, and swelling, not having slept for several nights. They want immediate relief and they are in a frame of mind to accept any measures that will accomplish this end. Acceptance of and introduction to analgesia under these circumstances is quickly accomplished. Another great advantage of sedation with nitrous oxide is the rapid recuperation and absence of after-effects, which make it unnecessary to have the patient accompanied by another individual.

ELECTRIC PULP TESTING

With extremely sensitive teeth electric pulp testing can be a painful experience. If local anesthesia is employed, differentiation of response is impossible. However, with the use of relative analgesia it is possible to diminish pulpal responses without eliminating them.

ACUTE APICAL ABSCESS AND CELLULITIS

In acute cases, effective local anesthesia is difficult to obtain because of the acidic condition in the inflamed tissues. With the use of a new bur in an ultra-high speed handpiece it is possible to penetrate into the pulp (in most cases) in less than 30 seconds. Using a high dose of nitrous oxide analgesia (3 liters of oxygen and 8 liters of nitrous oxide) for that short time permits a painless entrance. By the time the patient has returned to normalcy, drainage will have been established.

In cases of acute cellulitis where localization of exudate has occurred, incision and drainage can be swiftly executed with a new, disposable scalpel. The concomitant use of a high dose of nitrous oxide for 30 seconds or less permits a painless incision and drainage procedure.

TOPICAL ANESTHETIC SUBSTITUTE

Although topical anesthetics are useful, they may take a few minutes to become completely effective. Additionally, some may cause tissue necrosis or be allergenic. Nitrous oxide analgesia is effective rapidly, precluding the necessity of using topical anesthetics, with their possible drawbacks.

PAINLESS INJECTION

Relative analgesia is of tremendous value in eliminating the fear and pain of the injection needle and of the forcing of the fluid into the tissue.

POSITIONING OF RUBBER DAM CLAMP

The use of relative analgesia is helpful in relieving the usually moderate pain and discomfort of placing a rubber dam clamp on an intact crown with a cervical bulge. However, with a badly broken-down tooth crown, the gingival tissue will usually have to be impinged upon during the clamp application. Relative analgesia and local anesthesia are used synergistically when necessary.

PULPECTOMY

In the extirpation of a vital pulp it is essential that a local anesthetic be used. Nitrous oxide analgesia is a highly important adjunct in this procedure for its ataractic effect. When only pulpal tissue shreds remain, analgesia alone will usually suffice. In those instances in which the pulpal shreds are extremely sensitive, intrapulpal injections of a local anesthetic are frequently necessary. This is usually a very painful procedure unless relative analgesia is employed as an adjunct.

INSTRUMENTATION

It is extremely difficult to limit instrumentation to the confines of the root canal. Penetrating slightly beyond the apex can be a painful experience.

Inhalation analgesia helps to minimize the patient's perception of the pain. Where a periapical lesion is present deliberate instrumentation beyond the apex is done for fluid evacuation and possible cyst destruction. Granulomas and radicular cysts contain nerve tissue, so that penetration into these areas creates pain. Local anesthesia in combination with relative analgesia solves this problem.

POSTOPERATIVE APICAL PERIODONTITIS

Between visits an apical periodontitis (pericementitis) may develop. This may be the result of any of the following:
1. Overinstrumentation.
2. Application of irritating medicaments.
3. Antigen-antibody hypersensitivity reaction.
4. Microbes or their products interacting with the host.
5. Occlusal trauma.

As a result, a fluid exudate or transudate is produced which exerts pressure on the apical periodontal ligament and causes pain. A frequently indicated treatment is to open the canal under a rubber dam and allow the canal to remain patent for a few minutes. This relieves the pressure and permits the accumulated fluids to escape. If local anesthesia is used for the procedure, the patient cannot inform the doctor whether or not the pain has subsided. If relative analgesia has been administered, the doctor can readily ascertain whether the symptoms have been relieved.

ROOT CANAL OBTURATION

Filling of the root canal can be painful to the patient, especially when excess filling material or cement is expressed beyond the apex. The use of relative analgesia diminishes the patient's awareness so that the procedure is

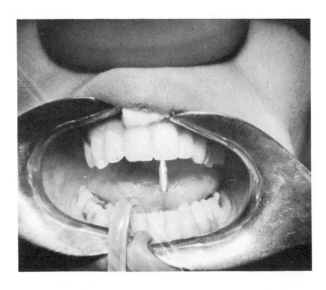

Figure 8–28 Emergency treatment: establishing drainage through the canal of a tooth with acute pericementitis while the patient is under analgesia (no local anesthesia is utilized).

tolerated much better. When endodontic implant obturations are being inserted it is essential that local anesthesia be employed in addition. Nerve fibers and blood vessels are present in periapical bone. The local anesthesia controls the pain, the incorporated vasoconstrictor controls the hemorrhage, and the analgesia controls the patient's reactions.

SURGICAL ENDODONTICS

Endodontic surgical procedures such as apicoectomy, periapical curettage, retrograde amalgam seal, hemisection, root amputation, transplantation, replantation, and implantation are often time consuming and involved. Even very good dental patients tend to become apprehensive and restless. The utilization of relative analgesia allows the patient's thoughts to travel beyond the confines of the office, so that the procedure becomes much more tolerable. With the use of a soft rubber nasal inhaler it is not necessary to remove it for the taking of roentgenograms. If a plastic rubber dam frame is employed it need not be removed for x-ray exposures. There is thus less opportunity for salivary contamination and for stimulating the gag reflex.

Frequently it is difficult to obtain complete anesthesia with a local anesthetic when injecting into a granulomatous area. Nitrous oxide analgesia helps in this procedure. It also diminishes the patient's response to the normally painful intraosseous injection. Should there have been some pain, the partial amnesic effect is of great value, especially with the child-patient.

POSTOPERATIVE TREATMENT

Removal of sutures and drains are considered minor procedures. They may be painful for the patient. Relative analgesia helps in alleviating the pain and the anticipation of pain.

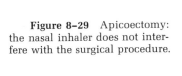

Figure 8–29 Apicoectomy: the nasal inhaler does not interfere with the surgical procedure.

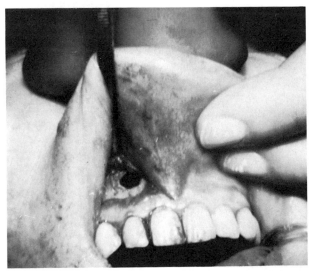

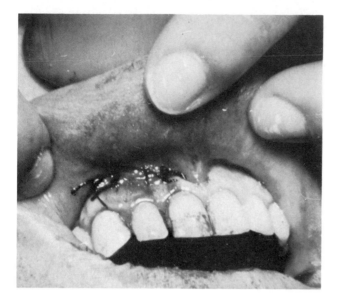

Figure 8–30 Suturing after apicoectomy: with analgesia less awareness means greater patient cooperation.

PROSTHODONTICS

In the preparation and fitting of dental prostheses, relative analgesia is recommended for all of the following procedures.

FIXED PROSTHESIS

1. The preparation of abutment teeth (Fig. 8–31).
2. Impression taking. In this procedure, analgesia is used to minimize the

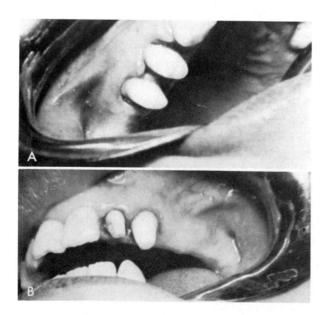

Figure 8–31 With relative analgesia, preparations for full coverage may be done on two quadrants at one sitting (very often without local anesthesia).

pain caused by band pressure against the gingival tissue, by heat and cold, and by retraction procedures for rubber base impressions. See also the section on the control of gagging.

3. The removal of temporary coverings at subsequent visits.

4. Grinding in and fitting individual abutments or the entire fixed prosthesis.

5. Sterilization of teeth and cementation.

PARTIAL AND FULL PROSTHESES

1. The preparation of abutment teeth to properly receive clasps or attachments.

2. Determining the centric relationship (Fig. 8–32). Frequently encountered is the patient on whom it is almost impossible to determine the correct centric relationship. He is either a tense individual or one who is so anxious to cooperate and help that he thrusts his mandible into every position but the centric relation. To counteract this, first see that the patient is under relative analgesia, and then tip the operating chair back slightly. Watch how easily the mandible slips back into the most relaxed, most retruded position.

Eliminating Premature Points of Contact. Relative analgesia is also helpful in the removal of premature points of contact, since keeping the patient relaxed permits him to give more authentic markings for correct spot grinding.

Fitting Immediate Full Dentures (Fig. 8–33). The initial insertion of an immediate full denture is traumatic to most people. For example, when the remaining teeth have been extracted from both sides of the jaw, local anesthe-

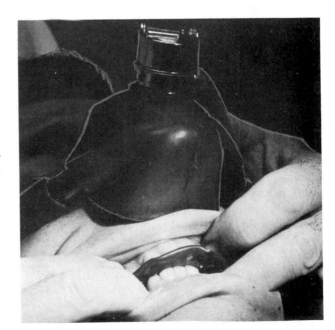

Figure 8–32 The taking of centric relationships under relative analgesia.

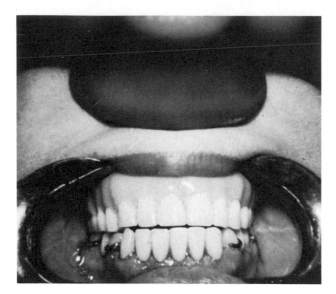

Figure 8-33 Insertion of immediate full upper denture: pain, trauma, and gagging are minimized with relative analgesia.

sia may have been employed bilaterally, or alveolectomy may have been needed, and either procedure makes the fitting difficult. Gagging may also be a problem, to say nothing of the psychological reaction to the loss of that last remaining tooth. When analgesia is used, the experience is far less traumatic and, if the remaining teeth are mobile, no local anesthesia is needed. Moreover, initial gagging is adequately controlled, and the lessened awareness of the entire procedure and of how long it is taking makes for a happier patient and a far happier dentist.

PEDODONTICS

The child's prerogative is to be a "child" in the dental chair. Just as the infant suffers a biological helplessness which induces anxiety, so the child-patient may become fearful of the state of immobilization necessitated by the dental procedure. The infant is dependent upon parental authority and, although the parent nurtures the child, he also causes discomfort through interference with the child's oral pleasure-seeking needs. Similarly, the child-patient is dependent upon dental authority and, although the dentist cares for the patient's oral conditions, he also probes the oral cavity and may thereby touch off profound feelings of impending danger. Since the dental situation readily lends itself to symbolization of early life situations, it can therefore evoke much of the threat which the patient experienced in the past.

The adult has the advantage of years to his credit, years which permitted him both to develop and to exercise some controls relative to overt emotional response. The child's immaturity restricts him primarily to acting out his feelings, a response which involves the additional threat of disapproval or retaliation from the individual in authority. Furthermore, the adult has free choice in regard to the care of his teeth, whereas the child has no alternative for, if he does not comply, he is forced into submission.

Fear of the dental experience in the adult arises from a broader background of experience. To the child everything is new and unknown, and the younger the child, the fewer the opportunities he has had to develop the capacity to "decentralize" himself. Consequently he is very close to his fears. In the early development of intelligence the child tends to divide the world of reality into the "good" and the "bad." His initial concept is that he is endlessly the object of the benevolent or malevolent thoughts and actions of others. For these reasons the child-patient may be overwhelmed when he perceives the dentist as a threatening, frightening figure.

Additional factors influence the child's response to the dental situation. These are the common stresses associated with basic needs that affect the individual at different age levels throughout life. Since growth and development occur with comparative rapidity from early childhood to adolescence, there is a succession of adaptations that the child is required to make. At the three to six year old level, the child experiences conflict between his need for extrafamilial contacts and cooperative play and the threat of entering school with its unfamiliar world of strange children and adults. These on-going difficulties in adjustment may enter into the child's relationship with the dentist.

Bell,[2] in her study of the dental treatment of children, points up the similarities between the child's school and dental experiences. In each situation, attendance is largely outside the control of the child and therefore demands a certain docility on his part. Secondly, each situation tends to restrict the activities of the child to a considerable extent. And finally, each situation furnishes an occasion for bringing the young child into contact with an adult in authority. The burden of responsibility for improved relationship between the child-patient and the dentist rests primarily with the dentist. When the dentist's behavior communicates sympathy and understanding, the patient is ready to relinquish his controls against anticipated pain and to give himself over to dental treatment. The dentist who is sensitive to the psychological significance of the oral cavity and its component parts will approach the child-patient with these thoughts in mind.

The Fearful Child-Patient[21] (Fig. 8–34)

Because the nervous and fearful child is usually a victim of maternal overprotection, treatment often involves the handling of the oversolicitous mother in addition to the child himself. By clinging to the child and by their show of exaggerated anxiety, these mothers suggest to the child that he is in for a terrible experience. In most instances it would be far better for such mothers to stay out of the treatment room. However, if either the child or the mother insists on her presence, permission should be granted but with the stipulation that the mother is not to enter into the conversation.

On the fearful child's first visit to the dentist, a great deal of patience and tact is necessary in order to begin the task of creating a good dental patient. Treatment should not be introduced immediately, but rather the dentist

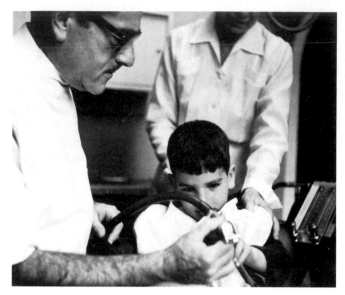

Figure 8-34   The fearful child-patient.

should get to know his patient. Play with him; talk with him; show him models, old dentures, and instruments; ride the chair up and down; let him marvel as the saliva ejector drinks a cup of water (Fig. 8–35). In short, get him to like you. Let him also handle the revolving handpiece. In this way he learns to play an active role as a dentist, which is the child's natural way of mastering anxiety derived from the passive, submissive position. Thus the dentist, by playing with the child, by coming down to his level, builds up a transference, a confidence, and the child does not feel that he faces an overwhelming situation.

OBJECTIVES IN TREATING THE CHILD-PATIENT

In the treatment of the child-patient, we must keep in mind three broad attainable objectives. First, we must quickly and effectively change the tense and often frightened child into one who will readily and, hopefully, enthusiastically accept our treatment. Secondly, once this has been achieved we must then perform the diagnostic, operative, surgical, prosthetic, corrective, or preventive measures without hurting, gagging, or frightening our patient. Thirdly, it is our obligation to the youngster to measure up to the best that dentistry can offer; that is, we must not permit any reduction in our high standards of dental treatment.

Relaxing the Patient. To accomplish the first objective of relaxing the child, reducing his anxieties, and preparing him to accept treatment, relative analgesia with nitrous oxide and oxygen is ideal. It rarely requires any special preparation of the child with respect to meals or premedication. Seldom is any work performed during the first visit, except on an emergency basis.

On the first visit, the primary discussion with the parent is an important factor not only in obtaining the essentials of the child's history but also in giving the parent a clear understanding of the reasons for this approach to child dental care. It is the first step in achieving our objectives. The clinical examination of the child's mouth is then done, followed by the taking of roentgenograms, if this is no trial for the patient. Should it create a problem, it would be wise to delay this part of the procedure until it can be done under analgesia.

In introducing analgesia, the nose-piece could be shown to the child, and if he allows it without too much protest, it should be placed on his nose. The dentist or the dental assistant could also don a nasal inhaler to demonstrate to the child how easy and interesting this is (Fig. 8–36). All this is done in a simple, quiet, matter-of-fact fashion, the child receiving the impression that this is the way things are always done in the dentist's office. Of course, we call upon all the props and word pictures mentioned previously. The extent of the discussion and its level will depend entirely on the child himself, his age, intelligence, and anxieties. As a rule, the younger the child the more readily are the dentist's suggestions accepted at face value.

Performing the Dental Procedure.   At the following visit, the nasal inhaler is a familiar instrument, and thus treatment can be begun. In most children analgesia induces a state of euphoria and a feeling of relaxation. The mouth opens freely, in a loose manner, and the child is susceptible to suggestion. Of course, the suggestions made are geared to his age level and intelligence. For example, the high-pitched sound of the airotor apparatus could be the sound of an airplane or "Whistling Charlie," and the squirting of water is to "wash the tooth" (Fig. 8–37). It is always wise to tell the young patient

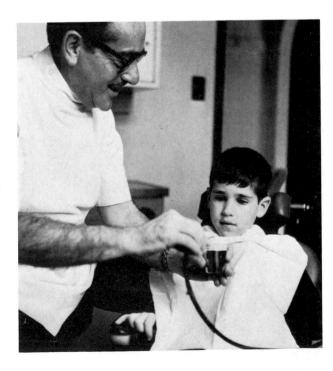

Figure 8–35 The saliva ejector magically drinks a cup of water.

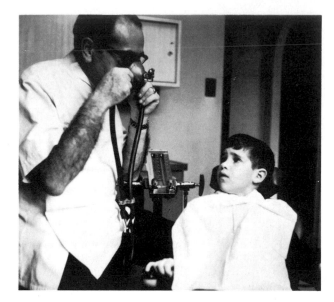

Figure 8-36   The dentist demonstrates the nasal inhaler.

what is about to occur, and to offer much praise for his performance. Once the child has accepted the procedure and the symptoms, he relaxes, and once he relaxes, the gases can take over and achieve the second objective of painless treatment. At this point, a remarkable change occurs in the patient's frame of mind.

To fulfill the pledge of complete painlessness, a local anesthetic injection will sometimes have to be administered. Every dentist is familiar with the child's reaction to this procedure. Indeed, when local anesthesia alone is employed for an extraction, the child's awareness of what is going on and his

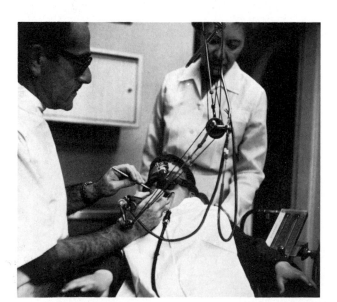

Figure 8-37   "Whistling Charlie" washes the tooth.

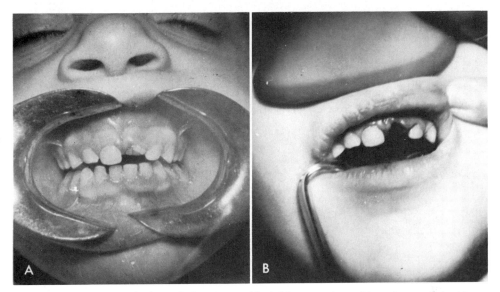

Figure 8–38 *A,* A frightened three year old child presenting with a shattered deciduous maxillary central incisor. *B,* Surgical removal of the fractured root done with care and deliberation, using analgesia and local anesthesia.

frequent fear and anxiety can often prevent treatment. With the child under analgesia, there is no problem. Relaxed under analgesia, with diminished awareness and effective local anesthesia, the patient has his tooth removed with dispatch (Figs. 8–38 to 8–40).

The Quality of Treatment. A fearful, uncooperative child-patient prevents the dentist from attaining the last objective, that of doing good dentistry. Properly introduced and administered analgesia with nitrous oxide and ox-

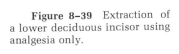

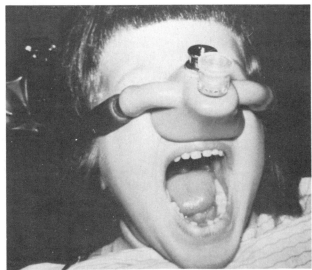

Figure 8–39 Extraction of a lower deciduous incisor using analgesia only.

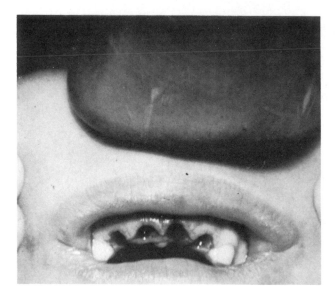

Figure 8–40 Multiple extractions for orthodontic purposes: future extractions will not be feared by this child.

ygen, by allaying fear and diminishing movement, makes it possible for the dentist to prepare difficult cavities and see to their proper filling. Moreover, the depression of the gagging reflex raises the patient's tolerance of cotton rolls, matrix bands, wedges, saliva ejectors, and water sprays. With analgesia, yet another benefit is realized: dryness of field, which is an absolute necessity for the placing of the restorative material. Without analgesia this is often a great, and sometimes insurmountable, problem. Finally, with analgesia, all four quadrants of the mouth can be treated at one sitting, if necessary.

In this manner it is possible to provide proper dental care for a child of any age, despite his fears, and to make of him a good dental patient. For most children analgesia alone is sufficient for all operative work, but for a few it will serve only as effective sedation for the local anesthetic injection. Even this is of great value, for the only other avenue of approach for this difficult management problem is premedication or co-medication. When this course is followed, the child leaves the office still under the effect of the sedative, an effect that probably lasts for many hours. Besides requiring that the child be accompanied by someone, this approach does not eliminate fear as effectively and consistently as the use of relative analgesia.

Analgesia and the Dentist's Approach to the Child-Patient

Many dental practitioners encounter difficulty in treating members of the younger generation, finding them uncooperative, restless, and fearful. Yet it is often the dentist who, by his unsympathetic approach and behavior, creates the uncooperative child-patient. It is true that some men are not emotionally constituted to successfully treat children; however, most dental practitioners have the necessary qualifications but do not employ them successfully.

In dealing with the child-patient, there is no medicament or anesthetic agent that can substitute for genuine kindliness, sympathy, and understanding. Many men faced with a recalcitrant, fearful child are themselves fearful and at a loss, and this reaction is readily imparted to the child. A sincere, friendly, and leisurely greeting, with a warm smile, can go a long way. At the same time, it is well to remember that the oral cavity has the potential for providing the child the most profound gratification and, for that reason, the deepest feelings of apprehension and threat.

Most youngsters do not want to behave in an uncooperative way. On the contrary, they welcome any assistance in controlling their fears and misgivings. This is not difficult to provide, since it calls for nothing more than gentleness, poise, and a little self-control on the part of the dentist.

Why then are some dentists fearful of the child-patient? Because they feel unequal to the task and do not know how to begin. They are afraid they will fail, and no one likes to fail. They have visions of much valuable time being wasted. Finally, they fear that their feeling of inadequacy and the wasting of valuable time will be repeated at every visit.

This frustration could be dissipated if the dentist were to have a definite modus operandi and a definite objective in mind. Most children are cooperative, although some require a little more patience and careful attention to their psychological needs than others. Only a small percentage are truly rebellious. But no matter what category the child may fall into, if the dentist will put his best foot forward and project his personality so that he gains the confidence of the child at the very first visit, he will easily solve his problem by making this child into a good analgesia patient. No longer will there be any floundering or feeling of frustration, when one has a definite objective in mind. The objective will be to introduce the child to analgesia. There will be no need for cajolery, threats, commands, or warnings.

A child accepts analgesia more readily and with less rationalization than an adult. Even though it is novel to him, if he has confidence in the dentist he

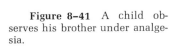

Figure 8–41 A child observes his brother under analgesia.

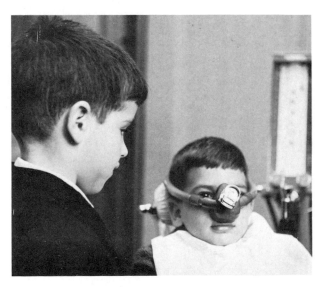

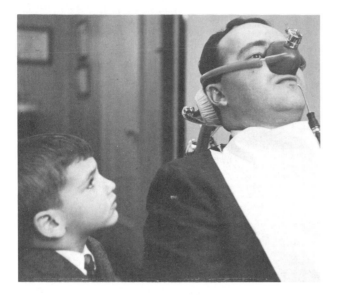

Figure 8–42 A child observes his father taking analgesia.

will not question the use of this instrument as much as would an adult. The ideal way to introduce analgesia to the child is to let him observe its use on someone else. If possible, this person should be another child, a relative, or a friend (Fig. 8–41). If one of his parents is an analgesia patient, the dentist and the dental assistant should engage the services of the parent in propagandizing the child so that he is favorably conditioned to the idea of taking analgesia at the subsequent visit (Fig. 8–42).

Once the child-patient has been introduced to analgesia, he is no longer a problem. Fear is gone. Tension and lack of cooperation are things of the past. In fact, children who are introduced to dentistry accompanied by analgesia become excellent patients. In many instances they look forward to their next

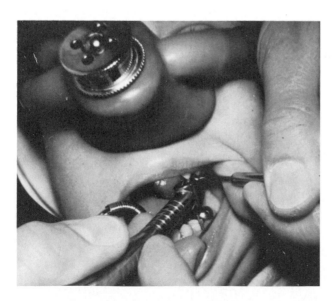

Figure 8–43 Preparations for stainless steel crowns for a five year old child are quickly and efficiently accomplished under analgesia (no local infiltration).

visit to the dentist with pleasant anticipation. Since they are cooperative, they are definitely not time-wasters. On the contrary, since preparations on deciduous teeth can be rapidly done by an experienced operator and since analgesia places no limit on the number of quadrants that can be worked on at one sitting, much work can be accomplished in a short time (Fig. 8–43).

PERPETUAL MOTION VERSUS SUSPENDED ANIMATION IN THE CHILD-PATIENT

The problems that analgesia can help solve for the dentist in treating the child-patient are not alone those of fear of pain and the pain itself. Children are, as a rule, more restless in the dental chair, their bodies moving around and their heads jerking to and fro. They would like to carry on a conversation with the dentist while he is working on the oral cavity. They salivate more, flooding the field which the operator is so desirous of keeping dry. Very often they cannot tolerate the cotton rolls, gagging as a result. And they also gag on impression taking. They want to expectorate and take a drink of water at half-minute intervals. All this may add up to a major problem for the dentist. With analgesia, however, the problem does not exist.

It is more than interesting to see the change that occurs in the child-patient under analgesia. It is best described as "suspended animation" (Fig. 8–44). The body does not move, and the head remains still. The tongue does not move around, attempting to push the cotton rolls out of the mouth or interfering with the bur. Salivation is decreased and there is no expectoration, rinsing, or drinking of water. These ideal results are obtainable if the patient is kept under analgesia until the filling operation is completed.

Once the child is under analgesia, it is well for the operator to remember that children, as a rule, are more open to suggestion than mature persons. It is therefore relatively easy to suggest good, positive thoughts to the child in the

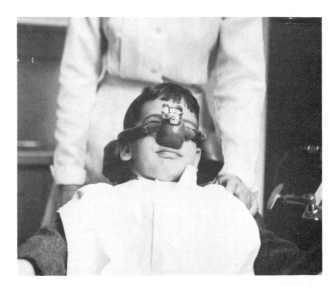

Figure 8–44 Suspended animation.

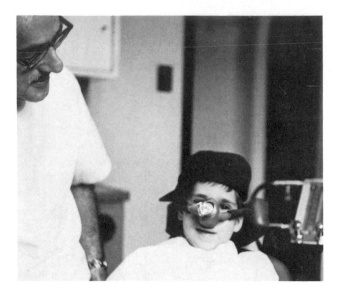

Figure 8–45 "Club member."

analgesic state. One may suggest that he is on a "Magic Flying Carpet" or that he is the pilot of an airplane and can travel to any pleasant destination he desires. He very often does take such an imaginary trip. The nasal inhaler is a pilot's mask or a space cadet's mask. He is getting space gas and is an astronaut flying to the moon. Or he is breathing peppermint air, sweet air. The approach to the child should, of course, be made on his age level. The services of a properly oriented dental assistant, secretary, or hygienist can be of great value here. The use of "props" may also be of help—for example, a Plexiglas helmet for the spaceman, a Mickey Mouse hat for the "club member," or a nasal inhaler and tubings that are painted with red and white stripes, suggesting a peppermint stick, and perhaps a tiny dab of oil of peppermint on the inside of the nasal inhaler. A touch of orange solvent could make it "orange air."

While the child is thus distracted, the dentist is doing his work with dispatch and no discomfort to the patient. This approach is economically sound in itself. In addition, parents most often become the patients of the dentist who can successfully treat their child.

By thus successfully treating the child-patient, the dentist ensures the preservation of the dental tissues and prevents the development of the patient into an adult with dental phobias. Children introduced to dental treatment via relative analgesia continue to be good dental patients in later life even without the use of relative analgesia if it is not available in their community. However, they continue to prefer dentistry with analgesia.

THE CHRONICALLY ILL OR AGED PATIENT

Until recently very little has been done to care for the oral health of chronically ill patients and the aged. Since many of these patients are confined to their beds at home, they could not expect proper dental care. Recently, however, ingenious home care instruments have been devised that are portable and can be set up at the patient's bedside in a matter of minutes. A gas machine with small cylinders of nitrous oxide and oxygen weighs very little and can easily be transported to and from a patient's home. Since the aged, the debilitated, and the chronically ill can take relative analgesia with great success, the author feels that the use of this modality would give great stimulus to adequate, effective, and expeditious treatment of this somewhat neglected segment of our society.

ORAL CANCER[18]

Because the dentist sees more apparently well patients than any other member of the health professions and because the mouth is readily available for examination, the dentist has a particular responsibility in oral cancer detection. Oral cancer is responsible for approximately 6000 deaths in the United States each year. The five year cure rate for oral cancer is less than one-third the cure rate for all cancers, constituting one of the lowest survival rates in any form of cancer. Yet, there is a potential for a high survival rate if oral cancer is diagnosed early enough. The number of victims surviving five years is doubled if treatment is initiated when the lesion is less than 2 cm. in diameter.

Dentists should perform periodic, uniform, and systematic examinations of the oral cavity of all patients, special attention being given to those 35 years of age and older. The complete oral examination should include both visual inspection and digital palpation of extra-oral areas as well as of intra-oral structures. Adequate lighting, a tongue blade or depressor, a dental mirror, gauze, and a rubber glove or finger cots are the only material requirements. Dentures should be removed before starting the examination.

Relative analgesia can be of great assistance in the performance of this examination because it allows greater ease of manipulation of the tissues and reduces the awareness of the patient. Furthermore, because the gag reflex is controlled and the musculature is more relaxed, a more thorough examination can be made of the base of the tongue and the areas posterior to it.

THE ORAL CANCER EXAMINATION

The following procedure (Figs. 8–46 to 8–65) for the detection of oral cancer has been recommended by the Oral Cancer and Detection Center of the St. Francis Hospital, Poughkeepsie, New York. The dentist should be thoroughly familiar with this procedure and, when any indication of cancer is in evidence, he should advise the patient to see his physician and, if possible, he should notify the physician himself.

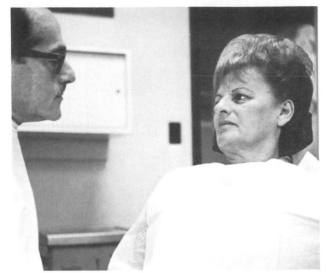

Figure 8–46 In the initial confrontation with the patient, observe generally for skin blemishes, pigmentation, moles, asymmetry, and swellings.

Figure 8–47 Palpate the preauricular, parotid, submental, and submaxillary chains of the head and the jugular and posterior cervical chains in the neck. One hand may be used to steady the head while the other palpates, in this case the submaxillary group.

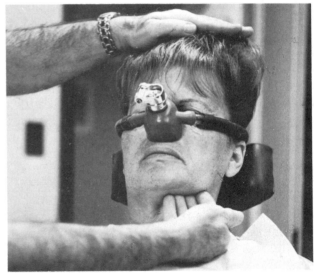

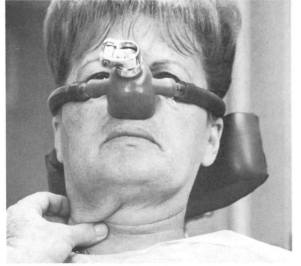

Figure 8–48 Palpate deeply with two fingers to identify the jugular chain, which includes the subdigastric group and lies beneath the sternomastoid muscle along the internal jugular vein.

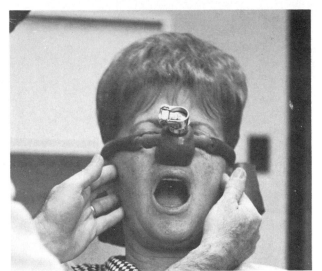

Figure 8–49 Palpate the temporomandibular joint bilaterally with the patient's mouth closed and then wide open. Note any tenderness, crepitus, or deviation.

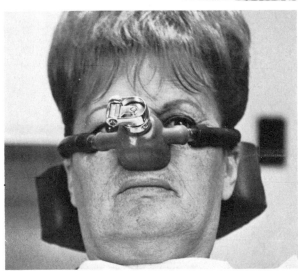

Figure 8–50 Examine the lips with the patient's mouth closed and then open. Note the color, texture, and any surface abnormalities.

Figure 8–51 Palpate the lips for any induration.

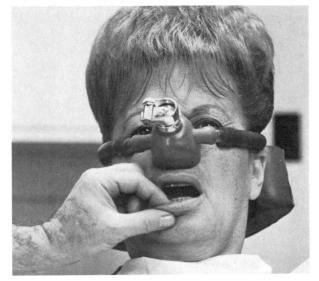

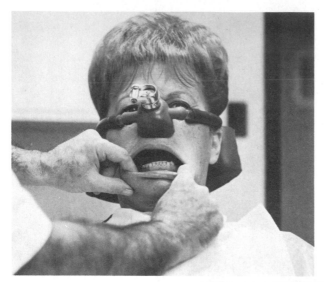

Figure 8–52 Examine visually and by palpation the mandibular mucobuccal fold (vestibule) and frenum with the patient's mouth partially open. Observe the color, character, and any swellings of the mucosa interproximally and in the vestibule.

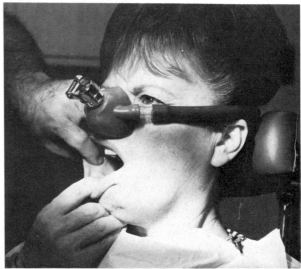

Figure 8–53 Using the fingers as retractors and with the patient's mouth wide open, examine the inner aspect of the cheek, Stensen's duct, and other areas covered by the buccal mucosa.

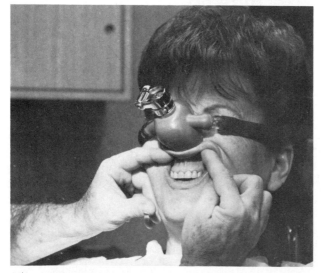

Figure 8–54 Visually and by palpation examine the maxillary mucobuccal fold and frenum with the patient's mouth partially open. Conclude by palpating the entire area.

272

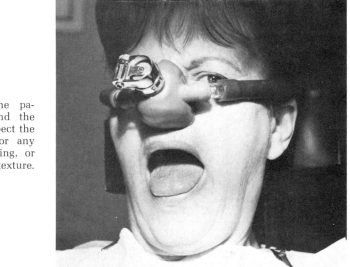

Figure 8–55 With the patient's tongue at rest and the mouth partially open, inspect the dorsum of the tongue for any swelling, ulceration, coating, or variation in size, color, or texture.

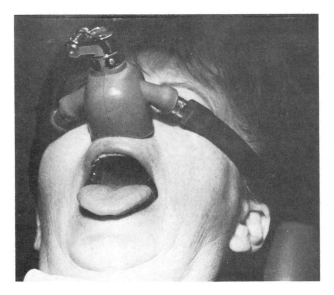

Figure 8–56 With the patient's tongue protruded, observe any deviation, tremor, asymmetry, or limitation of motion. Note any variations in texture, size, or color.

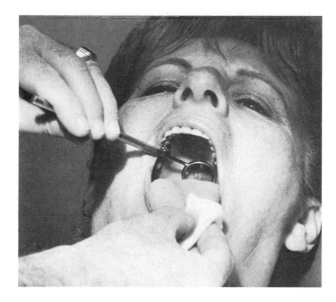

Figure 8–57   Wrap a 4 × 4 gauze square around the tip of the protruded tongue. Lightly press a warm mirror of proper size against the uvula and observe the base of the tongue and circumvallate papillae.

Figure 8–58   Holding the tongue with the gauze, gently move it to the patient's left and retract the right cheek. Observe the entire lateral border of the tongue and its attachments to the floor of the mouth back to the anterior pillar. Gently swing the tongue to the right and repeat the examination of the left lateral border.

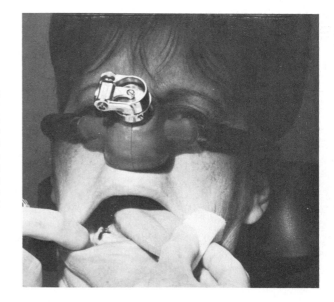

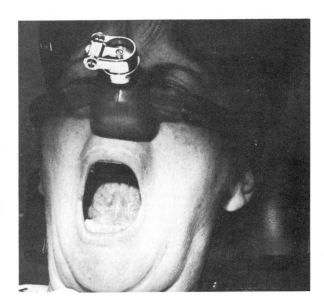

Figure 8–59 Release the tongue and instruct the patient to touch the tip of the tongue to the palate. Observe the ventral surface and note any varicosities and swellings. With the tongue still elevated, inspect the floor of the mouth for swellings or other abnormalities and note the condition of Wharton's ducts, the sublingual ridge with the openings of the sublingual ducts, and the lingual frenum.

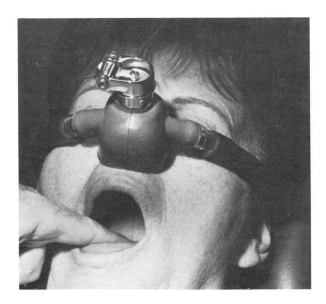

Figure 8–60 Carefully palpate the entire tongue, including the base, for any induration.

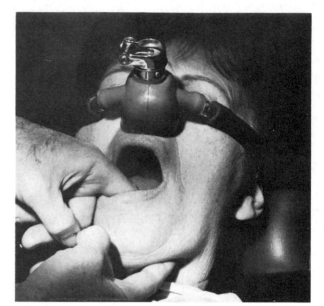

Figure 8–61 Palpate the entire floor of the mouth, and identify the submaxillary gland.

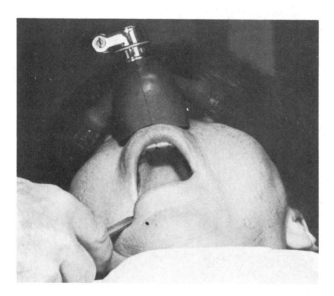

Figure 8–62 With the patient's mouth wide open and the head back, gently depress the base of the tongue with a tongue depressor or mirror. Inspect and then palpate the hard palate.

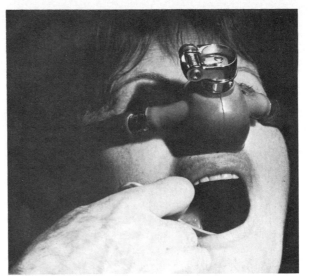

Figure 8–63 Observe and palpate the soft palate and uvula.

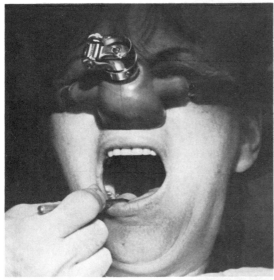

Figure 8–64 With the patient's tongue still depressed, inspect both fauces (tonsillar area) and the anterior pillars (glossopalatine arch). Instruct the patient to say "Eh," which will expose a wide area of the oropharynx for inspection.

Figure 8–65 Examine the nasopharynx by placing a mirror of suitable size behind the uvula. Tell the patient to breathe through his nose and mouth.

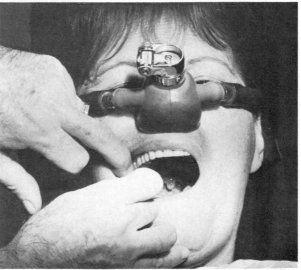

CLINICAL APPLICATIONS OF
RELATIVE ANALGESIA IN MEDICINE

Relative analgesia with nitrous oxide and oxygen has a multitude of uses for the physician. In order to make proper use of this modality and gain valid and valuable results, the physician (as with the dentist) must first properly introduce the patient to analgesia so that he accepts it and can relax under it. Once the physician has mastered the technique, he will find it useful in the following situations and procedures:

1. *Differential diagnosis in cardiac conditions.* It is sometimes difficult to differentiate between a so-called "nervous" heart and a heart with organic disease. Electrocardiogram readings cannot be taken at face value because of the erratic tracings produced by the overly tense individual. Since nitrous oxide itself causes no change in cardiac output or rate, it can be used to relax the patient, and the electrocardiogram reading can then be taken while the patient is in the state of relative analgesia.

2. *Patients with hypertension* (nervous high blood pressure). There are many people whose blood pressure rises when a blood pressure reading is being taken. In these cases also, a truer reading will be obtained if the patient (properly introduced) is under the influence of relative analgesia. Nitrous oxide itself has no effect on blood pressure when used for relative analgesia.

3. *Psychoanalysis and psychiatric care.* Because of its relaxing effect and its ability to produce a state of euphoria and to allow the subconscious mind to function more easily, relative analgesia can be of great help in psychoanalysis. It can also function with great effect in the treatment of psychiatric patients.

4. *Venipuncture.* Nitrous oxide inhalation makes the surface veins more prominent and thus more accessible for venipuncture.

5. *Postoperative analgesic.* Because of its analgesic capabilities and minimal irritation, nitrous oxide is used as an analgesic following thoracic or pulmonary surgery.

6. *Cystoscopy.*
7. *Changing and removing of dressings.*
8. *Incisions.*
9. *Suturing and removing sutures.*
10. *Removing foreign bodies.*
11. *Irrigations.*
12. *Insertion and removal of drains.*
13. *Injections.*
14. *Placing and removal of casts.*
15. *Painful or uncomfortable examination procedures.*
16. *Esophageal dilation.*
17. *Gastroscopy.*
18. *Proctoscopy.*

THE UTILIZATION OF RELATIVE ANALGESIA
FOR THE HYPNOTIC INDUCTION OF COMPLETELY
RESISTANT PATIENTS

Bleadon and Sugarman[3] had experienced the hypnotic trance countless times and thus, when they were exposed to relative analgesia with nitrous oxide and oxygen, they were struck by the similarity of sensations. They set about investigating the effects of utilizing hypnotic induction techniques on themselves while in the state of analgesia. The results were spectacular. Hypnotic induction was brought about almost immediately. A euphoric state with diminution of conscious awareness and muscular relaxation in excess of the degree usually obtainable with relative analgesia were evidenced, and this was brought about in 30 seconds. The nitrous oxide was then turned off and the investigators breathed only oxygen and air while the usual hypnotic induction procedure continued. Each investigator remained in a hypnotic trance much deeper than he had ever experienced before, and each remained in that state until the signal to come out of the trance was given.

The decision was made to try this approach on resistant patients with whom they had failed repeatedly with the usual hypnotic techniques. It was found that deep trances could now be induced in these patients as quickly as in good hypnotic subjects. Posthypnotic suggestion was then utilized: the subjects were told that subsequently they would go into a trance with the usual induction methods. This was also highly successful. One patient explained the results in this manner: "I always had my mind wandering with many thoughts, but with the combination of this gas and hypnosis I become completely calm, and my attention is completely fixed on your conversation."

Ten resistant subjects in whom no demonstrable hypnotic state could be obtained were asked to try this new approach. All 10 were easily induced into a deep trance with the aid of relative analgesia. The case reports of two of these patients are described below:

Case Report.   A 22 year old woman had a severe obesity problem; her weight was 272 pounds, her height 5 feet 2 inches. She complained of severe depression because of continual criticism by members of her family and friends. She had received some psychiatric counseling, which, however, did not solve her obesity problem.

Hypnotic induction was started with the aid of relative analgesia. Although previously no results were obtainable, the results were now both rapid and good. The patient related that formerly she felt herself fighting the doctor, but now she was able to relax and permit her attention to be completely fixed on the operator's conversation. She was repeatedly treated with this approach. As a result of ego-strengthening suggestions relative to dieting, she began to lose weight steadily and her feelings of depression completely disappeared. Her dietary control was so excellent that she lost 100 pounds in four months.

Case Report.   The patient was a 16 year old girl, a fairly good hypnotic subject in whom no traumatic events could be elicited on exploration. Subjected to the hypnotic technique with the aid of relative analgesia, she was unable to regress spontaneously on several occasions to the ages between two and five and to recall specific events of which she had no conscious memory, but her parents revealed that these events had taken place.

Bleadon and Sugarman believe that this field warrants further investigation. In their experience the arduous task of working with the resistant patient was made easy. Additionally, they were not confronted with the collateral problems that are raised when barbiturates and tranquilizers and the intravenous route are employed. They were at all times treating a patient who was awake and capable of speaking. Furthermore, the patient's recovery of all mental, muscular, and balancing faculties took no more than 1 minute.

Hypnosis has also become useful in dentistry as an aid in eliminating fear and anxiety. In this regard, the use of nitrous oxide as relative analgesia not only eliminates the long induction period in almost all cases but it also makes it possible to obtain hypnosis in nearly every case.

BREATHING CARDIAC PAIN AWAY[25]

Pain associated with acute myocardial infarction is currently alleviated by narcotic analgesics, such as morphine sulfate. However, it is well recognized that these agents, though effective, may create undesirable side effects, such as nausea or cardiac complications. This drawback has prompted a continuing search for more tolerable but effective analgesics. One recent observation is that nitrous oxide may be successfully used to relieve myocardial infarction pain, usually without side effects.

A study undertaken at the Peter Bent Brigham Hospital and the cardiovascular laboratories, Harvard School of Public Health, suggests that nitrous oxide is an effective sedative and analgesic for less severe pain and is a valuable adjunct to standard drugs for more recurrent pain.

Dr. Bernard Lown, associate professor of cardiology at Harvard, and Dr. Peter L. Thompson, a fellow in cardiology at Harvard, set up a controlled study.

A total of 108 patients were given inhalations of nitrous oxide over a $2\frac{1}{2}$ year period in the two-part study. One part compared the efficacy of a mixture of 35 per cent nitrous oxide and 65 per cent oxygen with 100 per cent oxygen in a double-blind study; the other part observed use of the gas mixture in conjunction with other analgesics.

Patients were asked to inhale the gas by face mask in an attempt to relieve pain. Both oxygen and the nitrous oxide mixture were given for 5 minutes; neither the nurse nor the patient knew the sequence of administration. Patients were asked to grade their pain from mild to agonizing, and nurses ranked patient appearance as asleep, comfortable, uncomfortable, or distressed. Pulse, blood pressure, and respiratory readings were taken.

Forty-five patients received 55 inhalations for relief of pain following this protocol, Dr. Thompson reported to the American College of Cardiology in Chicago. Forty-five per cent of patients obtained complete relief from pain after inhaling the 35 per cent nitrous oxide mixture; 35 per cent reported partial relief, and 20 per cent said there was no effect. In contrast, the oxygen administration gave partial relief to 30 per cent of patients and had no effect on 70 per cent.

A breakdown of the double-blind study showed that when oxygen was the first gas administered, no patients received complete relief of pain, 11 claimed partial relief, and 16 said that the gas had no effect. When nitrous oxide was substituted for the oxygen in the second 5 minute period, 13 patients felt complete relief, eight felt partial relief, and six felt no relief of pain.

When nitrous oxide was the first gas administered to patients in the study, nine received total and 11 received partial relief of pain; eight reported no effect. After oxygen substitution for the second 5 minutes, no patient reported complete relief, three felt partial relief, and 16 no effect.

Patient response was dependent on severity of pain, Dr. Thompson reported. According to the study, 70 per cent of episodes of mild pain were relieved, and only 20 per cent of moderate, severe, or agonizing pain was alleviated. No significant changes were observed in blood pressure or heart rates, and side effects were minimal. Administration had to be stopped only three times.

"Inhalation of nitrous oxide does not compromise needed oxygen supply for these patients, as the oxygen administered in the mixture is adequate." The Harvard group is also investigating the effect of longer periods of administration, as well as higher concentrations of nitrous oxide. A mixture of 65 per cent nitrous oxide has been used effectively.

"Nitrous oxide is not as potent or effective for stopping pain as narcotics," said Dr. Thompson, "but we have found it is effective for some pain and that we can administer the gas on top of an initial dose of the narcotic analgesic." He reported one example: Recurrent pain was a problem for a 72 year old female patient who had evolved an inferior infarct. Morphine sulfate (8 mg. intravenously) and 35 per cent nitrous oxide controlled the pain. When treatment was discontinued, pain returned, but it was subsequently controlled with the nitrous oxide. Small doses of morphine were ineffective the next time pain recurred, but 65 per cent nitrous oxide was effective immediately.

"By continuing inhalation of 35 per cent [nitrous oxide] and boosting concentration to 65 per cent for short periods when required, pain was adequately controlled," Dr. Thompson reported. "In general usage in the coronary care unit, it has not replaced usual analgesics; but nitrous oxide has proved a valuable aid to sedation and analgesia in persistent and recurrent pain."

This report is significant not only in pointing up another medical use for nitrous oxide–oxygen analgesia, but also in demonstrating its great safety and minimal side effects even in these very ill patients.

NITROUS OXIDE–OXYGEN ANALGESIA IN OFFICE GASTROENTEROLOGY[26]

Although nitrous oxide–oxygen analgesia is being used in increased frequency to control fear, allay pain, and comfort the patient in dental practice, the medical profession has been very slow in adapting this for office procedures. It appears that this is so because it is not taught, it is not discussed, and it is not written about, presumably since it is hardly being used. In my own case, my close friend, Dr. Norman Menken, had been suggesting it to me for years and I admit that I was reluctant to consider it. But finally, the kind loan of an analgesia machine by Dr. Harry Langa, Dr. Menken's continued persuasions, and my own personal experience with nitrous oxide–oxygen analgesia as a dental patient prevailed, and I began to use it in my practice.

The uncomfortable or painful procedures done in the practice of office gastroenterology are instrumental examination of the esophagus (esophagoscopy), of the stomach (gastroscopy), of the colon (colonoscopy), and of the rectum and distal sigmoid (proctosigmoidoscopy), and instrumental dilatation of strictures or other lesions of the esophagus or rectum.

The purpose of this paper is to present my experience with a series of 100 cases done at my office, using nitrous oxide–oxygen analgesia, compared with 100 cases done in the hospital by myself, using on the average 50 mg. of Demerol (meperidine) and 50 mg. Vistaril (hydroxyzine pamoate) administered intramuscularly for sedation and analgesia. Patients of both series were also given 1/150 gr. of Atropine intramuscularly and 5 per cent Cyclaine Topical Solution (hexylcaine) for topical anesthesia, exclusive of rectal and colonic cases. At the conclusion of each case treatment a record was made regarding the degree of suppression of the gag reflex and the total evaluation of the examination with regard to ease of introduction of the instrument, degree of satisfactory completion of the examination, and comfort of the patient, and these were classified as shown in Table 8–1.

The results indicated that good to excellent suppression of the gag reflex occurred in 99 per cent of the cases with nitrous oxide–oxygen analgesia, compared to 89 per cent with Demerol-Vistaril sedanalgesia. Good to excellent examination was made in 98 per cent of cases with nitrous oxide compared to 85 per cent with Demerol-Vistaril. There was only one instance or poor examination or failure using nitrous oxide–oxygen analgesia compared to poor results in 12 cases using drug sedanalgesia (Tables 8–2 and 8–3).

TABLE 8–1   Classification of Analgesia Response

CLASSIFICATION	GAG CONTROL	TOTAL EVALUATION
Excellent	No interfering gagging.	Complete ease of instrumentation. Minimal discomfort. Complete examination done.
Good	Slight gagging.	Moderate discomfort to patient. No interference with complete examination.
Fair	Frequent gagging during procedure.	Problems in passage or during examination, but successful.
Poor	Major gagging.	Major difficulties, but procedure completed with varying success.
Failure	Insurmountable gagging.	Unsuccessful examination.

TABLE 8-2 Gag Control—Comparison of 100 Cases with Nitrous
Oxide–Oxygen and 100 Cases with Demerol–Vistaril

CLASSIFICATION	NITROUS OXIDE–OXYGEN	DEMEROL–VISTARIL
Excellent	85%	64%
Good	14	25
Fair	1	5
Poor	0	6
Failure	0	0

Most of the procedures done consisted of various combinations of esophagoscopy with biopsy, gastroscopy with biopsy, cinephotography and esophageal dilatation (Table 8-4).

The method of nitrous oxide–oxygen analgesia used was that recommended and outlined by Dr. Langa. A continuous flow analgesia machine was used with the oxygen flow set at 3 liters per minute, the nitrous oxide flow at an average of 6 liters per minute, and the air (inhaling) valve at the 1/4 open position (Table 8-5). Occasionally the air valve was closed off by finger pressure for a few minutes to secure deeper analgesia. In no way did the nose-piece or connecting tubing interfere with the transpharyngeal passage of instruments into the esophagus or stomach. The valuable suggestions concerning proper psychological preparation and reinforcement, described by Menken, were followed and proved very helpful. The average duration of nitrous oxide administration was 9 minutes (Table 8-6). The ages of the patients ranged from 11 to 85 (Table 8-7), and many of the patients had compensated cardiovascular disease. There were no adverse reactions to nitrous oxide–oxygen analgesia.

Of special interest was a subjective comparison of the two methods of analgesia by patients who required a series of treatments and therefore were exposed to both methods more or less alternately. Twenty-one of 22 patients preferred nitrous oxide–oxygen analgesia to Demerol (Table 8-8). It was also noted that in the series there were five patients who described little or no sensation that they were receiving nitrous oxide, although the obtundation of their gag reflex and tolerance of the procedure were satisfactory. Of these, two were alcoholic and three had marked anxiety neuroses. In seven patients, marked anxiety was greatly relieved by nitrous oxide–oxygen analgesia, and

TABLE 8-3 Total Evaluation—Comparison of 100 Cases with Nitrous
Oxide–Oxygen and 100 Cases with Demerol–Vistaril

CLASSIFICATION	NITROUS OXIDE–OXYGEN	DEMEROL–VISTARIL
Excellent	80%	62%
Good	18	23
Fair	1	3
Poor	0	5
Failure	1	7

TABLE 8-4   Analysis of Procedures

PROCEDURE	100 CASES DONE WITH NITROUS OXIDE–OXYGEN ANALGESIA	100 CASES DONE WITH DEMEROL–VISTARIL
Gastroscopy and/or esophagoscopy with biopsy and cinephotography	48	95
Esophageal dilatation	36	2
Colonoscopy	7	3
Sigmoidoscopy	5	0
Rectal dilatation	4	0

TABLE 8-5   Dosages and Settings of Analgesia Machine
(100 Patients; Air Valve ¼ Open)

OXYGEN	NITROUS OXIDE	NO. OF PATIENTS
3 liters/min.	4 liters/min.	5
3	5–6	66
3	$6^{1}/_{2}$–7	22
3	$7^{1}/_{2}$–8	7

TABLE 8-6   Duration of Nitrous Oxide–Oxygen Administration
(100 Patients)

MINUTES	NO. OF PATIENTS
3–6	43
8–12	36
15–20	20
35	1

TABLE 8-7   Analysis of Ages of 100 Patients Receiving Nitrous
Oxide–Oxygen Analgesia

AGE	NO. OF PATIENTS
10–20	3
21–40	15
41–60	15
61–80	66
81–90	1

TABLE 8-8   Analysis of Patients' Preferences

PREFERENCE	NO. OF PATIENTS
Preference for Demerol	1
Preference for nitrous oxide-oxygen analgesia:	
Slight	2
Definite	3
Great	7
Very great	9

complete examinations were carried out despite their conviction that they could not tolerate the procedures.

Comment

This series of cases demonstrated that nitrous oxide–oxygen analgesia was more effective than intramuscular Demerol–Vistaril sedanalgesia in suppressing the gag reflex and in permitting a more comfortable and more thorough examination and treatment of patients undergoing various gastrointestinal intubation procedures.

Second, and of great importance to the author, was the very obvious fact that induction and recovery from nitrous oxide was a matter of a few minutes, allowing the patient to enter the treatment room immediately upon arrival, receive his examination or treatment, and leave after a few minutes with full faculties and coordination, ready for work or other activities. When Demerol was used for ambulatory patients, they had to be accompanied by others, they needed a room with a table to lie down upon for an extra half hour before and a half hour after the treatment, waiting for the effect of Demerol to begin and then to wear off. Also, they had to sit in the waiting room another half hour or more until it was felt that it was safe for them to leave; they had to be taken home by a relative or a friend, and then had to rest for a few hours until the drug effect was eliminated.

Third, and of even greater importance, was the relief felt by the author that the hazard of unexpected and unpreventable sudden adverse reactions from the injection of Demerol with or without Vistaril was removed. Demerol is known to produce sudden collapse with hypotension, syncope, and vomiting, especially in debilitated or ambulatory· cases, and this may require vasopressor therapy. Shock, cardiac arrest, and convulsions can occur. Respiratory depression and sudden death can take place in those with asthma or chronic obstructive pulmonary disease. Deaths have occurred in patients in whom the action of Demerol was potentiated because they were taking other drugs unknown to the physician, such as monoamine oxide inhibitors. Vistaril can also potentiate the effect of Demerol, and this was obvious in one of the hospital patients who became narcotized and comatose during a gastroscopy and required resuscitation. Cases of convulsions have been reported, also from Vistaril. On the other hand, when nitrous oxide–oxygen is used as an analgesic, "it has never caused morbidity or mortality." Its contraindications are practically none, excepting possibly psychoses, severe pulmonary diseases, and patients with nasal obstruction.

Summary

1. A series of 100 cases in which nitrous oxide–oxygen analgesia was used for uncomfortable or painful gastrointestinal intubation procedures was compared with a series of 100 cases in which intramuscular Demerol–Vistaril sedanalgesia was used.

2. Nitrous oxide proved superior in gag suppression (99 per cent good to excellent results versus 89 per cent) and in total evaluation (98 per cent good to excellent versus 85 per cent).

3. Patients who underwent both methods of analgesia preferred nitrous oxide to Demerol.

4. The greater additional advantages to the physician are considerable savings in office time and space when nitrous oxide–oxygen analgesia is used and the avoidance of the possibility of serious adverse reactions to Demerol or Vistaril.

APPLICATIONS OF RELATIVE ANALGESIA IN PODIATRIC MEDICINE[27]

Nitrous oxide–oxygen analgesia has been used with the following procedures:

1. Bunionectomy.
2. Metatarsal surgery.
3. Hammer toe surgery.
4. Ingrown nail repairs.
5. Excisions of soft tissue masses, such as cysts, verrucae, and so forth.
6. Heel surgery.
7. Achilles tendon lengthening.
8. Minor tendon lengthening.
9. Sesamoid removals.
10. Some implants at joints.

APPLICATIONS OF RELATIVE ANALGESIA IN DERMATOLOGY[28]

1. Surgical treatment of plantar warts.
2. Relieving the anxiety and pain of surgical draining of the large comedones and cysts of acne vulgaris.

REFERENCES

1. Adelson, J. J.: The effects of dental treatment on behavior of handicapped patients. J. Amer. Dent. Assoc., 71:1411, 1965.
2. Bell, J. O.: Psychological aspects of dental treatment of children. J. Exp. Educ., 1943.
3. Bleadon, S. B., and Sugarman, H.: Personal communication.
4. Blum, L. H.: Psychological aspects of dental practice and the child-patient. New York J. Dent., 34:59, 1964.
5. Brown, R. H., and Warren, S. A.: The handicapped child—a challenge to dentistry. New Zealand Dent. J., 66:3, 1965.
6. Cheyne, V. D., and Marsh, E.: Psychological problems in dental care of the feeble minded patient. A study of the behaviorism in 70 cases. Amer. J. Ment. Def., 53:582, 1949.
7. Cohen, E.: Some aspects of operative dentistry under analgesia. New York Dent. J., 32:212, 1966.
8. Colding, A.: Universal analgesia and universal anesthesia. J. Dent. Child., 32:124, 1965.
9. Emmertsen, E.: The treatment of children under general analgesia. J. Dent. Child., 32:123, 1965.
10. Fox, L.: Control of pain and apprehension and use of local anesthesia in periodontics. Dent. Clin. N. Amer., July, 1961.
11. Harvey, W.: Letter to the Editor. J. Am. Dent. Assoc. Anesthesiol., 12(No. 1), 1965.
12. Holst, J. J.: Use of nitrous oxide-oxygen analgesia in dentistry. Inter. Dent. J., 12:47, 1962.
13. Kirk, S. A.: Educating Exceptional Children. Boston, Houghton Mifflin, 1962.
14. Klock, J. H., and Tom, A.: Nitrous Oxide Amnalgesia. North Conway, N. H., Reporter Press, 1965.
15. Langa, H.: Analgesia for modern dentistry. New York J. Dent., 27:228, 1957.
16. Langa, H.: Analgesia for modern pedodontics. New York Dent. J., 28:58, 1962.
16a. Menken, N.: Nitrous oxide analgesia in dental practice. J. Am. Anal. Soc., 2:10, 1967.
17. Morse, D. R.: The use of analgesia in endodontics. J. Am. Anal. Soc. 2:6, 1964.
18. Pamphlet: Oral Cancer Prevention and Detection Center of St. Francis Hospital, Poughkeepsie, N. Y., 1966.
19. Roistacher, S.: Analgesia in dental practice. New York Dent. J., 32:163, 1966.
20. Seldin, H. M.: Practical Anesthesia for Dentistry and Oral Surgery. Philadelphia, Lea & Febiger, 1947.
21. Selden, H. S.: Children without fear. New Jersey Dent. Soc., Feb., 1962.
22. Sendax, V. I.: The Role of Analgesia in Oral Reconstruction. New York J. Dent., 36:81, 1966.
23. Snyder, J. R., et al.: Dental problems of non-institutionalized mentally retarded children. Northwest Dent., 39:132, 1960.
24. Wolf, W. C.: Dental care for the mentally retarded. Dent. Dig., 72:456, 1966.
25. Medical World News, 13:44e, 1972. New York, McGraw-Hill Book Company, 1972.
26. Sasson, L.: Nitrous oxide–oxygen analgesia in office gastroenterology. J. Am. Anal. Soc., 10:2–10, 1972.
27. DeHart, W. W., Jr.: Personal communication.
28. Wiegand, S. E.: Personal communication.
29. Morse, D. R.: Endodontics. J. Nat. Anal. Soc., 1:55–58, 1972.

RELATIVE ANALGESIA FOR THE HANDICAPPED CHILD

9

Harold Diner, D.D.S., M.A.

The dentist who has gained experience and proficiency in the administration of nitrous oxide analgesia is potentially a strong force for the extension of complete dental care to the handicapped or exceptional child. Indeed, he possesses a safe, effective, and relatively uninvolved instrument, one that is capable of broadening the scope and refinement of patient care, including the care of many patients hitherto considered "difficult" or "untreatable" in the average dental office. The utilization of nitrous oxide analgesia for the pediatric patient, as presented and clarified by Langa[10] and others, can be successfully applied with relatively little alteration to include the unusual child.

Under consideration is an inhalational technique with or without accompanying local or regional anesthesia and with or without occasional oral premedicative sedation—one that requires only unsupplemented low nitrous oxide and high oxygen ratios. Its utilization is directed toward the greater ease of management of the handicapped child in the general dental office, for it permits the dentist to incorporate the care of such patients into the regular office schedule without serious disruption. Admittedly the technique has limitations and is not universally applicable to handicapping conditions, most particularly to those in which severe mental retardation and/or emotional involvement accompanied by extreme fear are the main clinical features. However, there are few physiological and medical contraindications to its use. As a contributing element in establishing regular care in place of sporadic care and as an aid in eliminating inadequate care for the handicapped, it can enhance the operator's ability in several areas:

1. In performing more sophisticated services that may require multiple visits, that is, complex restorative procedures, involved pulpal therapy, periodontal treatment, and preventive, interceptive, and corrective orthodontic therapy.

2. In establishing a more regular and effective recall system, whereby the child may receive the full benefits of routine examination and prophylactic measures.

3. In performing operations with standard office personnel and equipment.

4. In inducing the analgesic state in the patient rapidly and in dismissing

289

him equally rapidly without prolonged recovery time, once initial operative rapport has been established.

5. In prolonging the per-visit treatment time, and consequently in achieving greater per-visit productivity, particularly in cases in which many visits may create some degree of hardship for both the parent and the child.

6. In performing operative procedures with complete safety.

CURRENT CONCEPTS IN MANAGEMENT

A review of the development of attitudes in the dental management of the handicapped child reveals a diversity of approaches and philosophies. First, there is the attitude that the handicapped child is not so remarkably different from the normal or average child in response to treatment and that *patience and understanding alone* can prove operatively adequate in the great majority of cases. That such efforts in many instances are successful is undeniable, but they frequently represent the results of laborious, time-consuming, and frustrating endeavor.

Secondly, there is the approach that attempts to further stabilize the child and to enhance the efficacy of usual pedodontic practice by means of *premedicative drugs*. A variety of such drugs and combinations of drugs have been explored. However, the effective correlation of the optimal effective dosage with the individuality of response is an inherent difficulty in premedication, frequently resulting in either extreme or inadequate sedation. The rules of age and weight in computing effective pediatric dosages from average adult dosages are often unreliable criteria for obtaining a single optimal dosage. Physiological, emotional, and metabolic differences, especially among handicapped children, are troublesome obstacles to standardization of drug dosage. A variety of peripheral factors, too, may affect the constancy of drug response in dental management problems. Nevertheless, premedicative drugs have certainly proved their supportive value in providing a more favorable treatment milieu. Yet, even in this role, their greatest value lies in their synergistic reinforcement of analgesic and anesthetic agents.

A third approach involves the effort to control the patient completely by utilizing *general anesthesia*. There are, certainly, instances in which this approach is obligatory, when it is justifiable as the only choice from the standpoint of management and operative care. It does, however, demand a highly refined and knowledgeable background, and a highly skilled team of several members, whether it is administered in the hospital or in the private office. It has frequently been described as the "last resort" in management problems, and it is in this context that many basic questions arise regarding its appropriate use.

Is there another approach to the dental management of handicapped children that falls somewhere between the extremes of strictly standard management and the use of general anesthesia? Within this range, are there tools and techniques that can make the child less fearful and apprehensive? And can these instruments function to instruct and educate the child in the routine acceptance of dental care? Most importantly, can this modality be incorporated into the practice of the general practitioner with unquestionable safety? All of these questions can be answered in the affirmative when the fourth approach is employed.

This approach involves the use of *inhalation analgesia with nitrous oxide and oxygen*. This is the "middle ground," an approach that has a wide range of applicability to dentistry for the handicapped. Its use can create the mildest of euphoric states or an analgesic level just short of loss of consciousness. Its greatest value lies in its ability to create a quiescent and cooperative patient who is at the same time physiologically awake.

INHALATION ANALGESIA: A GENERAL CONSIDERATION

The use of nitrous oxide and oxygen analgesia has been referred to in a variety of ways: relative analgesia, hypalgesia, general analgesia, universal analgesia, and amnalgesia. Let us review briefly the techniques, goals, and approaches of several clinicians in the administration of nitrous oxide analgesia. This will provide an opportunity to assess the scope and range of the analgesic stage and to determine, within that stage, the optimal level for our own particular needs.

In Seldin's description of analgesia,[11] as the deeper phases of analgesia are attained the awareness of pain disappears, but the ability to recognize touch and pressure is still present. Sounds seem distant and, should the depth of analgesia draw close to the excitement stage, sensations of flying or falling are experienced. In general, the patient is comfortable and warm, feeling as though he were in a pleasant dream. Yet, he still retains the ability to respond to a command to speak, and thus to reply to a question.

Seldin[11] has further stated that the exact dosage of nitrous oxide will vary for each child, depending on his age, weight, basic temperament, sensitivity to the gases, and mental or emotional state at the time of administration. He feels that, with the child under analgesia, local injection presents no problem, for the nose-piece blocks the child's view and, since he is in the euphoric state, it is possible to make the injection without his awareness. He concludes that nitrous oxide and oxygen analgesia is best utilized on a cooperative and comprehending patient; rarely is it effective when any force or coercion is employed.

Langa[9] has reported a high degree of success in the planes of relative analgesia, using relatively low nitrous oxide alveolar concentrations. He has been able to obtain amnesic as well as analgesic states, even with these relatively low minute flows. His primary premise is that analgesia is being used primarily to eliminate the fear of dentistry and that it constitutes a form of hypnosis. Stressing the need for genuine kindliness, sympathy, and understanding in administrations for children, he states that no matter what category the child may fall into, if the dentist would win the confidence of the child at the first visit, the child would become a good analgesia patient.

Emmertsen,[5] in her description of general analgesia, defines it as the first stage of general anesthesia, in which consciousness is retained although altered, the pain reaction threshold is raised, and the swallowing and cough reflexes are retained. Her administrations have numbered 15,000 on about 2000 children of 1 to 16 years of age, without serious complication. Many of these children were referred to her by colleagues as "too difficult to treat." Emmertsen utilizes as her initial dose 60 per cent oxygen and 40 per cent nitrous oxide, and over the course of 1 minute, she increases the nitrous oxide to 60 per cent, the level that is maintained during treatment. The desired level of analgesia is reached after 2 minutes, being characterized by muscular relaxation, steady nasal respiration, and a contented facial expression. If comprehensive treatment in one session is desirable, occasional reduction of the nitrous oxide concentration is recommended to avoid nausea and vomiting.

Emmertsen suggests that, in her analgesic range, analgesia can be used for pulpotomy in primary teeth after the ages of 7 to 8 years. It is also very suitable for cavity preparation in primary and permanent teeth, and she considers it, in concentrations of 75 per cent nitrous oxide, suitable for the extraction of incisors, cuspids, and severely resorbed molars in the primary dentition. A combination of analgesia and local anesthesia is used in such cases when analgesia does not raise the pain reaction threshold sufficiently or when the child is unable to carry on constant nose breathing. There are no contraindications, although it cannot be used if the desired level of analgesia cannot be obtained owing to the child's persistent aversion to the procedure.

Colding,[4] in describing universal analgesia and universal anesthesia, considers that different patients have different levels of cerebral activity and that the level depends on the individual's psyche as well as outside factors. Analgesia does not subdue this activity to the same degree in every patient, the induction being more difficult in a patient with high cerebral activity. This factor, plus the type of treatment to be carried out, helps to determine whether analgesia or anesthesia should be used.

Holst,[6] in his description of general analgesia, notes that respiration, size of the pupils, muscle tonus, and laryngeal and pharyngeal reflexes are not affected. Thus, there is no risk of laryngospasm or aspiration during analgesia administration. It is possible for the experienced operator to avoid the next, or excitement, stage of anesthesia. The passage into this stage is often attended by psychic and physical unrest, and dilation of the pupils and increased lacrimation are noted.

Klock and Tom[8] have reported the use of unsupplemented 80 per cent nitrous oxide and 20 per cent oxygen (amnalgesia). They describe the "amnalgesia" plane as comparatively narrow, occurring between the symptoms of analgesia and those of excitement. Their results imply a combined state of analgesia (without pain) and amnesia (without memory). They state that the respiratory and cardiac centers are not affected and that there can be no danger from failure of these centers. The essential requirement, they maintain, is the ability to distinguish between the symptoms of analgesia and those of excitement and to keep the patient somewhere between the two. It is also necessary to be familiar with all the symptoms of beginning hypoxia.

A variety of other techniques have been described, including the technique of the initial utilization of 90 to 100 per cent nitrous oxide for the induction of analgesia in the resistant patient and then a leveling off to analgesic ranges for maintenance, or, in order never to reduce the oxygen level below metabolic requirements (20 per cent), the supplementation of nitrous oxide and oxygen with small percentages of more potent inhalation anesthetics (halothane, and so forth).

Inhalation techniques combined with intravenous barbiturates, narcotics, and ataractics have also been described. Such techniques are not without risk for the inexperienced operator and should be in the province of trained anesthesiologists. The intramuscular injection of supportive drugs or, as is occasionally suggested, the inclusion of drugs into local anesthetic solutions can be readily accomplished once an effective analgesic level has been attained. However, an analgesic induction, successfully obtained and maintained, rarely requires any additional medicative support. It is the introduction of analgesia that may require adjunctive sedation, and toward this end, the preference is for oral administration.

This general review should make it apparent that administration of amnalgesia, general analgesia, and universal analgesia, because their use results in the induction of a state in proximity to the excitement stage and light surgical anesthesia, requires skills above those of the average dental practitioner. However, if we are to limit ourselves to relatively low nitrous oxide and high oxygen flows, safely below the excitement level (relative analgesia), we should supplement our administration, wherever necessary, by supportive medication. For care of the handicapped child, this makes obligatory a greater knowledge of his particular condition and an exploration and assessment of his potential as well as of his disability. The handicapped child usually needs supportive therapy, but this support must be based on his individual attributes as well as on those of the clinical group he represents.

THE HANDICAPPED CHILD: BASIC CONSIDERATIONS

In order to deal with the aberrations with which we are concerned, let us consider brain injury as the core of the problem. Brain damage, an all-inclusive term, is clinically manifested in motor and neurological impairment, as in cerebral palsy, convulsions, or epilepsy; mental retardation; and hyperkinetic behavior disorders on an organic basis (the Strauss syndrome, minimal brain damage, or brain injury). In addition, auditory, visual, and orthopedic handicaps are commonplace. Within these subclassifications, there is often an overlay of clinical features and a concomitant emotional disturbance. Thus, Kirk has stated:

> In many instances we find multiple handicaps or other combinations of divergences from the normal. A crippled child can be gifted. A deaf child can be blind. A cerebral palsied child can have many deviations; he may be partially seeing, hard of hearing, mentally retarded (or gifted), and defective in speech.[7]

It is important to realize that attempts to equate empirically any of these categories with success or failure in dental treatability may prove misleading. It would be a mistake to presuppose that all children who are clinically identical are emotionally identical as well.

PRELIMINARY ASSESSMENT

Observation of the child's waiting room behavior will offer a basic psychometric appraisal of his social, behavioral, and physical characteristics. His attitude toward and manipulation of waiting room toys and materials (Fig. 9–1) and appropriate response or lack of response to simple conversation will be helpful in making this appraisal. He may exhibit various degrees of shyness, apprehension, fearfulness, tenseness, hyperactivity, distractability, difficulty in communication, motor disorders, physical disability, impulsiveness, aggressiveness, emotional instability, intellectual inadequacy, or withdrawal. These observations should be related to overt physical stigmata, size and stature, and chronological age.

History taking should be directed toward the determination of individual features; previous dental experience; drug regimens and responses, past and current; medical status, past and current; and parental attitude and expectation. When, for any reason, the reliability of the parent as informant is doubtful or when questions concerning medical background or the use of potential premedications arise, consultation with the child's physician is advisable.

Unless obviously detrimental, the mother should be enlisted to play an integral role in the execution of her child's dental program. In the dental treatment of the handicapped child, she constitutes a valuable adjunct, and to inflexibly exclude her from the operating room procedure may serve to reduce effective management. After all, she is a reassuring force emotionally and the best interpreter of the child's speech and actions when they are difficult to comprehend. When communication is difficult or minimal, she can best convey what is intended. Moreover, the transition from waiting room to operatory is often best accomplished with her help, and the postural adjustment of braces, prosthetic devices, and wheelchair position may require her advice. A

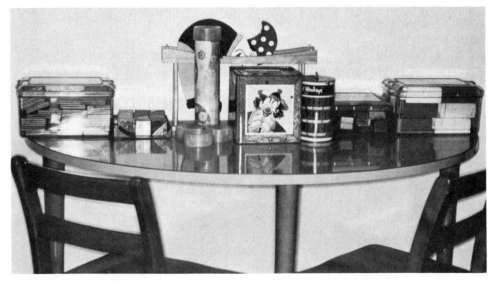

Figure 9–1 Observe the handicapped child-patient's attitude toward and manipulation of waiting room toys and materials.

physically small child, whether resistant or not, is usually best treated in her lap. She can also be supportive when coercive measures, physical or vocal, are indicated. In particular, when treatment needs are minimal or when analgesia is not totally successful, her physical assistance is welcomed. As a general rule, she is requested to attend through the induction of analgesia and is then dismissed unless her physical presence is necessary.

In most instances, the child will come into the operatory, although he may require gentle assistance. The physically large, older child who actively resists poses a special problem. The decision must be made whether to persist in forcing his entrance physically, whether to assess the possibility of pre-medication, or whether to recommend him for general anesthesia.

Once in the operatory, the child may still exhibit reservations in the form of open crying and parent-clinging. No immediate attempt should be made to force him into the dental chair, for many children will eventually sit in the chair of their own accord or with very little urging. Instead, the dentist, seated on an operating stool, can begin a demonstration on large tooth models. Such models always create some response, even from mentally retarded children. Since prophylaxis is the first consideration, this is demonstrated with the prophylaxis angle and rubber cup held in the hand, but not attached to the handpiece. As the dentist counts by number, the angle is rubbed over several teeth on the model. A sweet-tasting prophylaxis paste is then picked up on the rubber cup and applied to one of the child's upper anterior teeth. He must be held momentarily for this, even if he resists. Such resistance is generally of short duration, and the child will accept further application of the paste. The seating of the child can usually be accomplished with little difficulty. The angle is attached, demonstrated, and moved about the mouth. This permits a basically adequate clinical evaluation.

Next, the child can be introduced to x-ray examination by "shaking hands" with the x-ray cone. Periapical films can be better stabilized by the use of a plastic film holder. The use of occlusal film, intra-orally and extra-orally, should be considered for some patients, with the parent holding the film packets. Should the results prove unsatisfactory, they can be supplemented later by the use of the more usual intra-oral films, which analgesia will permit.

Very frequently, when the attention of the child appears sustained, an initial introduction to analgesia is made. In a matter-of-fact way, allusion is made to "magic air" and the "funny rubber nose." The child is encouraged to hold the nose-piece as 100 per cent oxygen is blown on his hand and cheek. The nose-piece is then touched to his nose and even momentarily seated. The procedure is casually referred to as "lots of fun," and no further trial is attempted.

The foregoing represents a fairly typical first visit. However, when the child presents with dental pain, sedative dressings should be placed with a minimum of manipulation. Only if the dentist is convinced that this palliative treatment is inadequate and more involved therapy is indicated should the administration of analgesia be attempted. Teeth which are obviously beyond redemption, causing great discomfort, and seemingly difficult to remove demand referral outside the office for extraction.

Great emphasis should be placed on keeping the initial visit a benign one. The most important single factor in analgesia for the handicapped child, and for the normal child as well, is the initial administration and its acceptance. The analgesic methodology which we prefer, with its low ratio of nitrous oxide to oxygen, is dependent in great part on the ability to establish a favorable interpersonal relationship. Frequently this may be established even when intellectual function is marginal, physical involvement severe, and emotionality high, on the basis of a sympathetic approach and manner and the effective use of inflection of voice and care in language. Yet analgesia, even though expertly and skillfully applied, may still prove unacceptable to an alarmed and frightened child. For such patients, consideration should be given to the use of supportive medicative drugs.

PREMEDICATIVE DRUGS

Since the literature on premedication for the difficult and handicapped child is extensive, it is recommended that the practitioner familiarize himself with a few drugs and combinations of drugs and learn to use them expertly. The chief reason for premedication in the use of nitrous oxide analgesia is to allay the fear, anxiety, and apprehension that sometimes accompany the initial administration. As a general rule, these fears and anxieties occur with greater frequency in the handicapped child. Even with the handicapped, however, it often happens that premedication may be used for the initial introduction to analgesia and then found unnecessary for future administrations.

The selection of drugs and their prescribed doses should be equated with the needs of the particular patient. It is important to remember that we are dealing with an outpatient whom we wish to discharge immediately following the completion of our procedure—that is, without the necessity for a prolonged recovery period. Therefore, drug selection and dosages should be directed toward obtaining minimal but effective sedation. Since extremely apprehensive children will usually require heavier sedation, it is imperative to impress upon the parent that a constant watch must be maintained over the child once he is dismissed from the office.

Because of the relative lack of potency and the rapid elimination of nitrous oxide, drugs can be recommended in somewhat larger than normal doses, which may, in turn, permit analgesia to be induced more easily and maintained more smoothly at lower levels of nitrous oxide. Another benefit of the larger doses is that inadequate premedication may prove to be a hindrance, with any previously established cooperation lost. This happens most frequently with the barbiturates. By the same token, heavy premedication, to the point at which the patient is roused with great difficulty, is equally undesirable. Such a situation will serve to create a very worried parent, as well as a very harried dentist. Competently controlled general anesthesia is preferable to the extremely deep depression produced by drugs.

As a prelude to nitrous oxide analgesia, the following drugs are most frequently used: Noctec Syrup (chloral hydrate), Vistaril (hydroxyzine pamoate) Oral Suspension, and the combination of Demerol and Phenergan. Chloral hydrate is generally given in doses of 7.5 to 15 grains one hour before the appointment; Vistaril is given in doses of 50 to 100 mg. the night before the appointment and 50 to 100 mg. 1 hour before the appointment; Demerol, 25 to 60 mg., is combined with half the Phenergan equivalent, 12.5 to 30 mg., and is taken 1 hour before the appointment. These are empirical dosages and should be altered according to the judgment of the dentist and the child's physician. The elixirs or syrups are preferred, and the use of straws, particularly for the cerebral palsied, will serve to reduce the amount spilled. The greatest disadvantage in oral premedication is the difficulty in determining the actual amount consumed. Of course, existing drug regimens and past responses to drug therapy must be carefully scrutinized to determine any contraindications.

ANALGESIA TECHNIQUE

The handicapped child with average comprehension and the capacity to attend requires remarkably little deviation from the usual analgesia technique. As with the normal child, the symptoms of analgesia are described in advance in language that the child can understand. Young or physically small children may be seated in the mother's lap, and the dentist can first place the nasal inhaler on his own nose. The flow of gases can then be demonstrated by directing the flow over the hand, arm, or cheek of the child. The nose-piece, or "funny or magic nose," can be rubbed gently on the tip of the child's nose. In doing so, the inhaler should be brought up from the chest, rather than slipped over the head, from above the line of vision. If there is no resistance to seating the nose-piece, slight pressure should be exerted on it to prevent a flow of gas to the eyes. To make the nasal inhaler more pleasant smelling, one of the floral scented air purifiers is sprayed on the nose-piece and wiped off before its use. One hundred per cent oxygen should be instituted, and then 5 per cent nitrous oxide, with the flow of the latter being increased gradually, 1 per cent for every two respirations, until an appropriate level is reached (usually 10 to 15 per cent). The doctor should speak simply, steadily, and monotonously to enhance the effect of the nitrous oxide (Fig. 9–2).

Gentle physical restraint may be attempted on the child who resists by pushing the nose-piece away or by constant head turning. To prolong his attention span and to discourage head movement, several distracting devices frequently prove helpful. One is a mobile that is suspended directly over the chair, to which sailboats or other toy items are attached (Fig. 9–3A). It is set is motion, and the child is requested to watch one article in particular. Another device found helpful is a pecking bird which moves steadily and slowly down a long metal rod (Fig. 9–3B). Conversation centered on these objects frequently produces a temporary cessation of activity. The concentration of nitrous oxide is then set to about 50 per cent, and the inhaler is not seated, but held close to the nostrils. It is important to pinch the nose-piece, so that the flow of gases may be directed away from the eyes. What is delivered is a mixture of nitrous oxide and oxygen diluted with air, yet sufficiently strong, even with mouth-breathing, to create a mild euphoric effect. Resistance may cease,

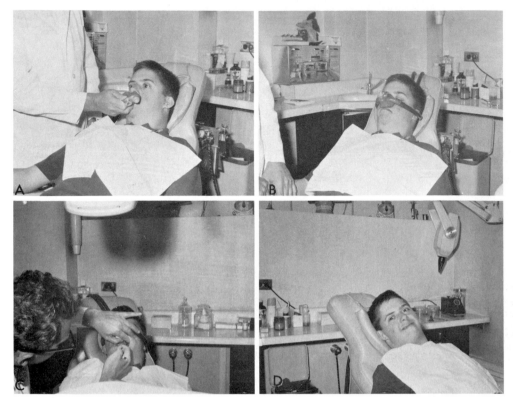

Figure 9–2 Acceptance of relative analgesia by the mongoloid child. *A*, Introduction. *B*, Induction. *C*, Supplementary local anesthesia. *D*, Procedure completed.

or become sufficiently diminished in a very short time to permit seating of the nose-piece. At this point, the concentration should be lowered accordingly.

It is often mistakenly assumed that, for analgesia to prove effective in dentistry for the handicapped, it must be maintained at very deep levels. What is more frequently the case is that lower levels are effective but that more frequent supplementation with local anesthesia is indicated. Stronger physical restraint is not the solution to continued resistance. Adjunctive premedication may be prescribed, and the procedure repeated. In instances of total management failure, continued violent resistance, and a heavy restorative schedule, the patient is almost certainly a candidate for treatment under general anesthesia.

An evaluation of this analgesic effect depends on observation of the patient, his reaction to treatment procedures, and his response to questioning. The diagnostic value of verbalization in determining the analgesic level is either altogether inappropriate or unreliable in some handicaps. It is obviously not valid in severe auditory involvement. On the other hand, it is extremely useful in evaluating the analgesic level in the visually impaired.

When speech is seriously involved, as in cerebral palsy, it may be difficult to interpret the response. In the brain-damaged and mentally retarded patient, the response may be totally inappropriate, or difficult to elicit, even in ordinary situations. It becomes highly important, then, in analgesia administration for the handicapped, to be able to judge the deviation from the patient's normal physical and emotional state, for the dentist must be less dependent on vocal response from the patient.

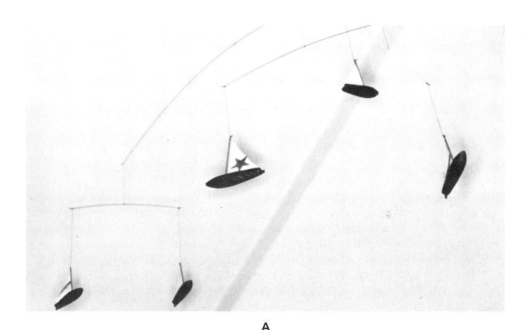

A

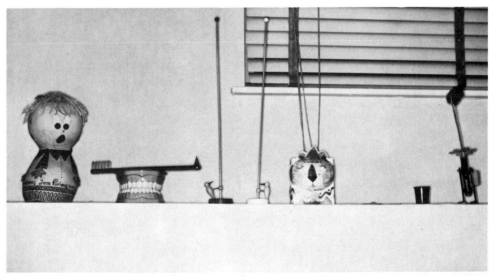

B

Figure 9–3 Distraction devices. A, A mobile is suspended over the chair. B, A large toothbrush and teeth model amidst pecking birds and other toys.

OPERATIVE CONSIDERATIONS

As Cohen[3] has so adequately expressed it, careful treatment planning must be accompanied by the deliberate consideration of the most effective utilization of materials and personnel. Much can be learned and borrowed from operative procedures that have been employed under general anesthesia. From the standpoint of the economic feasibility of treating the handicapped child in the general dental office, attention must be paid to the performance of treatment without the sacrifice of quality in as expeditious a fashion as possible. And toward this end, the use of relative analgesia can prove of tremendous value.

Dental restorative procedures should follow a graded stimulus sequence; that is, simpler procedures should precede more highly involved and complex procedures. It is suggested that, for the first analgesia session, low-speed instrumentation be used for operative procedures. For subsequent visits, high-speed equipment will find more ready acceptance. If local anesthesia is to be used, the syringe should be passed from behind the chair and brought up from chest level. The free hand can be utilized as an additional eye shield. The dental assistant should place his (or her) hands gently but firmly across the child to prevent any sudden arm movements.

Effective oral evacuation equipment is practically obligatory. Frequent toileting of the mouth will improve operating efficiency and reduce the incidence of coughing and vomiting. Vomiting occurs relatively rarely, and with good suction equipment it is rarely necessary to suspend treatment. Should vomiting occur, the child must be oxygenated, the vomitus suctioned off, and the analgesic level restored. The child is often unaware that anything has happened.

Skill in multiple matrix placement, in the adaptation of proprietary stainless steel crowns, and in the utilization of the rubber dam will all pay divi-

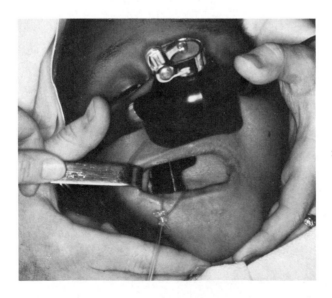

Figure 9-4 The rubber mouth prop.

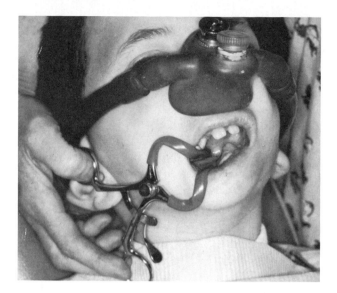

Figure 9-5   The ratchet mouth prop.

dends in the form of improved restorative service and reduced time expenditure. In using the rubber dam, which has a very definite place in analgesia administration, it is only necessary to remember that the usual dilution effect of an open mouth is lessened by the rubber dam, and therefore the proportion of nitrous oxide must be decreased appropriately. The administration of analgesia facilitates the use of the rubber dam, which in turn improves the quality of the restorative service.

Mouth props, of either the rubber or the ratchet type, are retained without frequent dislodgement under nitrous oxide analgesia (Figs. 9–4 and 9–5). Occasional resistance to their placement can be overcome by exerting gentle pressure with the thumb in the lower mucobuccal fold at the labial frenum or by inserting the forefinger behind the last lower molars and rotating. Both actions will result in sufficient mouth opening to insert the props.

In the handicapped child, macroglossia, hyperactive tongue movements, and pooling of saliva are frequent features. Although detrimental to good restorative results, they are considerably less frustrating under analgesia, since salivation is decreased, tongue movements are lessened, and deflection of the enlarged tongue is maintained more easily.

THE HANDICAPS: DESCRIPTIONS AND CASE REPORTS

It is important to describe the major handicapping conditions and to evaluate their differences and similarities as they affect the successful utilization of nitrous oxide analgesia. This can be better elaborated by the presentation of representative case reports which can serve to delineate the limitations as well as the advantages and versatility of the relative analgesia technique.

CEREBRAL PALSY

Children with cerebral palsy may have accompanying disorders of speech, hearing, and vision, as well as behavioral problems. Behavioral involvement may or may not be present in all handicapping conditions, but in cerebral palsy it serves to highlight the already exaggerated components. On the basis of neuromotor impairment, cerebral palsy may be differentiated as follows: spastic paralysis, athetosis, ataxia, tremor, and rigidity. The spastic and athetoid groups represent the greatest number of cerebral palsied patients.

In *spasticity* the balance between antagonistic muscles is absent, resulting in jerky, uncontrolled movements with spasmodic contraction of the muscles. Sudden involuntary contraction of the muscles of mastication can make dental procedures hazardous for both the patient and the dentist. In addition, the pooling of saliva, due to ineffectual swallowing mechanisms, is detrimental to many dental restorative procedures.

In *athetosis*, movements are not rhythmical and they appear uncontrolled. They are accompanied by squirming, writhing, and grimacing. During sleep, these movements disappear, whereas on conscious effort and excitement, they become exaggerated. Affected patients present a moving target to the dentist in the performance of his work.

Frequently, the spastic and athetotic movements of the victim of cerebral palsy give a false impression of mental retardation. Actually there is no real relationship between intellectual capacity and the degree of physical involvement. Statistically, it has been found that 58 per cent of children with cerebral palsy have an IQ below 70, compared to a distribution of 5 per cent in the unaffected population.

The ability of nitrous oxide analgesia to provide a very appreciable reduction in anxiety has proved to be highly important in the dental treatment of the cerebral palsied. With analgesia, there is a definite decrease in muscular spasticity and uncoordinated movement so that restraints are almost always unnecessary. There is also greater tolerance of mouth props and ratchets, and salivation is decreased. Posturally, there is less physical stress and discomfort for the child, and he can tolerate a much longer treatment period. Nevertheless, one does encounter resistance to nitrous oxide analgesia among such children. Paradoxically, it is frequently easier to induce analgesia in a child with severe physical involvement and approximately normal intelligence than in one with mild physical involvement and severe mental retardation. In any event, a severe disability acts as a natural restraining force, and the child who is intellectually sensitive to a kind and sympathetic approach will frequently respond in a highly cooperative manner.

Case Report: Cerebral Palsy (Mixed Spasticity and Athetosis). The patient was an attractive 13 year old girl with no impairment of sight or hearing. Of above average intelligence, her speech was relatively difficult to understand. She wore leg braces and arrived in a wheelchair. Although she was undergoing physical therapy, she was extremely reluctant to leave the wheelchair and use a walker. Her extreme apprehension was supposedly heightened by her mother's death the previous year. Previous dental treatment had been only partially successful, and the child had refused treatment at her last visit. Her movements were uncoordinated, with frequent arm flailing.

The Initial Visit. The patient was highly apprehensive and cried in the waiting room, so that premedication was given (Demerol, 40 mg., and Phenergan, 20 mg.). She seemed quieter after a half hour and was brought to the operatory. Although she refused to leave her wheelchair, she permitted a clinical examination. Occlusal x-ray films were taken, and nitrous oxide analgesia was explained and its supportive qualities described. A mixture of 50 per cent nitrous oxide was administered close to her nostrils for a few minutes, but no attempt was made to seat the nose-piece. The patient agreed that it was pleasant, but also had reservations.

Clinical Findings. All of the patient's permanent first molars were highly carious and badly broken down. Of her other teeth, only four had relatively uninvolved carious surfaces. It was decided to prescribe Vistaril, 75 mg. the night before the next visit, and the same dose 1 hour before the appointment.

The Second Visit. On her arrival the patient seemed more relaxed; therefore analgesia was induced in the previously attempted manner. The nose-piece was then seated and, because of mouth-breathing, analgesia was maintained at 25 per cent nitrous oxide. Local anesthesia was given without incident, and both right first permanent molars were excavated and sedated. All the work done during this visit, and indeed throughout the treatment series, was performed with the patient in the wheelchair, for she refused to leave it. There was marked reduction in athetotic movements, tongue movements were lessened, and a reduction in salivation was noted. The patient expressed no discomfort or fatigue, even though maintaining her position in the wheelchair appeared difficult.

Subsequent Visits. Premedication was discontinued, and local anesthesia was used for the treatment of all first permanent molars, each of which received stainless steel crowns. The remaining fillings were done under analgesia alone. The total number of treatment visits was seven, the last being used for polishing fillings, prophylaxis, and topical fluoride application.

Subsequent recall visits for this patient have presented no problems. Analgesia administrations have been utilized and accepted with no difficulty, and the teeth have been maintained in good condition.

Case Report: Cerebral Palsy (Mixed Spasticity and Athetosis). This 12 year old boy was of normal intelligence, but was affected with marked athetotic component. Although highly apprehensive, he was very anxious to cooperate. He showed a marked protrusion of maxillary anterior teeth.

The Initial Visit. The child was received as an emergency patient. A fall he had suffered several hours earlier had severely loosened his upper left central incisor. The mobility of the tooth was of such degree that it was elected to perform extra-oral root canal therapy and reimplantation.

This was the patient's first dental experience. Head movements became more extreme with the patient's attempts to cooperate. Analgesia was introduced and accepted with no resistance, and at a flow of 10 per cent nitrous oxide, the incisor was removed. No local anesthesia was used. Analgesia was discontinued while the tooth was treated endodontically but, for reimplantation and ligation, analgesia was renewed. To limit involuntary movement, the analgesic range was extended to 25 per cent nitrous oxide. Again, no local anesthesia was necessary. The tooth was reinserted to its original position and splinted to the adjacent tooth with stainless steel wire ligature. This was reinforced with self-cure plastic filling material and surgical cement.

Uncontrolled head movements would have made this procedure quite difficult, but it was accomplished with relative ease. A rubber mouth prop was used throughout and was well tolerated.

Subsequent Visits.   Analgesia in the range of 25 per cent nitrous oxide was used for routine treatment in subsequent visits. It was necessary to extract five permanent teeth, and analgesia supplemented by local anesthesia was used.

Three months later, the patient again suffered a severe fall, and the upper left central incisor, which had apparently reattached and was functionally comfortable, was knocked out and not recovered. It was decided to make a temporary splint. Under analgesia at 25 per cent nitrous oxide, anterior orthodontic stainless steel bands were fitted to the upper right central and lateral incisors, and the upper left lateral incisor. Impressions were taken and on the model the bands were joined and a pontic was fabricated. The appliance was cemented and at the last visit was functioning well.

Case Report: Cerebral Palsy (Spastic Paraplegia with Severe Mental Retardation and Epilepsy).   This 7 year old patient was of normal stature, and although the child could not speak, her hearing was unimpaired. The patient functioned on the infantile level, being totally dependent, and had been on Dilantin therapy, with an occasional change to phenobarbital, since the age of nine months. Physical therapy had been discontinued because of severe vomiting and screaming. Although institutionalization had been recommended, the parents refused.

The Initial Visit.   The child was held in the mother's lap. A mixture of 40 per cent nitrous oxide and 60 per cent oxygen was administered close to the nostrils. Crying, head turning, and mild arm movements resulted. The movements were easy to follow, and within 2 minutes the child smiled and babbled a few times. Nitrous oxide was reduced to 15 per cent, and the nosepiece was seated. Clinical examination was performed, and anterior periapical and occlusal (lateral exposure) films were taken.

Clinical Findings.   Only two primary incisors were actually visible, and both showed severe carious involvement. There was a heavy fibrous gingival hyperplasia due to the Dilantin therapy. It was decided to remove the incisors and to expose the remaining teeth by surgical means. The parent was made aware of the almost certain regrowth of tissue, but requested that treatment be attempted anyway.

Subsequent Visits.   For each subsequent visit (five in all), at the physician's suggestion, a Thorazine suppository (25 mg.) was given the night before the appointment. Nitrous oxide induction was performed as on the first visit, but before the reduction to 15 per cent nitrous oxide, local anesthesia was given. Excess tissue was removed, surgical packs were placed without any apparent discomfort or sequelae, and the indicated extractions were performed.

Analgesia was maintained smoothly and evenly during every visit. Recall has not been possible to evaluate the regrowth of tissue, for the child was subsequently institutionalized.

MENTAL RETARDATION

Mental retardation can be attributed to three major causes: organic, genetic, and cultural. Retardation from organic causes is attended by demonstrable nonhereditary central nervous system pathology. Aberrations in the brain or nervous system may occur pre-, peri-, or postnatally, as a result of injury, disease, toxicity, and so forth.

Prenatal and perinatal causes may include rubella in the first trimester of pregnancy, toxemia, syphilis, encephalitis, and other diseases. Birth injuries may also be included as potential causes of mental retardation. Postnatally, disease and injury immediately after birth and during infancy and early childhood may be contributory.

Genetic causes may include chromosomal aberrations (Down's syndrome), inborn errors of metabolism (phenylketonuria), and what has been described as familial mental deficiency.

Cultural causes center on factors in the social environment, child-rearing practices, and socioeconomic levels in the home and the community.

The totally dependent mentally retarded child (IQ of 0 to 25) almost always has an acquired organic or genetic defect. In most cases, the trainable mentally retarded child (IQ of 25 to 50) also demonstrates organic defects. Studies have shown that in this group one-third are children with Down's syndrome and one-third are brain-injured children, with the remainder having retardation of unknown etiology.[13]

The educable mentally retarded child (IQ of 50 to 75) may demonstrate mixed etiologic factors. A small number may have organic involvement, with minimal brain damage. The greatest number, however, present with causal hereditary factors and subcultural environments.

The slow-learning child (IQ of 75 to 90), in a small number of instances, may demonstrate organic causes, but the greatest number in this group come from subcultural homes and communities.

Snyder[12] attempted to correlate measured intelligence with treatment response, patient treatability, and the establishment of rapport. His patients were noninstitutionalized mentally retarded children. At IQ levels above 63, Snyder reported full cooperation and treatability in the private dental office.

In contrast, the study of Cheyne and Marsh[2] was performed on institutionalized patients. Their findings indicate that a definite trend in favor of initial and continued cooperation is associated with the approach to normal intellect; that is, positive behaviorism showed a significantly correlated increase with rise in IQ.

In our experience, normal or near normal intellectual capacity is not the essentially critical feature in nitrous oxide analgesia administration as is commonly supposed. After all, intellectually competent children have refused to accept analgesia. For the mentally retarded child, greater effort must be made to create a nonthreatening and benign atmosphere. This is necessary to compensate for his relative inability to be influenced by suggestion and his lack of effective verbalization. The analgesia induction should be structured around his mental rather than his chronological age. Language should be simple, couched in short phrases. It is inadvisable to attempt to seat the nasal inhaler immediately. On the contrary, this should be postponed until the effort has been made to achieve mild euphoria by blowing higher percentages of nitrous oxide across the nostrils. It is extremely important initially to maintain light analgesic levels for the slow-learning child. Sudden descent into deeper analgesic levels, unaccompanied by comprehensible verbal preparation, may prove too frightening, and strong resistance may ensue. Such resistance may make future attempts at administration unacceptable. Therefore, greater emphasis should be placed on careful observation rather than on machine dosage.

For children in the lower intellectual ranges, strong consideration should be given to supporting the initial analgesia administration with adjunctive premedication. Since organic defects are prominent clinical features in this group, drug regimens should be given careful evaluation, probably in conjunction with the child's physician.

Case Report: Down's Syndrome. A physically small 6 year old girl presented with all the clinical features of Down's syndrome (mongolism). Her intellectual capacity was in the low trainable range.

The Initial Visit. Clinical examination, during which the mother was highly supportive, was accomplished with only mild resistance, but attempts at obtaining adequate roentgenograms, even with the mother's assistance, were unsuccessful. Therefore, although the child had chronic upper respiratory involvement and was a habitual mouth-breather, nitrous oxide analgesia was attempted. When a mixture of 60 per cent nitrous oxide and 40 per cent oxygen was blown across the nostrils, euphoria was obtained, but the child resisted the seating of the nasal inhaler. The analgesic level was maintained, and intra-oral x-ray films were taken successfully. Prophylaxis and topical fluoride application were performed with ease.

Clinical Findings. The child was free of carious defects; however, severe crowding of the lower anterior segment and a lack of resorption of primary teeth were creating problems in the eruption of permanent teeth. Several permanent incisors were erupting lingually.

The Second Visit. At this visit, a similar analgesic level was obtained. The nose-piece was tolerated in close proximity to the nostrils, but was not seated. Local anesthesia was infiltrated around the four lower primary incisors, and the response to the initial insertion of the needle was extremely mild. The incisors were removed without incident, and the child remained completely placid.

Case Report: Minimal Brain Damage; Severe Mental Retardation. This 7½ year old boy had no gross neurological abnormalities and was functioning intellectually at the marginal totally dependent-trainable level. His speech was monosyllabic and essentially meaningless.

The Initial Visit. The patient was received on an emergency basis with severe pain in the lower right molar region. His waiting-room behavior was generally resistant. Premedication with Demerol (60 mg.) and Phenergan (30 mg.) was given and was consumed without loss. After one half hour, he was taken to the operatory with only moderate resistance. With gentle physical restraint, a mixture of 50 per cent nitrous oxide and 50 per cent oxygen was directed at the nostrils. Analgesia was obtained surprisingly rapidly, the nasal inhaler was seated, and nitrous oxide reduced to 25 per cent. An x-ray film of the lower right first permanent molar was taken, and a mandibular block performed. The nitrous oxide level was then reduced to 15 per cent. A vital pulpotomy was performed, and an amalgam filling was placed.

Subsequent Visits. For the second and third visits, the same procedure was followed, except that the premedicative doses were reduced to half the initial doses. Restorative procedures were performed with no difficulty, although it was necessary to utilize a ratchet type of mouth prop each time. Two more visits were necessary to complete all the restorative procedures. The same analgesia technique was employed, but without the use of premedicative drugs. Analgesia induction was accomplished easily and maintained smoothly.

Case Report: Mental Retardation; Low Educable Range. The patient was a highly apprehensive 12 year old girl, with minimal organic injury and retarded developmentally. Her dental age indicated a two year delay in normal maturation.

Clinical Findings. The orthodontic pattern was that of a mild disto-occlusion, open bite anteriorly, and maxillary space deficiency. Several dental restorations had been placed previously, but with laborious effort and with no reduction in the child's emotionality.

The Initial Visit. Premedication with Vistaril, 100 mg., the night before and the same dose 1 hour before the appointment made standard analgesia induction entirely acceptable. Fifteen per cent nitrous oxide and 85 per cent oxygen proved entirely adequate. Clinical and radiographic examination, prophylaxis, and impressions for study models were all performed.

Subsequent Visits. After the first visit, premedication was discontinued. Routine operative procedures were performed using nitrous oxide analgesia (15 per cent nitrous oxide) supplemented with local anesthesia. First, a fixed lower lingual arch was placed. Then, using analgesia and local anesthesia, the upper primary cuspids and first primary molars were removed. An upper twin wire labial arch was placed, with banding of the four permanent incisors. Subsequently, the upper first permanent bicuspids were exposed and extracted. Marked improvement in facial appearance was, by then, already apparent.

With this patient, nitrous oxide analgesia permitted a remarkable degree of dental manipulation. Her visits were multiple and the procedures performed were relatively complicated, demanding the continuous cooperation of the patient. Without analgesia this child could very easily have developed into a hopeless dental problem.

Case Report: Mental Retardation; Marginal Trainable-Educable. This 3½ year old boy with no apparent physical stigmata had been born prematurely at seven months and had a birth weight of 3 pounds, 3 ounces. He was fearful and absolutely reluctant to leave his mother's side. The mother was very much concerned about his badly involved upper incisor teeth, which exhibited severe hypoplastic defects, with carious lesions superimposed.

The Initial Visit.   Chloral hydrate, 7½ grains, was prescribed 1 hour before the appointment. With the child seated in his mother's lap, 40 per cent nitrous oxide and 60 per cent oxygen was blown across his nostrils. In spite of some head movement, sufficient euphoria was obtained to seat the nasal inhaler. No local anesthetic injection was attempted. The nitrous oxide level was then reduced to 15 per cent and maintained at this level. With a low-speed contra-angle, the upper right primary central and lateral incisors were disked interproximally. A round bur and hand excavators were used to complete the caries removal, with no attempt being made at definite cavity preparation. Anterior orthodontic bands were fitted and crimped appropriately. A fast-setting zinc oxide and eugenol paste was flowed over the most deeply excavated surfaces, and the bands were cemented with zinc oxyphosphate cement.

The Second Visit.   The same procedure was performed for the second visit, and the upper left central and lateral incisors were banded (Fig. 9–6).

AUDITORY HANDICAPS

Children with hearing handicaps may be totally deaf or only hard of hearing. They may have been born deaf (congenital), or they may have acquired deafness as a result of infection, drugs, or neurological change either before or after the acquisition of speech. Although they may be average in mental development, their achievement in language is often retarded. This difficulty in

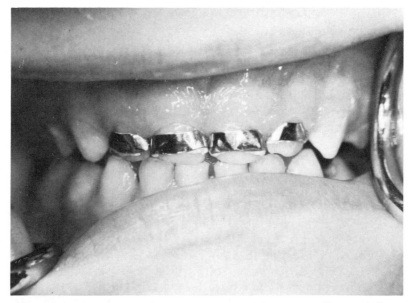

Figure 9–6   Relative analgesia made this dentistry possible in a mentally retarded youngster.

communication creates problems in interpersonal relations and prevents normal social maturity.

For the introduction of analgesia to these patients, the suggestions of Brown and Warren[1] are applicable and appropriate. It is important for the dentist to speak slowly and to make slow, purposeful gestures. For lip readers, directing the dental operating light on the dentist's lips may make comprehension easier. The mother is an important agent in communication, either by sign language or by familiar and usual gestures.

VISUAL HANDICAPS

The visually handicapped child may be blind or have partial sight, and may have defective vision even after corrective procedures. In introducing this child to analgesia, every procedure should be preceded by an explanation. He should be permitted to feel each piece of equipment that is to be used. Positional changes should be performed slowly and gradually, and unexpected changes, such as tipping the operating chair suddenly are to be avoided. I recall an entirely cooperative, partially seeing child, who, unprepared for a camera photoflash, temporarily became a severe management problem.

BEHAVIORAL DEVIATION

Behavioral deviations may assume various forms. The psychologically involved child may be hostile and aggressive, or withdrawn and restrained. He may demonstrate low or high intellectual capacity, and he may or may not have physical defects. Children showing behavioral deviation may include neurotic and psychotic children, and those with less severe emotional difficulties.

When confronted with the dental experience, many children with psychological involvement can be emotionally stabilized by nitrous oxide analgesia. There are, however, psychotic conditions such as the autism of childhood in which its application is rarely successful. Some psychotic, neurotic, and psychoneurotic conditions are characterized by swings in behavior in which a calm period may make them more amenable to analgesia application. We have children on our psychiatric ward who, with proper timing, are treated with relative ease.

There are no hard and clear-cut rules in the analgesia management of the behaviorally deviant child. However, it would be foolhardy to attempt to administer nitrous oxide analgesia to a historically psychotic child without previous consultation with the physician. Existing drug regimens may alter plans to premedicate or even to attempt any treatment at any given time. It is a basic premise that nitrous oxide analgesia serves to beneficially alter, reduce, and ameliorate disruptive behavior patterns. However, the decision as to when to use it must be based on the particular characteristics of each patient.

Case Report: Depression and Lack of Affect.   A 6 year old girl, small in stature and melancholy in appearance, the product of a full-term pregnancy, had a birth weight of 5 pounds. She was physically unstigmatized, although the mother stated that all her primary teeth erupted with severe hypoplastic defects. She was a completely withdrawn child, with total lack of affect; she attended all nine dental visits without uttering a single word, without a single smile, without a response of any kind. Her mother stated that she attended school, had many friends, and was entirely well behaved at home.

Her previous dental experience included the extraction under general anesthesia of all primary molars and all primary upper incisors. The child was entirely unresisting during the dental examination, which revealed four badly decayed primary cuspids, as well as primary lower lateral incisors that were moderately mobile. All the permanent first molars and lower permanent central incisors were actively erupting.

The treatment plan involved the insertion of upper and lower partial dentures. Since the child had a very severe gag reflex, 10 per cent nitrous oxide and 90 per cent oxygen was used for all restorative procedures as well as for the taking of impressions. Without supplementation with local anesthesia, all four primary cuspids were excavated and banded (Fig. 9–7 A). Bands with buccal lugs were also placed on the lower permanent first molars. Upper and lower partial dentures were inserted, which were worn daily but sporadically (Fig. 9–7 B).

It was felt that, with this child, midtreatment explosion and resistance could have occurred at any time within the treatment period. It was difficult to fathom this child because of the total lack of communication and affect. In any event, it was felt that analgesia provided a stabilizing factor in her treatment.

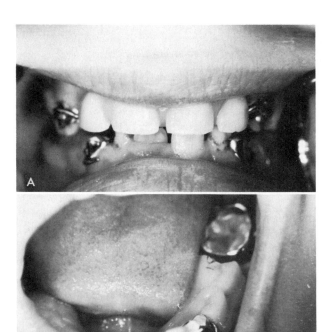

Figure 9–7 Depression and lack of affect. A, Primary cuspids excavated and banded. B, Partial dentures inserted.

BRAIN INJURY

There is another type of brain damage which manifests itself in certain behavioral disorders, errors in perception, and the inability to form adequate concepts. This comprises a variety of organic brain injuries, sometimes referred to as "minimal cerebral dysfunction" or the "Strauss syndrome," but now usually referred to as "brain injury." In the brain-injured child, the subcortical area, which is a stimulus-filtering mechanism, does not function properly, thus causing confusion and disorder. Swings of mood, easy distractability, low impulse control, inability to conceptualize, short attention span, and perseveration are characteristic of this condition. The afflicted child is typically hyperactive, destructive, easily sidetracked, and slow and clumsy. He is behaviorally difficult, restless, and uninhibited in speech and action. He may frequently show a pattern similar to that in emotional disturbance. His intellectual capacity can range through all levels.

This child may exhibit many of the factors that militate against effective dental management. Yet he has the ability to respond to a benign and sympathetic approach. If stimuli are kept to a minimum and if advantage is taken of his perseveration, it is frequently possible to make him a good analgesia patient. In treating such a child, it is important to avoid sudden and unusual movements, for his faulty spatial perception may, for example, give him the impression of falling when an abrupt chair change is made. Distracting devices, such as a 'mobile, may fix his attention long enough to permit analgesia induction. He will not listen to any prolonged explanation. Sometimes a single phrase or action will keep his attention long enough to permit the application of the nasal inhaler, or at least to permit its application close to his nose. Once a euphoric level is established and sounds and movements are kept to a minimum, he will frequently remain quiescent. He may not require the deeper analgesic levels but, in our experience, prolonged treatment periods are usually not possible. Local anesthesia and premedication obviously should be considered when strong operative stimuli are anticipated.

Case Report: Brain Injury. The patient was a physically small 5 year old boy who was physically unstigmatized and who vocalized constantly, albeit inappropriately. His history was essentially negative, and the mother attributed the child's hyperactivity to his general "brattiness." A recommendation for consultation with a pediatric neurologist had been made, but was never pursued.

The Initial Visit. The child exhibited many of the features of brain injury, but his small physical size and relative cooperation made his transfer to the operatory uncomplicated. He was obviously in pain from a badly broken lower right first primary molar. His attention was drawn to a mobile directly over the chair, and the nose-piece was placed with ease. Because of severe gagging and the necessity for giving a mandibular block for the extraction of the offending tooth, a mixture of 50 per cent nitrous oxide and 50 per cent oxygen was administered. The injection was then given and the patient promptly entered the excitement stage. Reduction and elevation of nitrous oxide levels was performed several times, and the tooth was finally removed. The entire session was stormy, and the child emerged with obvious nausea and discomfort.

Subsequent Visits.   After the first visit, Vistaril (50 mg.) the night before and again 1 hour before the appointment was prescribed, and food consumption was prohibited in the four hours before the appointment. Fortunately, the ill effects of the first appointment were apparently forgotten, so that he was easily maintained on 20 per cent nitrous oxide and 80 per cent oxygen with no difficulty. The dental procedures included routine fillings, another extraction, and the insertion of a fixed lower space maintainer.

CONGENITAL MALFORMATIONS

Cleft Palate.   Maintenance of teeth, both primary and permanent, is extremely important for the child with cleft palate. Orthodontic therapy assumes major importance in the rehabilitation of this patient, and its success depends on the ability to use teeth as appliance abutments. This is also true in prosthetic reconstruction.

The oronasal communication, depending on its extent, may affect the efficacy of analgesia administration. The possible dilution of the gaseous mixtures because of the impossibility of practicing strict nasal breathing may necessitate slight increases in the nitrous oxide ratio. It may also be advisable, if the communication is large, to limit the use of the heavy water spray in operative procedures or to occlude the opening with moist gauze.

Analgesia can prove highly effective in impression taking for this patient. Although the gag reflex is notably reduced, adjustments and alterations require the dentist to make frequent returns to the mouth. Such stress, especially for this child, can be reduced considerably with the use of analgesia.

Case Report: Micrognathia.   A 7 year old boy of normal stature was stigmatized by the "Andy Gump" type of facies. His speech was unintelligible, but his intellectual functioning was unimpaired. The child was attending school, and was in a grade appropriate to his age. He was highly apprehensive but otherwise cooperative.

Clinical examination revealed a remarkably small mandible, with opening of the mouth being severely limited. Surgery for the inclusion of a cartilaginous graft had been performed to increase the length of the mandible, but this had elevated, making intra-oral examination even more difficult. The tongue was rudimentary in size, and there were several carious teeth, some requiring extraction and several requiring restorations. Radiographically, partial anodontia was evident. In the past, several teeth had been extracted under general anesthesia.

The child's apprehension and limited mouth opening, further complicated by the cartilaginous hump, made management difficult. The administration of 15 per cent nitrous oxide and 85 per cent oxygen, in conjunction with local anesthesia, effected a considerable reduction in anxiety and permitted the necessary restorations and extractions to be done. Equally important was the ability to use a ratchet type of mouth prop, which was ordinarily painful for the child, in order to obtain the access necessary for treatment.

Eventual dental reconstruction, pending possible further surgery and the eruption of the permanent teeth, will be a highly complicated task.

Case Report: Congenital Heart Disease. A slightly obese, highly apprehensive 6 year old girl had a history of congenital truncus arteriosus, accompanied by defects of the interventricular and atrial septa, and was obviously intensely cyanotic. The child had never undergone dental treatment, and clinical examination revealed a severely involved dentition, requiring multiple fillings and several extractions. Consultation with the pediatric cardiologist offered the following: absolute contraindication to general anesthesia; procaine or lidocaine HCL with 1:100,000 solution of epinephrine permissible; premedication and low nitrous oxide analgesia permissible; and mandatory cover with antibiotics for three days after each dental visit.

For the initial two visits, Demerol (50 mg.) and Phenergan (25 mg.) were given 1 hour before the appointment. Ready acceptance of nitrous oxide analgesia (10 per cent nitrous oxide and 90 per cent oxygen) was obtained. The analgesic effect and the high oxygen level produced a remarkable reduction in cyanosis as well as a highly beneficial personality change in this child. Local anesthesia injection was performed without her perception. It was possible to restore several involved teeth at each visit.

It was elected to reserve the necessary extractions for the last visit. The teeth were removed at one sitting, with analgesia at the aforementioned levels and local anesthesia. Analgesia permitted, without objection, intramuscular bilateral deltoid injections, 600,000 units each of aqueous penicillin G. Subsequently, a fixed lower space maintainer was fabricated. In addition, a removable upper appliance was inserted for the dual purpose of space maintenance and reduction of a severe tongue thrust habit.

This report illustrates the effective utilization of nitrous oxide analgesia in a patient highly sensitive to a variety of factors, which would otherwise have created many treatment problems.

SUMMARY

It has been the purpose of this section to present a variety of handicapping conditions in which the utilization of relative analgesia can contribute greatly to successful dental management. It is suggested that the dentist who is successful in analgesia administration for his normal pediatric patients can extend the use of this instrument to include the treatment of many handicapped children. It is of great significance to know also that handicapped children who are treated successfully with relative analgesia return readily for recall appointments. Although an intermittent flow machine was employed for the cases recorded, continuous flow machines can be equally effective.

REFERENCES

1. Brown, R. H., and Warren, S. A.: The handicapped child—a challenge to dentistry. New Zealand Dent. J., 66:3, 1965.
2. Cheyne, V. D., and Marsh, E.: Psychological problems in dental care of the feeble minded patient. A study of the behaviorism in 70 cases. Amer. J. Ment. Def., 53:582, 1949.
3. Cohen, E.: Some aspects of operative dentistry under analgesia. New York Dent. J., 32:212, 1966.

4. Colding, A.: Universal analgesia and universal anesthesia. J. Dent. Child., *32*:124, 1965.
5. Emmertsen, E.: The treatment of children under general analgesia. J. Dent. Child., *32*:123, 1965.
6. Holst, J. J.: Use of nitrous oxide-oxygen analgesia in dentistry. Inter. Dent. J., *12*:47, 1962.
7. Kirk, S. A.: Educating Exceptional Children, Boston, Houghton Mifflin, 1962.
8. Klock, J. H., and Tom, A.: Nitrous Oxide Amnalgesia. North Conway, N. H., Reporter Press, 1965.
9. Langa, H.: Analgesia for modern dentistry. New York. J. Dent., *27*:228, 1957.
10. Langa, H.: Analgesia for modern pedodontics. New York. Dent. J., *28*:58, 1962.
11. Seldin, H. M.: Practical Anesthesia for Dentistry and Oral Surgery. Philadelphia, Lea & Febiger, 1947.
12. Snyder, J. R., et al.: Dental problems of non-institutionalized mentally retarded children. Northwest Dent., *39*:132, 1960.

RELATIVE ANALGESIA: EQUIPMENT AND GASES

10

EQUIPMENT

CYLINDERS

A gas dispensed at a gauge pressure exceeding 25 lb. per square inch at 70° F. is termed a compressed gas. In the United States, the Department of Transportation has promulgated regulations for construction and handling of cylinders containing such gases.

1. Gases used for anesthesia and inhalation therapy are dispensed in steel cylinders whose walls are ⅜ inch thick.

2. Anesthetic gases may be piped to treatment rooms through copper tubing. If the source of gas (cylinders) and the gas machine are in the same room, and no partitions, walls, or floors have to be traversed, high-pressure rubber tubing may be utilized.

3. The dentist should never attempt to refill a small cylinder from a large one, for there are serious hazards involved. The Compressed Gas Association, Inc., and the National Fire Protection Association, in its pamphlet No. 56 G 1975 recommend that cylinders be returned to charging plants for refilling under recognized safe practices.

4. *Retesting cylinders.* In conformance with Department of Transportation regulations, cylinders are subjected to a test by interior hydrostatic pressure at least once in 5 years. These retests are made at a pressure specified in DOT regulations for each of the types of cylinders. Each cylinder that passes the test is plainly and permanently stamped with the month and year of the test.

5. *Color code.* A color code to aid in the identification of medical gas cylinders has been adopted by the medical gas industry, the American Society of Anesthetists, and the American Hospital Association. This code has been published by the U.S. Department of Commerce as *Simplified Recommendation R176-41 of the Bureau of Standards.* Copies can be obtained from the Superintendent of Documents, Washington, D.C. The Department of Commerce, as well as the medical profession, recommends that anesthetic gas cylinders approximately 4½ inches in diameter by 26 inches long or smaller, which are intended for use on anesthesia machines, be marked with standard identifying colors.

6. Several large cylinders may be attached to a manifold system. This eliminates the necessity for frequent changing of cylinders, for when one cylinder becomes empty, the other cuts in (Fig. 10–1).

7. Cylinders designed to withstand pressures exceeding 450 lb. per square inch are constructed to resist a pressure 1.66 times the usual or service pressure. Since large cylinders designed for anesthesia are intended to be used at a service pressure of 2000 lb. per square inch or less, they are required to possess a tensile strength that is able to withstand a pressure of 3400 lb. per square inch.

8. The shoulder of each cylinder bears the dates of commissioning and testing, the service pressure, the insignia of the testing laboratory, and identification of ownership.

9. Cylinders should be stored in an upright position.

10. At high pressures, when their oxidizing properties are enhanced, oxygen or nitrous oxide can form an explosive mixture in the presence of grease or oil. These, as well as other organic materials, may oxidize with explosive speed and melt contacting metal.

When the pressure regulator is attached to the cylinder and the cylinder valve is opened suddenly, the escaping gas is immediately reduced from 2000 or more pounds per square inch to atmospheric pressure. This sudden expansion chills the gas to subzero temperature, but almost instantly, as more gas rushes into the confined space, pressure and temperature increase. The temperature may increase to a value sufficient to melt steel and ignite any com-

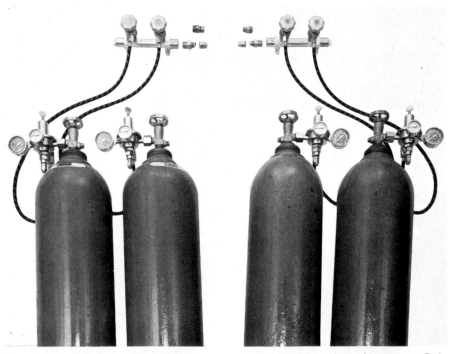

Figure 10–1   Large cylinders attached to a manifold system. (Courtesy of McKesson Co.)

bustible material present. Consequently, grease or oil is never to be used on valves, gauges, or other equipment for measuring or storing compressed gases.

11. Before attaching a cylinder to anesthetic equipment, carefully open it a little to blow out any small particles of dust that may obstruct the outlet of the valve. This will also facilitate the subsequent operation of the cylinder valve. (This is called "cracking.")

12. Never place cylinders near a source of heat.

13. Never drop a cylinder.

14. *Cylinder valves.* Cylinders are equipped with valves for filling and sealing the contents. Each valve stem is equipped with a hollow bolt packed with an alloy having a low melting point (93° C.). This fusible metal will melt in the event of fire, releasing the contents of the cylinder. The valve of an empty cylinder should always be closed to prevent contamination with dirt and moisture. Since the valve is the part of the cylinder most easily injured, the valves of large cylinders are protected by metal caps that are screwed over the top when the cylinder is not in use. These caps should not be removed until the cylinder is connected.

15. The dentist will find that using large cylinders is more economical and more practical, since small cylinders empty too quickly.

Nitrous Oxide Cylinders

The pressure in a full cylinder is usually between 800 and 900 lb. per square inch. In a full cylinder, nitrous oxide is present in liquid form. One ounce of the liquid will produce about 3.88 gallons of gas. The color code of the cylinder is light blue.

The various types of cylinders are listed in Table 10–1, and their relative sizes are shown in Figure 10–2. Of these, the following are most frequently used for dental analgesia and anesthesia.

Type	Volume
D	250 gal.
E	420 gal.
M	2000 gal.
G	3200 gal.

TABLE 10–1 Approximate Cylinder Weights and Dimensions

CYLINDER STYLE	APPROXIMATE DIMENSION (INCHES)	APPROXIMATE WEIGHT OF EMPTY CYLINDER (LB.)
A	3×10	$2^{3}/_{4}$
B	$3^{1}/_{2} \times 17$	8
D	$4^{1}/_{4} \times 20$	12
E	$4^{1}/_{4} \times 29^{1}/_{2}$	21
M	$7^{1}/_{8} \times 46$	74
G	$8^{1}/_{2} \times 55$	130
H	9×55	130
HH	$9^{1}/_{4} \times 59$	136

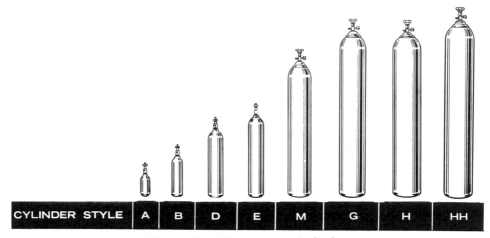

Figure 10-2 Various sizes of cylinders.

The D and E cylinders are attached directly to the gas machine. The M and G cylinders are the larger ones that are placed away from the gas machine. They connect to the machine by means of regulators and tubings.

In cylinders containing liquefied compressed nitrous oxide gas and vapor in equilibrium, the pressure in the cylinder is determined by the vapor pressure of the liquid at the existing temperature. Regardless of the amount of liq-

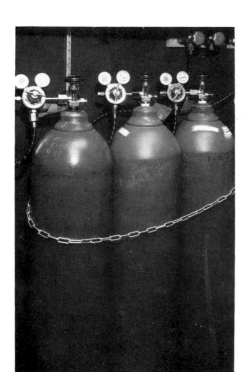

Figure 10-3 Manifold setup with chain around cylinders to minimize accidental tipping or falling. (Courtesy of McKesson Co.)

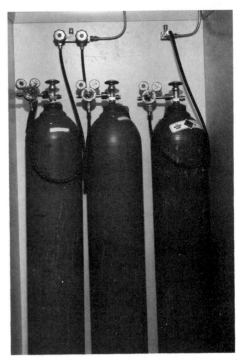

Figure 10–4 McKesson tank room setup: Double oxygen manifold with flexible hoses hooked to two oxygen pressure regulators on oxygen tanks. One nitrous oxide connection with flexible hose and nitrous oxide regulator. Both oxygen manifold and nitrous oxide manifold have built-in relief valves. (Courtesy of McKesson Co.)

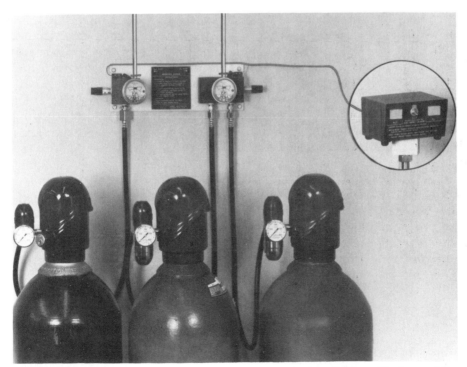

Figure 10–5 Manifold setup of oxygen and nitrous oxide cylinders. (Courtesy of Fraser Sweatman, Inc.)

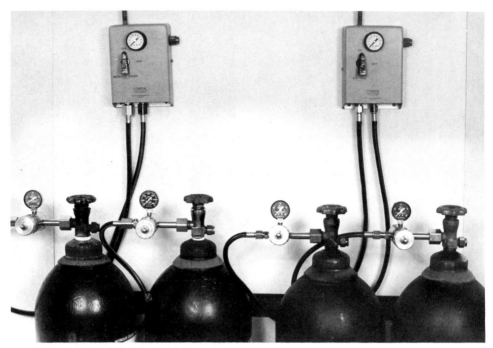

Figure 10-6   Coastal manifold system. (Courtesy of Coastal, Division of Chemetron.)

uid remaining in the cylinder, at a given temperature the pressure in the cylinder will remain constant until seven-eighths of the liquid has been withdrawn. Subsequently, the pressure drops in relation to the rate at which the remaining gas is withdrawn. So long as any liquid remains in the cylinder, the true contents can be determined only by weight.

The dentist will thus find that he will use the G cylinder of nitrous oxide for a considerable period of time before the pressure gauge shows any drop in pressure, because some of the liquid is still in the cylinder. As the liquid is withdrawn, the needle of the pressure gauge will fall very slowly. When it reaches the 500 mark, the liquid content of the cylinder is almost completely exhausted, with only gas remaining. From here on, the pressure indicator needle will fall much more rapidly than it did above the 500 mark. When the needle registers zero, the cylinder still retains 100 lb. pressure (not gallons). From this point, the regulator dial showing the pressure under which the gas is flowing to the machine is the indicator. When it begins to fall below the optimum pressure, the cylinder must be replaced. A spare cylinder should always be readily available.

Oxygen Cylinders

Oxygen for dental use is delivered in a gaseous state. In a full cylinder the pressure varies between 2000 and 2500 lb. per square inch. One ounce of the gas is equal to 5.22 gallons. The color code of the cylinder is green.

Type	Volume (gal.)
D	95
E	165
M	800
G	1400

In cylinders containing nonliquefied compressed gas, the pressure in the cylinder is related to the temperature as well as to the amount of gas in the cylinder. Thus, the contents of an oxygen cylinder can be determined by the pressure. At a given temperature, when the pressure indicator has dropped 50 per cent, the cylinder will be approximately half full.

The Pin-Index Safety System

The Pin-Index Safety System for preventing erroneous interchange of medical gas cylinders with flush-type valves is built around the matching of pins and holes (Fig. 10-7). Two pins are installed in the yokes of the apparatus, and two holes are drilled in the body of the cylinder valves. For any one gas there is only one combination of pins and holes. Unless the right cylinder is used, the holes and pins will not match and the two parts will not fit together.

The Pin-Index Safety System provides for 10 combinations of gases, each using two position holes on the cylinder valve and two corresponding pins on the yoke. Eight medical gases or gas mixtures are in use at present, leaving two position combinations available for future assignment. The recommendations of the medical profession were followed in selecting the various pin positions for the various gases, particularly in the case of the gas mixtures.

With this two-pin system it is impossible for a cylinder of one gas to be unintentionally attached to a yoke pin-indexed for any other gas. For example, a carbon dioxide yoke has pins so spaced as to receive only a carbon dioxide cylinder, the valve of which has holes matched to the spacing of the carbon dioxide yoke pins.

The Diameter-Index Safety System

The Diameter-Index Safety System (DISS) was developed by the Compressed Gas Association, Inc., to provide noninterchangeable threaded connections. DISS applies where make-and-break threaded connections are employed in conjunction with medical gas-administering equipment at pressures of 200 lb. per square inch or less, such as threaded outlets and connections of the medical gas regulators for anesthesia, resuscitation, and therapy apparatus.

Each connection of the Diameter-Index Safety System consists of a body, nipple, and nut (Fig. 10-8). The system is based on two concentric and spe-

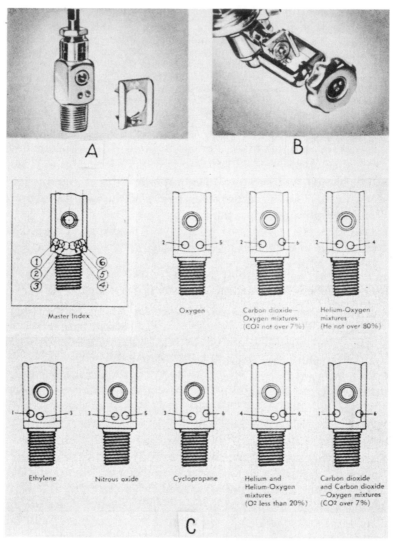

Figure 10–7 The Pin-Index Safety System for flush-type cylinder valves. *A*, On the right, a typical adapter with pins, to be installed on gas machine yoke, and on the left, a cylinder valve correspondingly drilled. Observe the identifying gas symbol (N_2O for nitrous oxide) on adapter. *B*, Yoke with adapter installed. *C*, Master index and eight assigned combinations of holes in cylinder valve bodies. Numbers indicate the standard designation for each hole. (Courtesy of Ohio Chemical & Surgical Equipment Co., Madison, Wisc.)

cific bores in the body (*A* and *B*), and two concentric and specific shoulders on the nipple (*C* and *D*). To achieve noninterchangeability between different connections, the two diameters on each part vary in opposite directions; i.e., as one diameter increases, the other decreases. Only properly mated parts fit with each other. Attempts to connect unintended parts result in interference at either the large or small diameter, which prevents thread engagement.

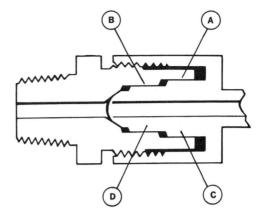

Figure 10-8 The Diameter-Index Safety System provides a noninterchangeable connection for each gas.

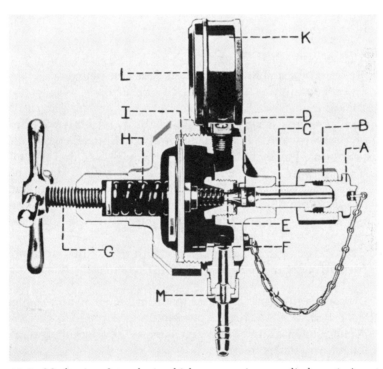

Figure 10-9 Mechanism for reducing high pressure in gas cylinders. A, A metal plug replacing cylinder threads when regulator is not in use, to prevent the entrance of dirt and to protect threads from injury; B, a threaded nut for attachment to the gas cylinder; C, gas under same pressure as cylinder contents; D, conical male element of valve which high gas pressure forces into valve seat E, preventing the escape of gas to reduce pressure chamber F. When screw G is advanced against spring H, flexible diaphragm I transmits force to male element D of the valve, allowing gas to enter chamber F until pressure in F is greater than the force exerted on I by spring H; diaphragm I thus releases pressure on D and the valve closes. Spring gauge K registers pressure in chamber F on dial L; if outlet M is small, spring gauge K can be calibrated to serve as a flowmeter and be read in cubic centimeters or liters of outflow per minute. An extra spring and pointer can be added to dial L and connected to C so as to register cylinder pressure, or a pressure gauge can be added for that purpose. (From A.M.A. Fundamentals of Anesthesia. 3rd ed. Philadelphia, W. B. Saunders Co., 1954.)

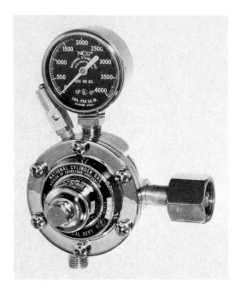

Figure 10–10   Regulator. One is used to control nitrous oxide and another to control oxygen. (Courtesy of Coastal, Division of Chemetron.)

Cylinder Regulators and Pressure Gauges

Large cylinders (M and G) must have a *regulator* (reducing valve) to step down the high pressure of the gases going to the gas machine to slightly above atmospheric pressure, and a *pressure gauge* to indicate the pressure of the gas within the cylinder. The regulator also ensures adequate delivery of gas to the machine. The pressure gauge, which is usually attached to the body of the regulator, indicates the *pressure* of the cylinder contents, not the *amount.*

Regulators (Figs. 10–9 and 10–10).   By maintaining constant gas pressure to the machine, regulators permit the following conditions to be achieved.

1. For any fixed setting of the flow control valve of the machine, the flowmeter reading will remain constant, regardless of the gas pressure in the cylinder.

2. The flow control valve of the machine can be adjusted more accurately. At a consistent, relatively low pressure (compared with cylinder pressure), the valve can be turned through a relatively large turn to achieve a small change in flowmeter reading.

3. The use of constant, relatively low pressures throughout the system precludes the possibility of a dangerous pressure build-up that could cause damage to the machine. Most systems in dental offices work at a pressure range between 35 and 50 lb. per square inch.

In high-pressure systems, regulators are usually equipped with pressure relief valves. These are preset to open at a specific pressure, depending on the system and gas used. They provide extra safety against the possibility of excessive pressure being delivered by the regulator. Such pressure may be created by a foreign particle that becomes wedged under the regulator valves or by a valve seat failure.

Pressure Gauges.   Pressure gauges, which show the pressure of gas in the cylinders, are connected to the circuit between the machine and the regulators, most often as a dial mounted on the regulator assembly (Figs. 10–9 and 10–10). Each gauge is especially calibrated, color coded, and identified by symbol according to the particular gas it monitors, for each kind of gas requires a gauge of special mechanical characteristics to provide maximum gauge sensitivity for the pressure range used with that particular gas. Oxygen pressure gauges usually range from zero to 3000 lb.; nitrous oxide pressure gauges range from zero to 1500 lb.

Nitrous Oxide-Oxygen Analgesia: Matching Technical Safety to Clinical Safety[10]

With the benefit of the knowledge gained over very many years as to the clinical safety and the effectiveness of nitrous oxide-oxygen analgesia in controlling apprehension and pain, the dental profession has found a myriad of applications to every phase of dental practice. In addition, physicians are using relative analgesia for many and diverse therapeutic and diagnostic procedures. Where state practice acts permit, podiatrists have been adding this instrument to their armamentarium. With this growth, some few but serious technical problems have been revealed. *They must be eliminated!*

A few years ago there were two explosions in dental offices in California due to faulty piping systems for nitrous oxide and oxygen. In both cases investigation revealed that a stainless steel mesh-covered Teflon manifold and nylon check valve had been used, which ignited as a result of the heat of recompression. Oxygen at over 2000 lb. per square inch in a full cylinder surges into the manifold when the cylinder valve is opened. When it reaches the reducing valve or pressure regulator, the pressure will drop to 50 lb. per square inch. This resulting backup causes recompression of the gas and a tremendous increase in temperature (1500° to 2000° F.). Such a temperature can ignite any organic contaminants such as grease, oil, and (in these two cases in question) the Teflon tubing used in the manifold.

As a result of these events, the American Analgesia Society was requested to send representatives to a meeting of the Sectional Committee on Inhalation Anesthetics, a part of the Hospitals Committee of the National Fire Protection Association.

After two years of work standards have been devised, published in a booklet entitled *Inhalation Anesthetics in Ambulatory Care Facilities* (NFPA No. 56G 1975). This booklet is obtainable by writing to the National Fire Protection Association at 470 Atlantic Avenue, Boston, Massachusetts 02210. In addition to fire hazards, it covers toxological hazards, mechanical hazards, electrical hazards, and *crossed-piping hazards* – this last item having been the reported cause of more than one tragic accident in the past few years.

Among the most pertinent provisions regarding central piping systems for small, non-hospital facilities having no more than six use points are the following:

1. The system shall have not more than 2000 cubic feet total capacity of all gases connected and in storage at one time. Since a G cylinder of oxygen contains 188 cubic feet and a G cylinder of nitrous oxide contains 488 cubic

feet, an office could have an ample supply on hand—five G cylinders of oxygen and two G cylinders of nitrous oxide.

2. A pressure regulator should be directly connected to each cylinder, which will effectively reduce the pressure to the pipeline to a working pressure of 50 to 55 lb. per square inch.

3. Cylinders and gases should be obtained from sources that strictly observe the United States Department of Transportation (DOT) specifications and regulations.

4. The enclosure for the storage of cylinders must have a lock so that the gases cannot be used by unauthorized personnel. No compressors, evacuation systems, storing of supplies, open electrical conductors, or sources of heat are permitted in this enclosure. The door to this enclosure shall be provided with a louvered opening having a minimum of 72 square inches in total free area.

5. There shall be an alarm on the main oxygen supply line which will be activated when the line pressure drops 20 per cent below normal operating pressure. The alarm shall be audible and loud enough to be heard in all treatment rooms.

6. Where the central supply is remote from the system use points, the main supply lines shall be provided with shut-off valves labeled to indicate the gas controlled, and be accessible from use point locations in an emergency.

7. Installation of the piping system is to be done according to the NFPA regulations: fittings; method of cleaning them; the tools used to work on the system; type of brazing alloy and sealing compounds. Additionally, methods of testing for leaks and cross connection are detailed and should be followed not only on installation, but also after any repair or change in any part of the system.

8. Equipment should be obtained from and installed under the super-

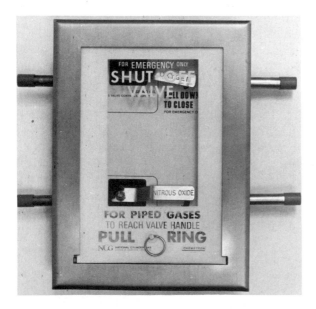

Figure 10–11 Coastal zone valves. (Courtesy of Coastal, Division of Chemetron.)

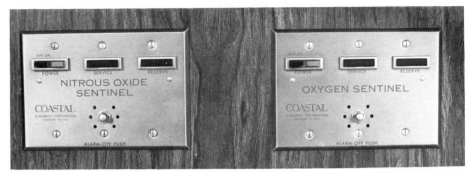

Figure 10–12   Coastal alarm panels. (Courtesy of Coastal, Division of Chemetron.)

vision of a manufacturer or supplier familiar with proper practices for its construction and use.

9. Special precautions concerning the handling of oxygen and nitrous oxide cylinders:

   a. Keep all petroleum products and other organic contaminants away from cylinders, regulators, fittings and lines.

   b. Clean particles of dust and dirt from the cylinder valve before applying any fitting to the cylinder.

   c. Open cylinder valves slowly with the gauge on the regulator pointed away from any person.

   d. Close cylinder valves when not in use.

GAS MACHINES

It must be clear to the reader of this text that, initially, successful administration of relative analgesia depends on the proper psychological conditioning of the patient. In most instances, the machine cannot initially create good analgesia; a proper relationship between patient and doctor must first be created. Then, and only then, can the machine take over and function properly. The gas machine is simply a convenient device for delivering a controlled proportionate flow of nitrous oxide and oxygen.

Any gas machine that delivers both nitrous oxide and oxygen can be employed successfully for the administration of relative analgesia. An anesthesia machine can be used to administer analgesia, although an analgesia machine does not usually function as an anesthesia device because of the smaller volume flow of gases per minute.

Basic Elements of Gas Machines

Yokes. Yokes hold the cylinders of compressed gas tightly in contact with the nipples of the gas machine. In the pin-index system, prongs or studs in the collar of the nipple fit into holes in the head of the cylinder to prevent

TABLE 10-2 Precautions in Handling Cylinders For Oxygen-Nitrous Oxide Analgesia Systems*†

GENERAL RULES	STORING CYLINDERS	WITHDRAWING CYLINDER CONTENT
Never permit oil, grease, or other readily combustible substance to come into contact with cylinders, valves, regulators, gauges, hoses, and fittings. Oil and certain gases such as oxygen or nitrous oxide may combine with explosive violence.	Storage rooms should be dry, cool, and well ventilated. Where practical, storage rooms should be fireproof. Storage in subsurface locations should be avoided. Storage conditions should comply with local and state regulations.	After removing valve protection cap, slightly open valve an instant to clear opening of possible dust and dirt. This should not be done with cylinders containing flammable gas.
Never lubricate valves, regulators, gauges, or fittings with oil or any other combustible substance.	Cylinders should be protected against excessive rise of temperature. Do not store cylinders near radiators or other sources of radiant heat. Do not store cylinders near highly flammable substances such as oil, gasoline, waste, etc. Keep sparks and flame away from cylinders.	When opening valve, point the outlet away from you. Never use wrenches or tools except those provided or approved by the gas supplier. Never hammer the valve wheel in attempting to open or to close the valve.
Do not handle cylinders or apparatus with oily hands or gloves.		
Fully open the cylinder valve when cylinder is in use.	Large cylinders should be placed against a wall to offer some protection against being knocked over. They should not be placed along an aisle used for trucking traffic. The best practice is to provide means for a chain fastening of large cylinders to the wall.	After attaching regulator and before cylinder valve is opened see that the regulator is turned to the off position in the case of regulators equipped with a pressure adjusting screw. This is accomplished by turning the screw counterclockwise until it turns freely.
Never tamper with the safety relief devices of valves or cylinders.		
	Cylinders should be protected against tampering by unauthorized individuals.	Never permit gas to enter the regulating device suddenly. Always open the cylinder valve slowly.
	Valves should be kept closed on empty cylinders to avoid entry of atmospheric contaminants.	Before regulating device and cylinder are disconnected close the cylinder valve and release all pressure from the device.

*The information presented herein includes some of the significant safety precautions given in CGA Pamphlet P-2 and represents only a partial listing of the safety rules which should be observed by anyone handling or using compressed gases. Pamphlet P-2 may be obtained from Compressed Gas Association, Inc., 500 Fifth Avenue, New York, New York 10036.

†Courtesy of Puritan-Bennett Corporation.

TABLE 10-3 Gas and Cylinder Data*

GAS	NITROUS OXIDE (N₂O)			OXYGEN (O₂)		
Cylinder Size	E	G	H	E	G	H
Pounds/Square Inch Pressure When Full	750 PSI @ 70°			1950 PSI		2200 PSI
Cylinder Size and Weight	30" High 4½" Wide 22 lb.	55" High 8½" Wide 156 lb.	55" High 9" Wide 174 lb.	30" High 4½" Wide 17 lb.	55" High 8½" Wide 115 lb.	55" High 9" Wide 135 lb.
Color of Cylinder	Blue			Green		
Physical State in Cylinder	Liquid and Gas			Gas Only		
Capacity (liters)	1590	13,839	15,899	625	5300	6909

*Courtesy of Puritan-Bennett Corporation.

the wrong cylinder from being placed in the yoke. Of course, if large cylinders are being used, the end of the tubing system nearest the machine has the same attachments as the heads of the cylinders themselves.

Control Valves. From each nipple gas passes directly to a fine control valve, or through an automatic pressure-reducing valve and then to the fine control valve.

Flowmeters. The gas then passes through a meter that indicates the rate of flow. Three types of flowmeters are available for use in dentistry (Fig. 10–13).

Each flowmeter is calibrated only for the gas that it is to measure; hence the substitution of one gas for another may result in inaccurate measurement of volumes. The flow is gauged at atmospheric pressure (76 cm. Hg) and room temperature (25°C.). Each meter must have a reducing valve interposed between it and the cylinder valve in order to deliver the gases at a safe pressure and a constant rate. Gases may be measured in terms of the metric system, in

TABLE 10-4 Flow Chart for Standard Cylinders* of Oxygen U.S.P.†

	READING ON CYLINDER CONTENTS GAUGE				
		FULL	¾	½	¼
READING ON FLOW INDICATOR IN LITERS PER MINUTE	244 cu. ft. 2200 lb. pressure 6909 liters	220 cu. ft. 2000 lb. pressure 6000 liters	165 cu. ft. 1500 lb. pressure 4500 liters	110 cu. ft. 1000 lb. pressure 3000 liters	55 cu. ft. 500 lb. pressure 1500 liters
	APPROXIMATE REMAINING HOURS OF SERVICE				
2	57½	50	37½	25	12½
4	28¾	25	18¾	12½	6¼
6	19	16½	12¼	8¼	4
8	14¼	12½	9¼	6¼	3
10	11½	10	7½	5	2½
12	9½	8¼	6	4	2

*This chart is based on a full cylinder content of 244 cu. ft. For 220 cu. ft.-capacity cylinders, use appropriate columns. For 122 cu. ft.-capacity cylinders, divide hours of service by 2.
†Courtesy of Puritan-Bennett Corporation.

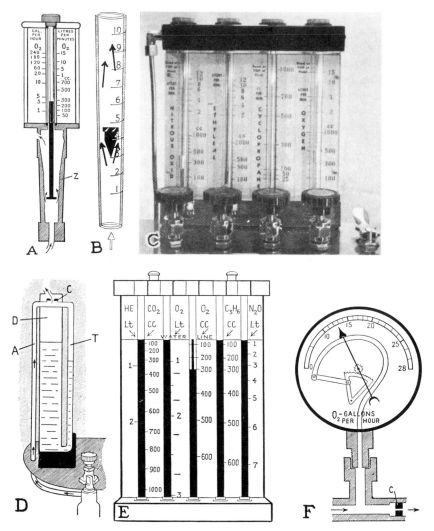

Figure 10–13   Flowmeters. *A, B, C,* Dry flowmeters. A small body floats in the stream of gas that flows upward through a tapered tube. The greater the flow, the higher the float rises. Taper can be varied to give fine readings at slow flows, coarse readings at higher flows. *A,* Diagram showing principles involved. *B,* Tapered cylinder is metal; reading is taken at top of floating rod. *C,* Set of four meters. A fine control valve is at the base of each meter. Floats show nitrous oxide and oxygen flowing. Valve at lower right is for rapid unmetered flow of oxygen. Gas leaves meters through pipe at left.

D, E, Water depression meters. Flow of gas is resisted by a small orifice. Before passing through the orifice, it depresses a column of water. The greater the pressure, the greater is the flow through the orifice, and the farther the water column is depressed. Gives undesirable coarse reading at slow flow, fine reading at rapid flow. Clogging of orifice decreases flow, yet meter indicates greater flow. *D,* Diagram showing principle involved. Gas passes in through *A,* exerts pressure on water at *T,* and escapes through orifice *C. E,* Set of five meters; central meter indicates a flow of 300 cc. of oxygen per minute.

F, Bourdon-gauge meter. Flow of gas is resisted by a very small orifice, *C,* exerting pressure in the flexible tube geared to the pointer, which indicates flow of over 12 gallons per hour. Inaccurate for the slow flows used in modern anesthesia. (Drawings from R. Macintosh et al.: Physics for the Anaesthetist. 3rd ed. Oxford, Blackwell Scientific Publications Ltd., 1963.)

liters or fractions of liters per minute or, in terms of the English scale, in gallons per minute or hour.

Gauge Type.   A constriction in the inlet tube increases the pressure of flowing gases. The increased pressure is transmitted to a diaphragm that works a clockwise mechanism and records the flow of gases in liters or gallons per minute.

Dry Flowmeters.   In the dry flowmeter, a small float is suspended by the stream of gas that flows upward through a tapered tube. The greater the flow, the higher the float rises. The taper can be varied to give fine readings at slow flows, coarse readings at higher flows. The float may be a rotor (a cone-shaped aluminum bobbin) or a ball made of plastic or metal. After passing the float, the streams converge and pass to the inhaling apparatus. The dentist will see this type of flowmeter more frequently than any other, especially on analgesia machines.

Hydraulic Flowmeters (Wet Flowmeters).   A constriction in the inlet tube causes an increase in the pressure of the flowing gas that is transmitted to a column of water in a calibrated tube which is depressed in proportion to the flow of gas.

Fail-Safe Mechanisms.   The machine is equipped with an auxiliary attachment that precludes the possibility of administering nitrous oxide without oxygen during the administration of analgesia. When the oxygen flow pressure falls below 15 pounds, the flow of nitrous oxide ceases.

Oxygen Switch.   Some machines can be turned on only by means of a switch which provides a minimal flow of oxygen. This, together with a controlled maximal flow of nitrous oxide, precludes the administration of a mixture containing less than 20 per cent of oxygen, or of a flow of nitrous oxide without oxygen.

Types of Gas Machines

Two types of gas machines are well suited for the administration of analgesia: continuous flow machines and intermittent flow machines. Each has advantages and disadvantages in relation to the other.

CONTINUOUS FLOW MACHINES

In the United States several types of continuous flow machines are available. Among them are: the McKesson Analor (Figs. 10–14 to 10–20), the Quantiflex RA and MDM analgesia machines (Fraser Sweatman, Inc.) (Figs. 10–21 to 10–24), the Coastal analgesia machine (Coastal Dynamics Corp.) (Figs. 10–25 to 10–30), the Starflite Dentatron (Star Dental Manufacturing Co.) (Figs. 10–31 to 10–34), the Heidbrink analgesia or anesthesia machine (Fig. 10–35), the Foregger analgesia machine (Foregger Co.) (Figs. 10–36 to 10–38), the Adec analgesia machine (Fig. 10–39), the Sedatron analgesia machine (Parkell) (Fig. 10–40), the Pelton and Crane analgesia machine (Fig. 10–41), the Simplaire analgesia machine (Hampton Research & Engineering Co.) (Fig. 10–42), and the Veriflo NRC-2 analgesia machine (Veriflo Corp.) (Figs. 10–43 and 10–44).

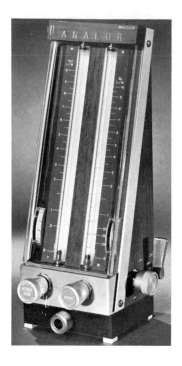

Figure 10–14 The McKesson Analor II for administering dental analgesia.

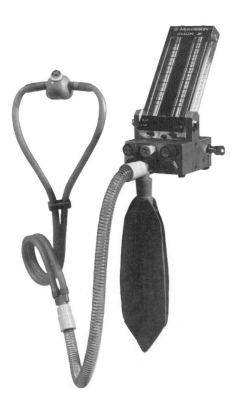

Figure 10–15 Analor II analgesia machine. (Courtesy of McKesson Co.)

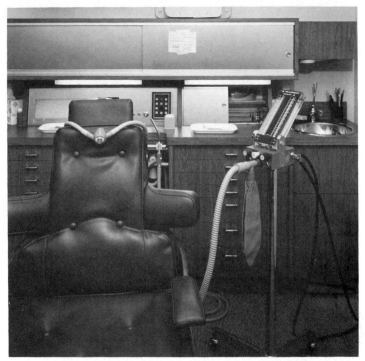

Figure 10–16 Analor III analgesia machine mounted on a mobile stand with casters. Machine is equipped with rubber parts and flexible hoses. (Courtesy of McKesson Co.)

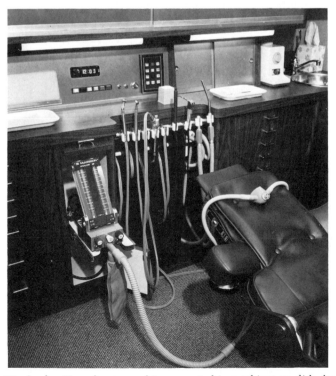

Figure 10–17 Analor III analgesia machine mounted in a cabinet on slide drawer. (Courtesy of McKesson Co.)

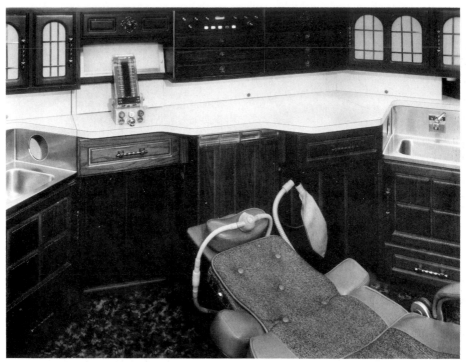

Figure 10–18   Analor III analgesia machine with special installation. Analor is mounted on top of cabinet, and outlet tubing is run down into cabinet and concealed until rubber parts are connected. Note that the rubber tubing and the reservoir bag are remote from the analgesia machine. This permits the machine to be placed in an optimal position and eliminates the annoyance of having the reservoir bag in a cumbersome and unsatisfactory position. (Courtesy of McKesson Co.)

There are other analgesia machines manufactured in other countries. They all function on the same principles.

Continuous Flow Principle.   Nitrous oxide and oxygen are fed into a reservoir bag by separate flowmeters. The proportions of the mixture in the reservoir bag are determined by varying the flow rate of each gas; the flow of one gas can be altered independently of the other gas. The patient inhales from this bag and exhales into the atmosphere through an exhaling valve placed in the circuit. Pressure equal to that of the gases is obtained by partial closure of the weighted exhaling valve, which results in distention of the reservoir bag.

A continuous flow gas machine is so called because the gases flow continually at the volumes and proportions set by the operator on the flowmeters and do not vary with any variations in the subject's respiration. The subject may breathe more rapidly, more slowly, more shallowly, or more deeply, but the output from the machine will be constant. A continuous flow machine is a quiet machine; usually the patient cannot tell whether or not gases are flowing. There is no blowing of gases under pressure against the nose and face. Since the gases flow from this type of machine under lower pressures, less gas

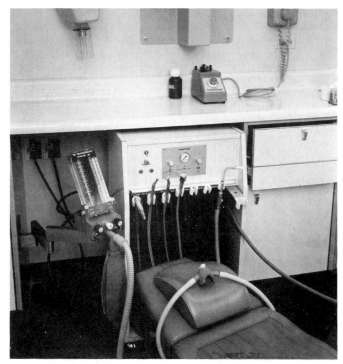

Figure 10–19 Analor III analgesia machine, wall mounted with extension arm. Analor is supplied from McKesson quick-connect outlet boxes. (Courtesy of McKesson Co.)

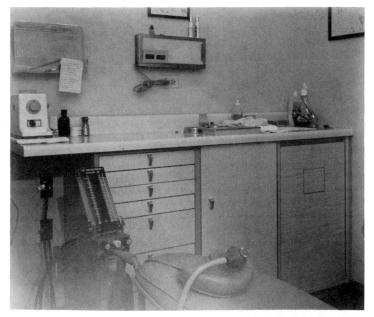

Figure 10–20 Analor III analgesia machine. The variety of mountings available places the machine exactly where you want it to be. (Courtesy of McKesson Co.)

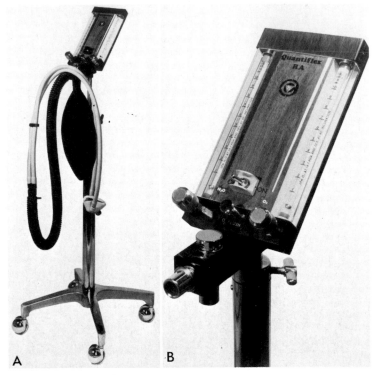

Figure 10–21   Quantiflex RA analgesia machine. (Courtesy of Fraser Sweatman, Inc.)

is consumed. A direct flow oxygen lever may be attached to a continuous flow machine.

Advantages of Continuous Flow Over Intermittent Flow Type. The continuous flow machine is superior to the intermittent flow type in that less gas is consumed, flowmeters show the exact output of the machine, there is less blowing of gas against the patient's face and nose, and there is less noise. The last two points are psychologically advantageous when administering relative analgesia for the first time. After the patient has become accustomed to the procedure, the noise and blowing of gas do not disturb him.

Nasal Inhalers for Continuous Flow Machines (Figs. 10–45 to 10–47). Inhalers are devices from which a subject breathes gases. For inhalation analgesia the semiclosed inhaler is used. Nasal inhalers for continuous flow machines have two valves.

Air Valve.   This valve, which is also called the inhaling valve, is the uppermost or innermost valve. Its function is to mix atmospheric air with the gases flowing from the machine. Very often the total volume of gases delivered for relative analgesia is less than the patient's minimal requirement (7500 to 8000 ml. per minute), and the air flowing through the air valve supplies the subject with sufficient volume to make breathing smooth and easy. This valve also provides a means of diluting or concentrating the analgesic mixture without changing the flowmeter readings. Of course, if the total output from the

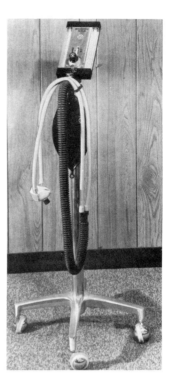

Figure 10–22 Quantiflex MDM analgesia machine on mobile stand. (Courtesy of Fraser Sweatman, Inc.)

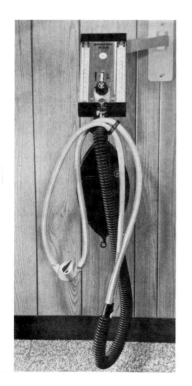

Figure 10–23 Quantiflex MDM analgesia machine, wall mounted. (Courtesy of Fraser Sweatman, Inc.)

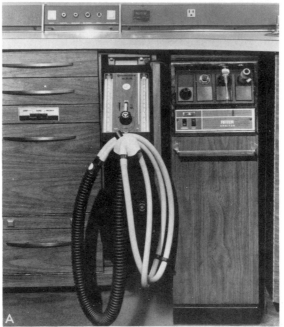

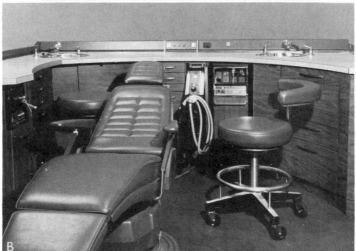

Figure 10–24 Two views of the Quantiflex MDM analgesia machine wall-mounted in cabinetwork. (Courtesy of Fraser Sweatman, Inc.)

machine is sufficient and a greater analgesic depth is desired, the valve may be closed completely. However, for routine procedure it is usually open to a greater or lesser degree.

Rebreathing Valve. This valve, also known as the exhaling valve, is below or outside the air valve. When it is completely closed, most of the patient's exhalations are forced back into the tubing instead of being expelled into the atmosphere. They are then rebreathed (see section on rebreathing,

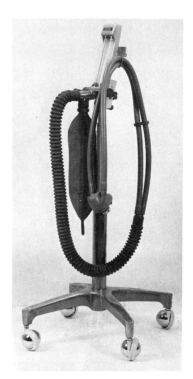

Figure 10–25 Coastal analgesia machine on mobile stand. (Courtesy of Coastal, Division of Chemetron.)

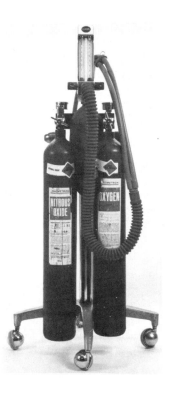

Figure 10–26 Coastal analgesia machine on mobile stand with E cylinders attached. (Courtesy of Coastal, Division of Chemetron.)

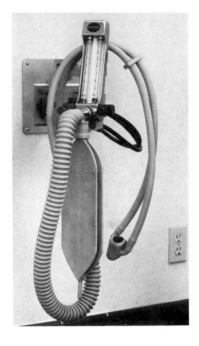

Figure 10–27 Coastal analgesia machine, wall mounted (front view). (Courtesy of Coastal, Division of Chemetron.)

Chapter 7). When this valve is open, the greatest portion of the gases is exhaled into the atmosphere.

Rebreathing Bag; Reservoir Bag. Continuous flow machines have a rubber bag attached to the machine or to the tubing. If the bag is attached to

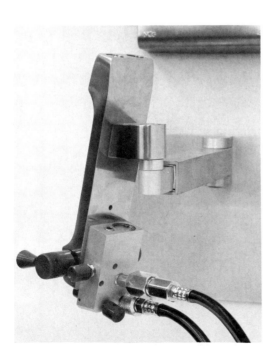

Figure 10–28 Coastal analgesia machine, wall mounted on swivel arm which also extends outward. (Courtesy of Coastal, Division of Chemetron.)

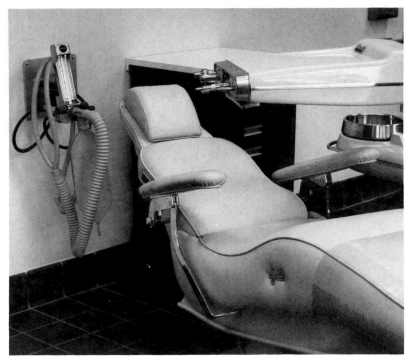

Figure 10–29 Coastal analgesia machine, wall mounted in optimal relationship to dental chair. (Courtesy of Coastal, Division of Chemetron.)

the tubing immediately behind the patient's head, it is a true rebreathing bag. The subject's inhalations will be forced back into this bag (when the rebreathing valve is closed) and then be rebreathed from there. If the bag is attached to the machine itself, it is too far away to function as a true rebreathing bag. It is rather a reservoir bag. Gases are stored up in this bag so that the patient will

Text continued on page 346

Figure 10–30 Coastal analgesia machine, wall mounted. (Courtesy of Coastal, Division of Chemetron.)

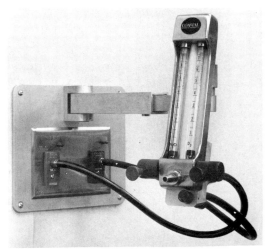
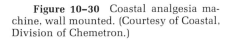

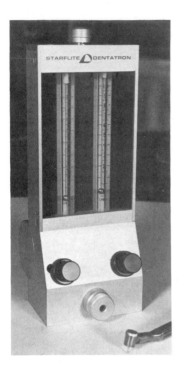

Figure 10-31 Starflite Dentatron analgesia machine. (Courtesy of Star Dental Manufacturing Co., Inc.)

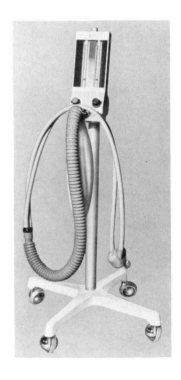

Figure 10-32 Starflite Dentatron analgesia machine on mobile stand ready to be attached to a central source of gas. (Courtesy of Star Dental Manufacturing Co., Inc.)

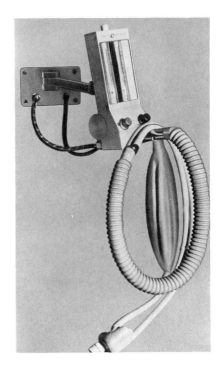

Figure 10–33 Starflite Dentatron analgesia machine on wall mount. (Courtesy of Star Dental Manufacturing Co., Inc.)

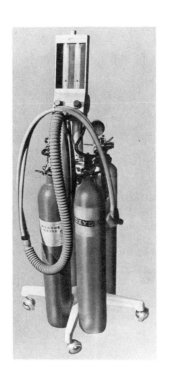

Figure 10–34 Starflite Dentatron analgesia machine on mobile stand with E cylinders attached. (Courtesy of Star Dental Manufacturing Co., Inc.)

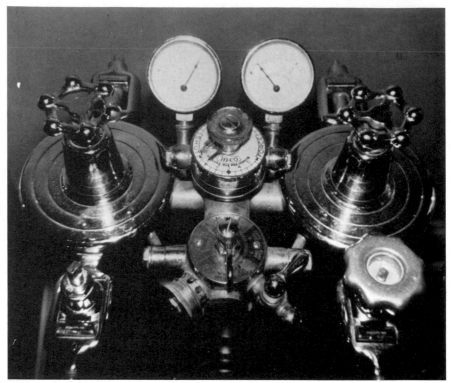

Figure 10–35 The Ohio Heidbrink anesthesia machine (Model T). (Courtesy of the Ohio Chemical Company.)

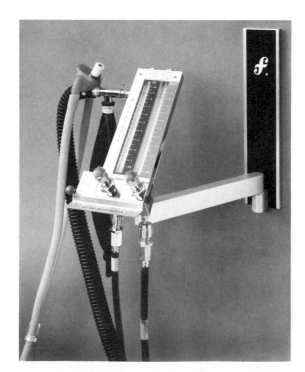

Figure 10–36 Foregger analgesia machine on wall-mounted swivel arm. (Courtesy of Foregger Co.)

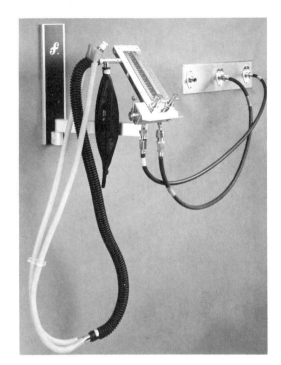

Figure 10–37 Foregger analgesia machine, wall-mounted and attached to quick-connects. (Courtesy of Foregger Co.)

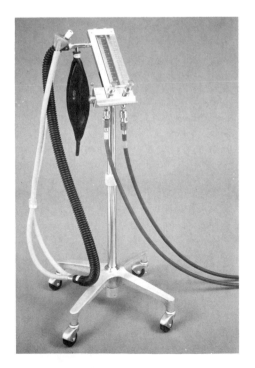

Figure 10–38 Foregger analgesia machine on mobile stand. (Courtesy of Foregger Co.)

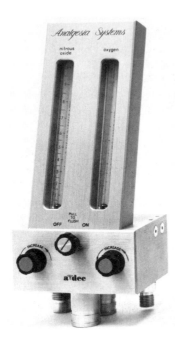

Figure 10–39   Adec analgesia machine. (Courtesy of Adec Co.)

always have a plentiful supply against which he can draw, should he require it. This will avoid the sense of suffocation that heavy breathers sometimes experience. At the commencement of administration, the operator should make certain that the reservoir bag is not collapsed, but that it contains some gas.

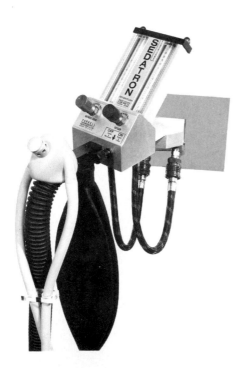

Figure 10–40   Sedatron analgesia machine on wall mount. (Courtesy of Parkell Co.)

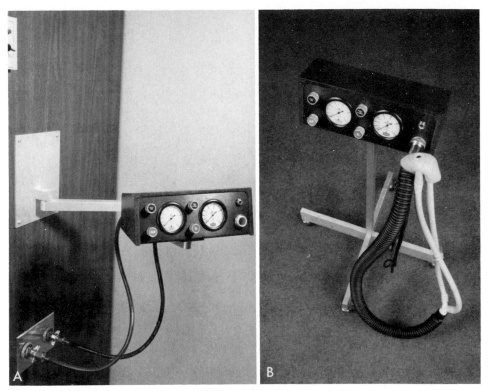

Figure 10–41   Two views of the Pelton and Crane N200 analgesia machine wall mount and floor models. (Courtesy of Pelton and Crane Co.)

Rebreathing bags are usually composed of rubber, are usually ovoid in shape, and vary between 1 and 5 liters in capacity, depending upon the type of inhaler for which they are designed. The rubber is of a light type that will not offer resistance to respiration. The bags are placed at some convenient point in the inhaling system and act as reservoirs for mixtures of gases. Each bag has a wide outlet at one end (2.5 cm. or more in diameter) and, for the semiclosed inhaler system used for inhalation analgesia, an inlet nipple may be furnished at the other end.

INTERMITTENT FLOW MACHINES

There are three types of intermittent flow machines: the McKesson Euthesor (Fig. 10–48), the McKesson Nargraf (Fig. 10–49), and the McKesson Narmatic. The first is an analgesia machine and the latter two are anesthesia machines. They are equipped with a semiclosed type of inhaler and have the following features:

1. An automatic mixing device that supplies preformed mixtures of nitrous oxide and oxygen.

2. An automatic feeding device that is activated by the reduced pressure in the inhaler caused by escape of gas or inspiratory negative pressure. It replaces gas lost from the inhaler.

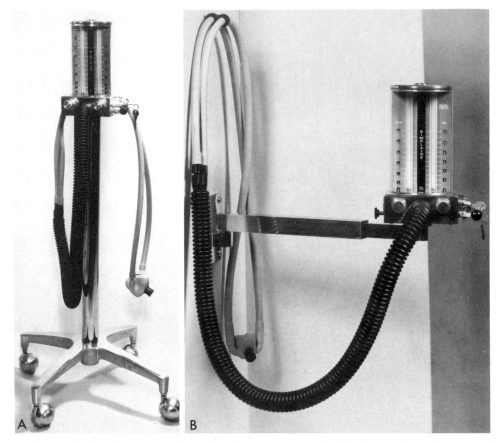

Figure 10–42   Simplaire analgesia machine. *A*, Mobile unit. *B*, Wall mount unit. (Courtesy of Hampton Research & Engineering, Inc.)

3. A device for adjusting pressure in the inhaler.

4. Gauges for indicating the pressure of oxygen and nitrous oxide supplied to the mixing meter.

5. An exhalation valve.

6. A direct flow oxygen button or lever.

7. A rebreathing (reservoir) bag.

Intermittent Flow Principle.   Intermittent flow machines are so called because the gases do not flow at a constant rate, but vary with the rate and depth of respiration and cease to flow during expiration. If the subject breathes rapidly or deeply, the intermittent flow machine will pour forth enough volume to supply his needs. If his breathing becomes slower or more shallow, the output of gas will decrease. Since the output varies with the patient's respiratory needs, this type of machine does not register the volume flow per minute, but simply the proportions of the two gases and the pressures at which they are being emitted. These pressures are registered in millimeters of mercury and can be varied. Any reduction in nitrous oxide

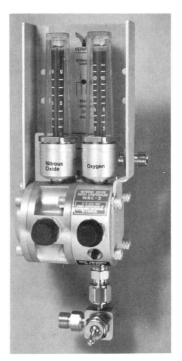

Figure 10–43 Veriflo NRC-2 analgesia machine, wall-mounted. (Courtesy of Veriflo Corp.)

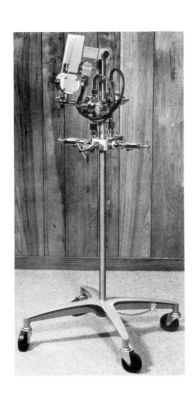

Figure 10–44 Veriflo NRC-2 analgesia machine on mobile stand. (Courtesy of Veriflo Corp.)

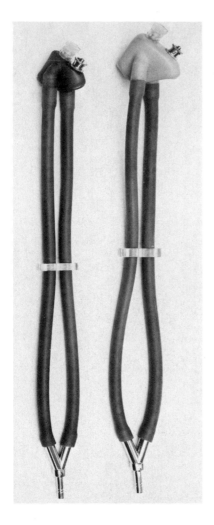

Figure 10–45   Nasal inhalers for continuous flow machines.

flow automatically increases the oxygen flow, and, by the same token, any reduction in oxygen flow increases nitrous oxide flow. The higher pressures under which gases are emitted by such a machine make for a greater consumption of gas, especially of oxygen.

   Advantages of Intermittent Flow Over Continuous Flow Machines. Because the gases can be forced into the respiratory system, this type of machine is advantageous when these conditions prevail: the patient cannot breathe easily or smoothly, the patient is a chronic mouth-breather, and the patient suffers from a nasal block in the form of polyps, deviated septa, and so forth. A further advantage is that a single manipulation adjusts the proportion of both oxygen and nitrous oxide.

   Nasal Inhalers for Intermittent Flow Machines (Fig. 10–50). Nasal inhalers for intermittent flow machines have but one valve, the rebreathing, or exhaling, valve. The extent to which the valve is opened is registered in degrees of spring tension. For analgesia administration, the spring is set at

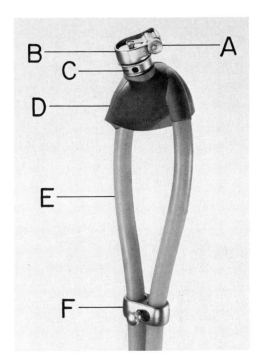

Figure 10–46 The McKesson nasal inhaler (continuous flow). *A*, Valve control (0 to 5 mm.); *B*, exhaling (rebreathing) valve; *C*, inhaling (air) valve; *D*, hood; *E*, connecting tubes; *F*, slide assembly.

zero tension. This setting provides for the greatest ease of exhalation and is tantamount to the wide open position of the exhaling (rebreathing) valve of the continuous flow machine. Rebreathing is initiated by increasing the spring tension.

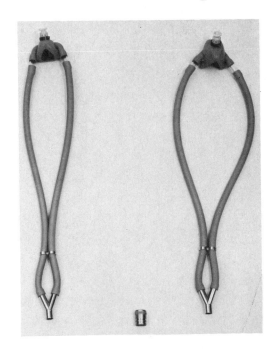

Figure 10–47 Nasal inhalers (continuous flow).

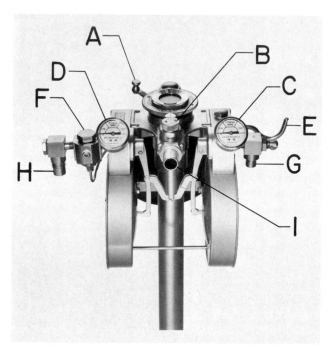

Figure 10–48 The McKesson Euthesor. *A*, Selector; *B*, pressure setting; *C*, oxygen gauge; *D*, nitrous oxide gauge; *E*, inhaler hook; *F*, Safe-T-Lok; *G*, DISS oxygen inlet; *H*, DISS nitrous oxide inlet; *I*, tube connector.

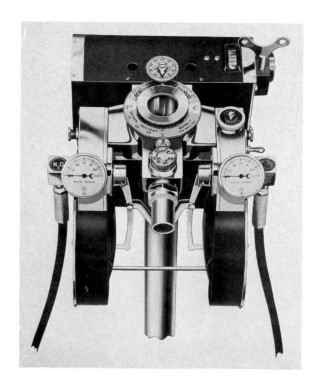

Figure 10–49 McKesson Nargraf anesthesia machine.

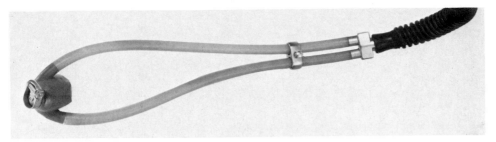

Figure 10–50 Nasal inhaler for an intermittent flow machine.

The air valve of the intermittent flow machine may be on the machine itself, instead of on the nasal inhaler. A numerically graduated scale indicates the degree to which the valve is opened. Each level progressively adds approximately 10 per cent air to the gas mixtures flowing from the machine.

Nasal inhalers for all machines come in sizes usually designated as child size and adult size. They are better called small and large, since they can be interchanged and used on both child and adult, depending on the size of nose and the facial contour.

THE PHYSICAL SET-UP OF THE GAS MACHINE AND CYLINDERS

The dentist who uses relative analgesia successfully keeps constantly in mind that his primary reason for making it a part of his equipment is the elimination of fear of the dental experience. It follows quite logically that he will do all in his power to allay fear and anxiety, even in the arrangement and placing of machines and cylinders, for the sight of these instruments frequently raises thoughts of life, death, emergency, operations, and so on.

THE GAS MACHINE

In setting up the gas machine, both the response of the patient and the convenience of the doctor should be considered. Several arrangements are suitable:

1. The machine can be mounted on a pedestal. If so, it should be a short pedestal, not a tall one, so that it is not overwhelming to the patient (Fig. 10–51). With this arrangement it is also easier for the doctor to read the flowmeters and to make the necessary adjustments, whether from a sitting or standing position.

2. If space is at a premium, the machine can be mounted on the wall (Fig. 10–52).

3. It can be located in a strategically placed drawer or cabinet, where it is hidden from view when not in use (Fig. 10–54).

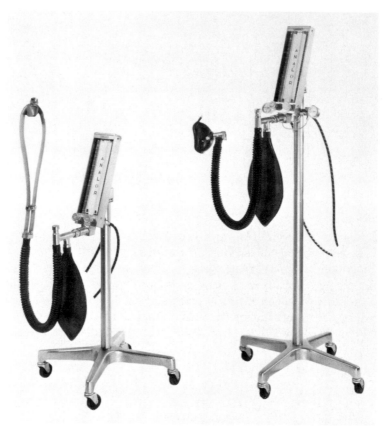

Figure 10–51 A machine mounted on a short pedestal is less frightening than one on a tall pedestal.

CYLINDERS

One disadvantage of small cylinders is that they are attached to the machine and cannot be hidden (Fig. 10–55). Other disadvantages in the use of these cylinders have already been pointed out. Large cylinders (M or G), on the other hand, can be hidden in many ways:

1. Place the cylinders behind a door. When the door is open, the cylinders are hidden (Fig. 10–56).

2. Cover the cylinders with a plastic drape.

3. Hide the cylinders behind a screen.

4 Build a cabinet around the cylinders.

5. Keep the cylinders in a room or closet outside the dental treatment room.

6. Store the cylinders outside the building proper: in the cellar, in a crawl space under the building, or in a shed connected to building.

Note: *Extremes of temperature will not affect cylinders. However, they must be stored in a vertical position and never next to a source of heat or electricity.*

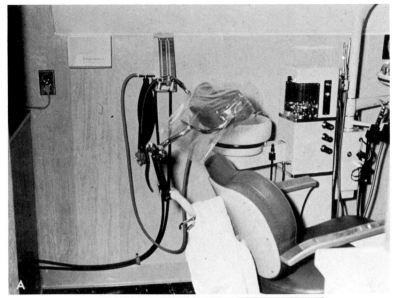

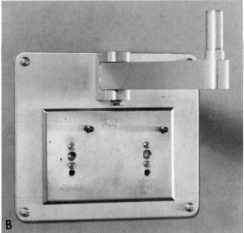

Figure 10-52 *A,* Machine mounted on wall. *B,* Wall mount with swivel arm. (Courtesy of Coastal, Division of Chemetron.)

TUBING AND QUICK-COUPLERS

When cylinders are stored in the dental treatment room, regulation high-pressure tubing can be connected directly to the machine (Fig. 10-57). When longer distances are involved, copper tubing ⅜ inch outside diameter is used, but this is a plumber's job. The gas from one set of cylinders can be piped into several rooms, with outlets for nitrous oxide and oxygen in each room.

The ideal type of outlet is a quick-coupling that permits rapid hookup and disengagement of the machine without the need for unscrewing bolts or

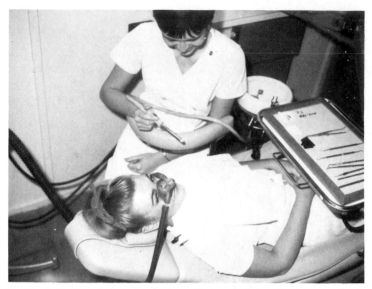

Figure 10–53 Patient under analgesia in reclining position. Equipment does not interfere with operator or chairside assistant.

using tools. The advantages of this type of outlet are that one gas machine can be used for several treatment rooms and that machines can be quickly interchanged. There are three kinds of quick-couplers:

1. The Schrader flush type, with one central control with which the gases can be shut off (Fig. 10–58).

2. The McKesson valve type, with control valves at each outlet (Fig. 10–59).

3. The NCG type (Figs. 10–60 and 10–61).

Auxiliary equipment and accessories (Figs. 10–65 to 10–73) are also available.

NITROUS OXIDE-OXYGEN SEDATION IN CONJUNCTION WITH AUDITORY MODIFICATION*

Ambient noise, inherent within each dental operatory, has a psychologically disturbing effect upon dental patients. Combined with the almost medieval perception most patients have about the dental experience, ambient noise magnifies any fear a patient has into real or imagined pain, and finally into distress.

Chemical sedation, using oxygen and nitrous oxide, will relieve fear and anxiety—but disturbing sounds may counteract the complete relaxation we are striving for. Distress, reinforced by constant ambient and vibratory noise sensations and lack of prescribed distress control, can lead to a serious intrusion into the patient's comfort and confidence.

*Courtesy of Sense Modification Research Institute.

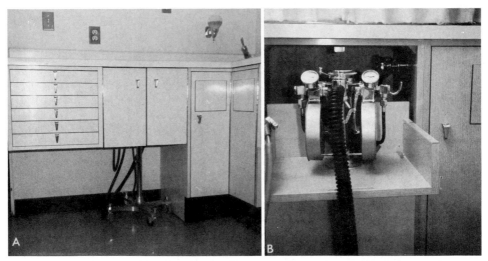

Figure 10-54 *A*, Machine stored behind swinging doors when not in use. *B*, Machine in a sliding drawer.

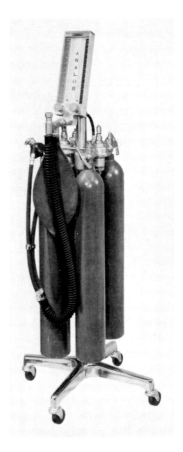

Figue 10-55 Small cylinders attached to a machine are uneconomical and frightening to the patient.

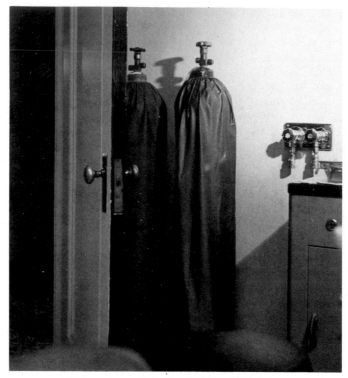

Figure 10-56   Cylinders hidden behind door.

Preselected taped music and utilization of progressive relaxation techniques, combined with soothing sounds of surf or rain, can provide maximum sound attenuation and create the ultimate relaxation atmosphere possible for the dental patient. In this relaxed atmosphere, the dentist may reduce the amount of chemical agent required to bring about the desired state of tranquility. During chemical sedation, the patient's sense of hearing becomes more acute, and increased acuity is being interpreted by higher brain centers that are chemically depressed. As a result, misinterpretation of sounds and words can lead to a psychologically disturbing atmosphere.

Chemical sedation in conjunction with phonic modification will result in a more controlled and relaxed environment.

The Phonic Mood Modifier (PMM) (Fig. 10-72 A to C) has been designed to mask ambient noise sensations, reduce dental vibratory noises conducted through the maxilla and the mandible, entertain the patient during operatory procedures, and provide a complete coordinated communication system between the dentist and his patient. The Surf Synthesizer (a filtered white sound within the PMM) functions as a sound absorber which masks out ambient noise interference by establishing a controlled sound energy field. The masking sound is delivered in two modes: the sound of an intermittent surf or a constant rain tone. This same sound is used to reduce vibratory sounds caused by tooth preparation and bone reduction procedures. The PMM is not used for pain reduction.

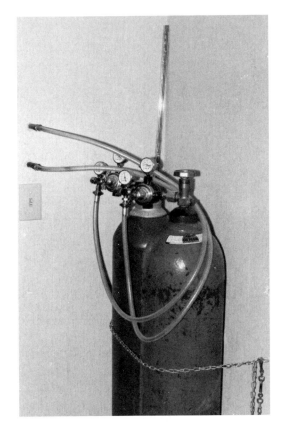

Figure 10-57 High pressure rubber tubing suffices for short distances as long as no part of the building structure is traversed. This figure shows rubber tubing going through a wall. Such installment is illegal; copper tubing should be utilized.

A separate music source is used in conjunction with the PMM. The PMM will automatically transform ordinary monaural or stereophonic music or taped program materials into a balanced symmetrical sound. A high fidelity speaker housed within the unit allows the dental team to electively enjoy the music selection. Cassette, eight-track, reel to reel, or radio is added for mood modification and entertainment.

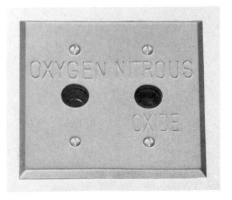

Figure 10-58 The Schrader quick-connect flush mounting.

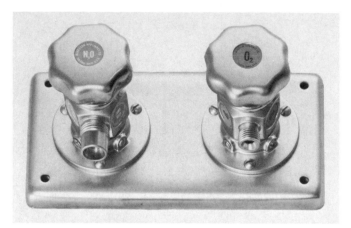

Figure 10-59 Quick-couplers with control valves.

To facilitate the various patient head positions used in the operatory, stethoscope or small sponge earphones are usually recommended. The mixer-signal transport is a specially designed, hand held, patient alert button and sound mixer device. The patient can electively listen to the surf synthesizer and mask vibratory procedures or listen to preselected music for entertainment. This dial proportioning device lets the patient determine his needs. The dentist must always control the volume of the input masking sound and music

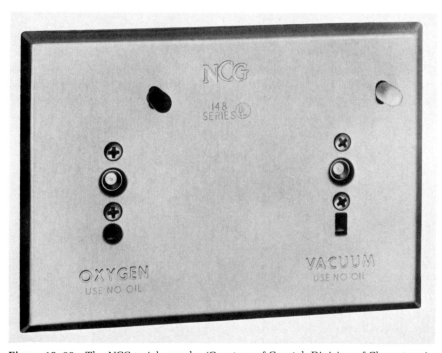

Figure 10-60 The NCG quick-coupler (Courtesy of Coastal, Division of Chemetron.)

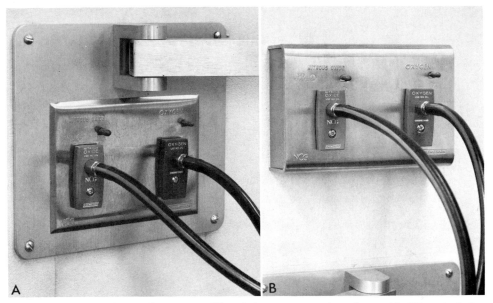

Figure 10–61 NCG quick-connects. All male inserts are non-interchangeable (Diameter Index Safety System). (Courtesy of Coastal, Division of Chemetron.)

source for auditory safety. It is essential that the sound pressure level always be within normal auditory tolerance limits.

If large cushioned or liquid filled earphones are used to completely eliminate ambient noise, an Operator Override Communication and Voice Resonant Modifier System Component may be added to the Phonic Mood Modifier and Music Source previously described. This will allow for a complete coordinated communication system. A foot control and internal microphone enables the dentist to communicate with the patient at any time. The voice

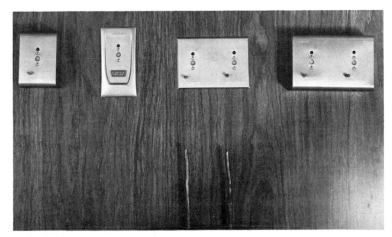

Figure 10–62 Coastal outlet stations showing different types of quick-connects. (Courtesy of Coastal, Division of Chemetron.)

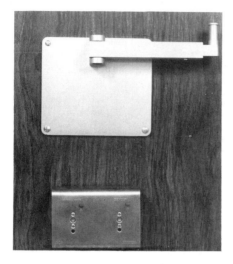

Figure 10–63 Coastal wall mounting plate with exposed outlet station. (Courtesy of Coastal, Division of Chemetron.)

resonant modifier automatically enriches the operator's voice by enhancing its mellow and pleasant tonal qualities. Auditory sensing of closeness or distance is electronically controlled.

Patient comfort and cooperation are readily achieved with chemical sedation and controlled auditory modification.

MAINTENANCE OF EQUIPMENT

Machines should be checked for proper performance about once a year by a representative of the manufacturer.

Text continued on page 372

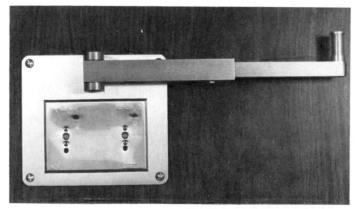

Figure 10–64 Coastal wall mounting plate with concealed outlet station. (Courtesy of Coastal, Division of Chemetron.)

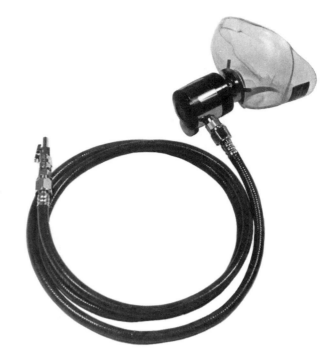

Figure 10–65 Resuscitator which can be attached to the head of the analgesia machine by means of rubber tubing and a quick-connect. (Courtesy of Fraser Sweatman, Inc.)

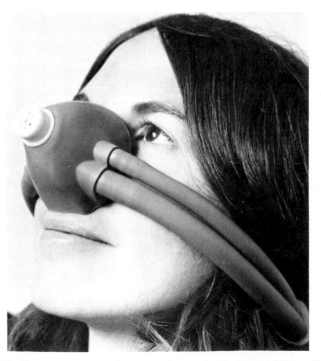

Figure 10–66 Brown nitrous oxide scavenging mask. (Courtesy of Summit Services.)

Installation of the

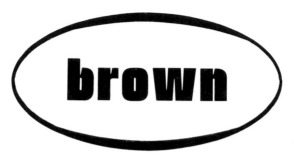

N₂O Scavenging Mask

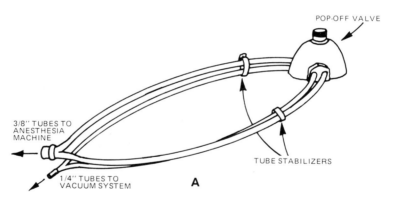

POP-OFF VALVE

3/8″ TUBES TO ANESTHESIA MACHINE

TUBE STABILIZERS

1/4″ TUBES TO VACUUM SYSTEM

A

Figure 10–67   *A,* The Brown scavenging mask is easily installed. It is supplied with a pair of tubes coming off each side. The ³/₈ in. breathing tubes connect to the anesthesia machine the same way as conventional masks; the smaller ¼ in. tubes connect to the suction. The central vacuum system must be in continuous operation when the mask is in use and it must be vented outside the building. *Caution: Do not connect mask to a vacuum pump in which motor is exposed to gas mixture; this could be a fire hazard, easily eliminated by installing a modern pump.* This mask comes with a pair of tube stabilizers, which can be positioned to curve the tubing conveniently over the back of the chair.

Connection to the Vacuum System

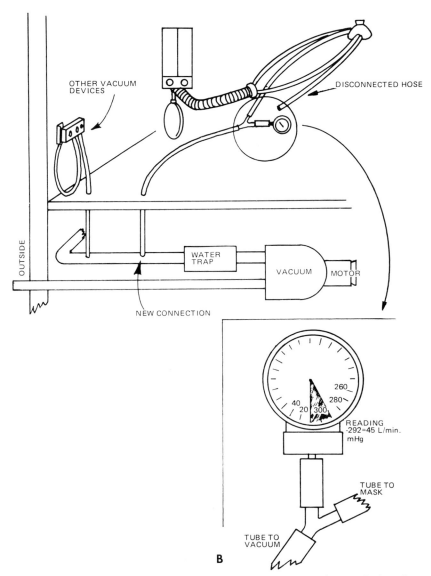

OTHER VACUUM
DEVICES

DISCONNECTED HOSE

OUTSIDE

WATER
TRAP

VACUUM   MOTOR

NEW CONNECTION

260
280
40
20 300
READING
-292=45 L/min.
mHg

TUBE TO
MASK

TUBE TO
VACUUM

B

Figure 10–67 *Continued. B,* The Brown scavenging mask can be attached to the existing central vacuum system if (1) it has adequate capacity, (2) motor is not exposed to the gas mixture, (3) system is vented outside the building away from air intakes, windows and personnel areas. If your vacuum system does not meet these criteria, a self-contained vacuum unit for gas scavenging only is available from Clarke Pharmaceutical. A separate vacuum line for the mask must be attached to the main vacuum pipes downstream from the operatory inlets to ensure adequate, stable suction both for the mask and for the removal of secretions. Do not attach the mask suction line directly to the existing vacuum lines located in the operatory.

Illustration continued on the following page

Vacuum Flow Required for Operation

The minimum vacuum flow for efficient scavenging is 45L/min. Flow is estimated from the negative pressure reading on an aneroid blood pressure gauge. Pressure should be checked periodically to verify the adequacy of suction.

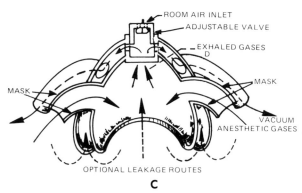

Figure 10–67   *Continued. C,* Pop-off valve (general and pediatric dentist's model). The Brown scavenging mask has a room-air inlet valve so that the patient's tidal volume will always be satisfied. When this valve is turned clockwise it progressively covers the suction vent holes, reducing the vacuum applied to the nasal cavity of the mask. This adjustment controls the size of the breathing bag.

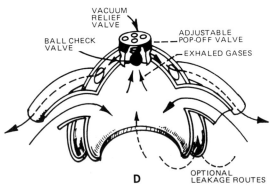

Figure 10–67   *Continued. D,* Pop-off valve (oral surgeon's model). The Brown scavenging mask has a ball check valve through which exhaled gases pass to reach the suction cavity. When this valve is turned clockwise, the spring tension of the ball is increased. This adjustment controls the size of the breathing bag. The holes in the top of the valve are to ensure that the vacuum source cannot exert excess pressure on the system.

Care & Cleaning

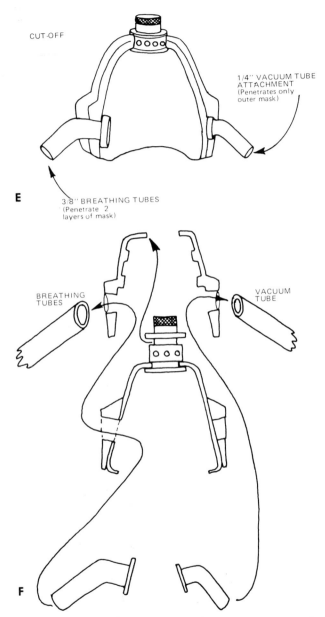

CUT-OFF

1/4" VACUUM TUBE
ATTACHMENT
(Penetrates only
outer mask)

E

3/8" BREATHING TUBES
(Penetrate 2
layers of mask)

BREATHING
TUBES

VACUUM
TUBE

F

Figure 10–67 *Continued. E, F,* The Brown N₂O scavenging mask is easily disassembled for cleaning. It is compatible with the usual antiseptics and autoclaving, or with gas sterilization. Reassembly is shown above. Note that large bore plastic connectors for breathing tubing are inserted through both layers of the mask. Small bore plastic connectors for scavenging are inserted only through the outer layer. Inner and outer mask shells fit into grooves in the pop-off valve.

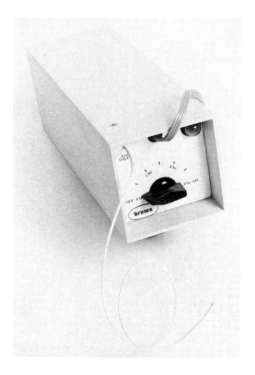

Figure 10-68 Brown Air Monitor. This instrument takes a three-hour air sample in the working environment. The air sample is then evaluated by laboratory analysis for levels of nitrous oxide and mercury vapor. (Courtesy of Summit Services.)

N₂O LEAK TESTING

Standard Four Part N₂O Dental System

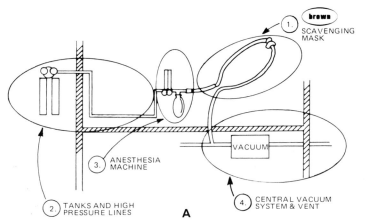

Figure 10-69 A, To achieve low N₂O room concentration, all four sections of the N₂O system must be leak free.

Tanks & High Pressure Lines

Your tanks and high pressure lines should hold pressure overnight. To test for high pressure leakage turn off tanks after office hours and note the pressure on the cylinder gauges. The next morning before the tanks are turned on check the pressure again. If the pressure has dropped more than 10%, excessive leakage is present. High pressure gas leaks can cause high N_2O room levels and are expensive. Call your gas service representative.

Anesthesia Machine & Connections

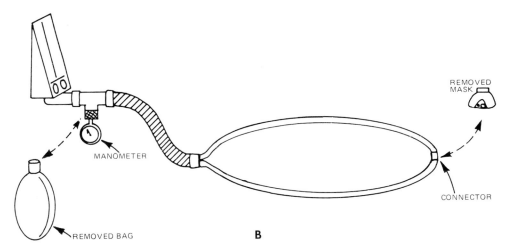

Figure 10–69 *Continued* B, To make your anesthesia machine gas-tight, first replace any rubber and plastic goods that are in poor condition. Check and tighten any loose connections and fittings related to the bag connector, mask adapter and N_2O line. Following these procedures, leak-test the machine: Remove the breathing bag and insert the blood pressure manometer into the bag adapter using the one-hole rubber stopper provided in the kit. Disconnect the 3/8 in. tubing from the mask and connect the two tubes together using the short length of plastic tubing provided in the kit. Using the oxygen flow meter, slowly fill the system to a maximum pressure of 30 mm Hg. (*Caution: Do not overpressurize the system or your gauge will be damaged*). Turn off oxygen valve and look for a loss of pressure. The machine should not lose more than 10 per cent of its pressure over a 30 sec. period. In case of more rapid loss, recheck the rubber goods, possibly immersing them under air pressure. Use a soap solution to check flow meter seals and joints, watching for bubbles. If leakage cannot be corrected contact your service representative.

Illustration continued on the following page

Vacuum System

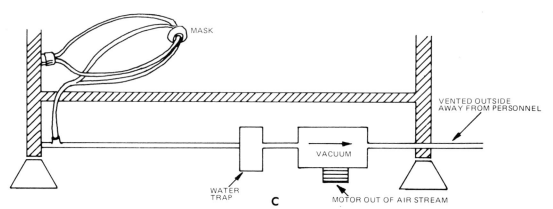

Figure 10–69 Continued   C, Waste N_2O is vented outside the building via continuously-operating suction.

Cautions: (1) Use a pump rated for continuous operation. (2) Do not vent gas through a pump motor exposed to gas flow because of a possible fire hazard. You must determine whether vacuum motor is safe and in compliance with all fire codes. (3) You must also determine that the effluent from the vacuum is vented outside the building away from all personnel areas and air intakes. (4) Suction for scavenging must operate without appreciable pressure variations. Connect as shown in installation instructions or install a separate vacuum pump. (5) Check suction flow from mask periodically (45 liters/min).

Illustration continued on the following page.

OTHER ENVIRONMENTAL CONSIDERATIONS

1. N_2O leakage from adjacent operatories may cause high gas levels in your office if adjoining dentists fail to scavenge their waste gas or vent their anesthesia gas near the intake of your heating and air conditioning inlets.
2. The patient himself is a potential source of N_2O in room air because of the large amount (up to 30 L) stored in his body. Most of this will be scavenged if the mask is left on the patient's face for a few minutes after N_2O is turned off.
3. N_2O leaks can occur from the patient's mouth during conversation. Some of this may be necessary in assessing the depth of anesthesia but talking should be held to a minimum.
4. A small percentage of patients are mouth-breathers. No nasal mask is effective in delivering analgesia to such patients.
5. Further reduction of occupational exposure may be achieved via a small fan (25 CFM) directed toward the patient's face. This reduces inhalation of the possibly high concentrations of N_2O coming from the patient's mouth.

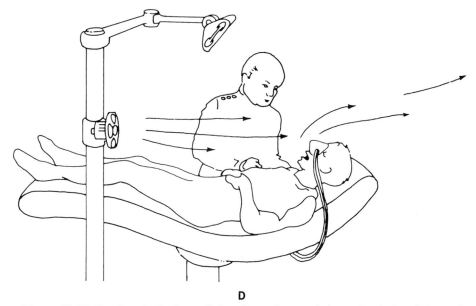

D

Figure 10–69 *Continued* *D*, A small fan directed toward the patient's face helps reduce occupational exposure to the possibly high concentrations of nitrous oxide coming from the patient's mouth.

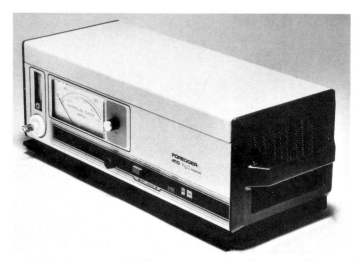

Figure 10–70   Foregger 410 N₂O trace gas monitor. (Courtesy of Foregger Co.)

The machine should be tested for leaks by painting a soap and water solution on all suspected places while the gas is flowing. The appearance of bubbles signifies a gas leak (Fig. 10–74).

Oil or grease should never be used on any part of the machine tubings, valves, regulators, or cylinders. In the presence of oxygen under pressure, these lubricants may form an explosive mixture.

GASES

PROPERTIES OF GASES

In order to understand how respired gases and inhalation anesthetics act in the body one must be familiar with the simple properties of gases and liquids. Basic to this discussion is the kinetic concept of fluids. Fluids are composed of particles (molecules) that are continually in motion, continually colliding with each other and with the vessel in which they are contained. The pressure exerted by a fluid is equal to the total impact force of the molecules against the confining wall.

Although the molecules of liquids move around a great deal, they are so close together that they are subject to strong intermolecular attractive forces. Therefore liquids have a volume independent of the container, and they can exert both pressure and tension in a closed space.

In contrast, the molecules of gases are far apart, and the attraction of one particle for another is very low. Thus, the incessant motion of the particles of a gas causes it to completely fill all the available volume of a container. Gases

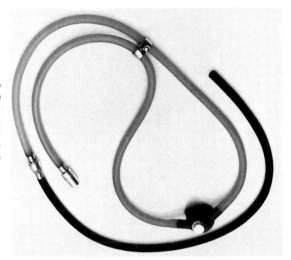

Figure 10–71 *A*, Anavac system. The purpose of the Anavac system is to carry away the exhaled gases from the dentist's and assistant's breathing areas. *B* illustrates the flow in the system. Nitrous oxide, being heavier than air, will flow out at floor level, where it can be attached by means of tubing and fed to the outside or to a suction system. (Courtesy of McKesson Co.)

A

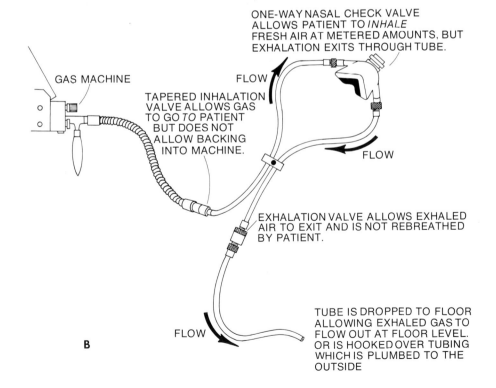

ONE-WAY NASAL CHECK VALVE ALLOWS PATIENT TO *INHALE* FRESH AIR AT METERED AMOUNTS, BUT EXHALATION EXITS THROUGH TUBE.

GAS MACHINE   FLOW

TAPERED INHALATION VALVE ALLOWS GAS TO GO *TO* PATIENT BUT DOES NOT ALLOW BACKING INTO MACHINE.

FLOW

EXHALATION VALVE ALLOWS EXHALED AIR TO EXIT AND IS NOT REBREATHED BY PATIENT.

FLOW

TUBE IS DROPPED TO FLOOR ALLOWING EXHALED GAS TO FLOW OUT AT FLOOR LEVEL. OR IS HOOKED OVER TUBING WHICH IS PLUMBED TO THE OUTSIDE

B

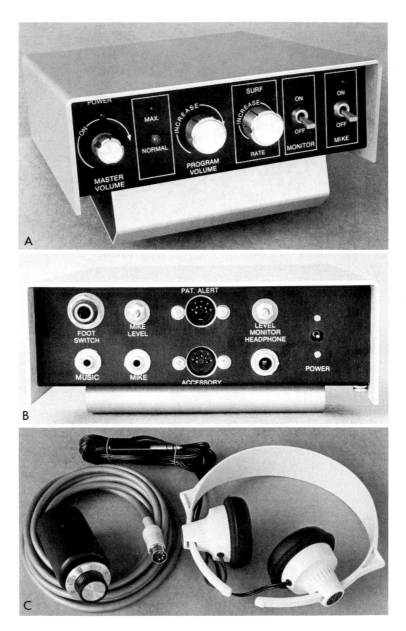

Figure 10–72   *A,* Front view of phonic mood modifer. *B,* Rear view of phonic mood modifier. *C,* Accessories for phonic mood modifier.

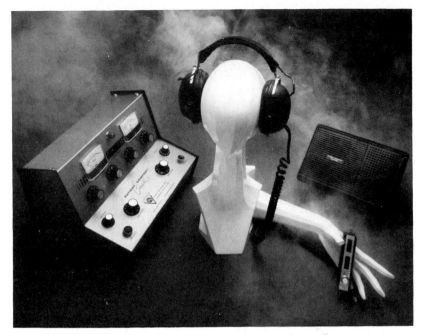

Figure 10-73 Patient Comfort Console. Sound and music may help in the administration of relative analgesia. (Courtesy of Fraser Sweatman, Inc.)

therefore exert only pressure. The behavior of gases may be explained by simple laws and principles:

Pressure of Gases (Boyle's Law). The pressure of a gas is inversely proportional to its volume (temperature remaining constant). Decreasing the volume of a gas increases the number of particles per unit volume and thus the number of collisions against the walls of the container; the result is an increase in pressure.

The Measurement of Gas Pressure. The pressure of a gas may be indicated by (1) the height to which the gas forces a liquid (water or mercury) in a tube, and (2) the force exerted in terms of weight per unit area (pounds per square inch, grams per square centimeter). Data essential to the measurement of a gas are its temperature, pressure, and volume. Pressure in excess of atmospheric pressure is termed positive pressure; pressure at less than atmospheric pressure is negative pressure. The volume of a gas is usually indicated at standard conditions: 0° C. and 76 cm. Hg pressure. In gas exchange within the body, pressure is also referred to as tension.

Two instruments used in the measurement of gas pressure are:

Manometers. There are two types, closed and open, each consisting of a calibrated U-shaped tube partially filled with mercury or water.

Pressure Gauges. In these instruments, the gas exerts a force directly upon a metal diaphragm which extends and contracts with variations in pressure. These changes are then amplified by a system of levers which control the position of the indicator of a dial. Pressure gauges, which are usually

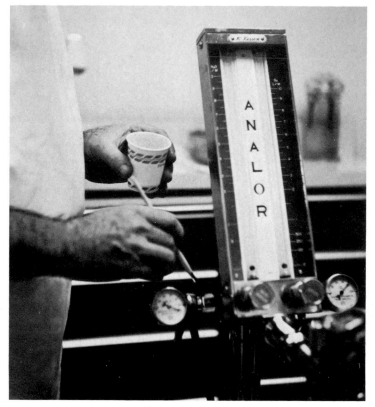

Figure 10–74   Testing for leaks with soap solution (at machine only).

calibrated in pounds per square inch, are suitable for measuring high pressure.

Expansion of Gases (Charles' Law).   The pressure of a gas is directly proportional to its absolute temperature (volume remaining constant). Increasing the temperature of a gas causes an increase in the velocity of the molecules, and thus an increase in the total number of collisions against the walls of the container.

Molecular Weight of Gases (Avogadro's Principle).   At equal temperatures and pressures, equal volumes of gases contain the same number of molecules.

Dalton's Law of Partial Pressures.   In a mixture of gases, each gas behaves as if it alone occupied the total volume and exerts a pressure (its own partial pressure) independently of the other gases present. In any one container having a mixture of several gases, the sum of the partial pressures is equal to the total pressure.

Solubility of Gases (Henry's Law).   The quantity of gas physically dissolved in a liquid at constant temperature is directly proportional to the partial pressure of the gas.

Diffusion of Gases (Graham's Law).   The rate of diffusion of one gas compared to another varies inversely as the square root of their molecular weights. The molecules of a gas or vapor in a closed space distribute equally throughout the space and exert an equal pressure upon all surfaces of the enclosure. The process of distribution of the molecule of a gas in a space is called diffusion.

Pressure Gradient. A gas or vapor diffuses from an area of higher concentration to one of lower concentration. The difference between the two levels of pressure is called the pressure gradient.

Joule-Thompson Effect. When a gas passes from a higher pressure to a lower pressure through a porous plug, there is a change in temperature (either a heating or a cooling), depending on the interactions of the molecules of the gas.

Bernoulli's Principle. The pressure of a fluid in motion through a tube of varying cross sectional areas is least at the narrowest portion, where speed is greatest, and is greatest at the widest portion, where speed is least. Gases behave like fluids but, because they are compressible, they deviate somewhat from this principle.

Liquefaction of Gases. As a gas is compressed, its molecules are forced into a smaller volume of space. They are thus packed closer together and move faster, so that energy in the form of heat is liberated. Because of the reduction of intermolecular distances, cohesive forces are intensified and, if the compression is continued, condensation occurs and the substance becomes liquid. Certain gases, however, do not liquefy regardless of the pressure applied unless they are cooled. The temperature above which a gas cannot be liquefied by pressure is called the critical temperature.

Differences Between Gases and Vapors. Gases and vapors behave similarly in most respects, the essential difference being that a gas is a vapor existing at a temperature above the critical temperature, whereas a vapor exists at about the critical temperature of the liquid from which it is derived and therefore may be liquefied by pressure without cooling.

Heat Capacity of Gases. Gases absorb and conduct heat, their heat capacity varying directly with their molecular weight. The number of calories required to heat a molecule of gas 1°C. is called the molal heat capacity.

NITROUS OXIDE

Nitrous oxide is prepared by heating ammonium nitrate crystals at 190°C. until they are fused. Further heating to 240° C. yields nitrous oxide of about 95 per cent purity.

PROPERTIES

Nitrous oxide, the anhydride of hyponitrous acid, is a colorless, tasteless, nonirritating inorganic gas with a faint, sweetish odor. Having a molecular weight of 44.01 and a specific gravity of 1.53, nitrous oxide is soluble in alcohol and highly soluble in blood and water. It liquefies at 0°C. at 460 lb. pressure and solidifies at −102°C. Above 450°C. nitrous oxide decomposes to nitric oxide. Although itself not combustible, it is a good supporter of combustion.

NITROUS OXIDE AS AN ANESTHETIC[9]

Nitrous oxide is administered as a gas, and it produces its effect by being absorbed into the bloodstream by the mechanics of respiration. Being a gas, it behaves pursuant to the kinetic action of gases as explained by Boyle's law, Dalton's law of partial pressures, and Henry's law on the solubility of gases. According to these laws, oxygen and nitrous oxide dissolve in the blood serum independently of each other. In other words, nitrous oxide creates no obstacle to the solution of oxygen, nor does oxygen interfere with the solution of nitrous oxide. Each gas dissolves in proportion to its own partial pressure. Nitrous oxide dissolves in the blood serum and forms no chemical combination with hemoglobin.

Gas molecules, which are in constant motion and tend to spread in all directions, enter or leave the bloodstream by the process of diffusion. Since, in a mixture of gases the diffusion of one gas occurs independently of the concentrations of other gases present, nitrous oxide and oxygen each diffuse through the alveolar membranes of the lungs without regard to the presence of the other until the tensions of the components on each side of the membrane are equal.

The quantity of a gas that can be absorbed by 1 ml. of liquid at standard temperature and pressure is called the absorption coefficient of that gas. The absorption coefficient varies directly with pressure changes and inversely with changes of temperature. Applying the laws of gases, it can be seen that the rate of diffusion of one gas in a liquid medium is independent of the presence of another gas dissolved in the same medium. It is therefore seen that nitrous oxide creates its effect as an analgesic or anesthetic agent without relation to the behavior of oxygen. Gellhorn[7] states:

> A complete parallelism between anoxia and anesthesia is not to be expected for the reason that anesthetics are usually distributed in all cells and tissues, and consequently may influence their function independent of their action on the oxidative metabolism. That narcosis is not based on a reduction of oxidative process is clearly shown by the fact that anaerobic organisms can be narcotized.

Nitrous oxide, of itself, possesses an anesthetic action, although a very weak action compared to that of the more potent agents such as ether and cyclopropane. The manner in which it produces narcosis is, as yet, unknown.

In 1948 Faulconer[6] and his associates at the Mayo Clinic set out to determine the effects of nitrous oxide under pressure on a human being. The subjects were placed in a pressure chamber and nitrous oxide and oxygen in equal concentrations were piped into the chamber. Continuous oximeter records were made of arterial blood saturation, and electroencephalographic tracings were made to determine the level of anesthesia. This mixture was administered first at two atmospheres (730 mm. partial pressure of nitrous oxide and 730 mm. partial pressure of oxygen), and then at one atmosphere. At one atmosphere the subjects remained conscious at all times. At two atmospheres, surgical anesthesia resulted, based on electroencephalographic findings. Continuous oximeter studies showed a normal state of arterial blood oxygenation. This again showed that nitrous oxide acts as an anesthetic agent in the presence of ample oxygen. It also demonstrated that, if nitrous oxide could be administered in a hyperbaric chamber, its usefulness could be extended to many situations in which this near-perfect anesthetic agent cannot now be used because of its lack of potency.

For a discussion of the pharmacologic action of nitrous oxide, see *The Analgesic Action of Nitrous Oxide* (Chapter 3).

OXYGEN

Discovered by Priestley in 1774 and prepared by Scheele in 1775, oxygen is a nonmetallic chemical element found almost everywhere in nature, either in a free state or in combination with other elements. As a constituent of water, oxygen forms approximately 89 per cent of its weight and 33 per cent of its volume. Oxygen constitutes about one-fifth (20.99 per cent by volume) of the atmosphere and, it has been roughly estimated, nearly one-half by weight of the various rocks that form the crust of the earth. A liter of oxygen at 1 atmosphere pressure and at a temperature of 0°C. dissolves in about 20 liters of water and in about seven volumes of alcohol at 20°C. at 760 mm. pressure. In the liquid state, oxygen is a pale steel-blue color. It can also be solidified. Nearly all the known elements will combine chemically with oxygen under suitable conditions.

Oxygen is widely used in the commercial field, in conjunction with acetylene and other fuel gases, for the production of flame for the cutting and welding of metals, for use in high explosives, and for the production of low temperatures, as in refrigeration. In the health field, it is used for anesthesia in conjunction with gases such as nitrous oxide, ethylene, and cyclopropane, and for resuscitation and the treatment of pulmonary, cardiovascular, and other diseases.

PREPARATION

Electrolysis of Water.   A direct electric current is passed through water to which a small quantity of acid or alkali, such as caustic potash, has been added. The electric current causes the decomposition of the water into hydrogen and oxygen. The oxygen liberated is accumulated at the positive pole, the hydrogen at the negative pole.

Chemical Method.   This involves the removal of oxygen from a chemical compound holding an oxygen excess, such as barium dioxide. Heating barium dioxide breaks it up into barium oxide and oxygen.

Liquid Air Method.   This is the most commonly used method. Because liquid oxygen has a boiling point different from other gases in the air, it can be separated from them. Liquid air separation takes place at extremely low temperatures, and these temperatures serve to cool and liquefy additional incoming air, thus making possible a commercially feasible process.

REFERENCES

1. Adriani, J.: Techniques and Procedures of Anesthesia. Springfield, Ill., Charles C Thomas, 1960.
2. American Medical Association: Fundamentals of Anesthesia. 3rd ed. Philadelphia, W. B. Saunders Co., 1954.
3. Clement, F. W.: Nitrous Oxide—Oxygen Anesthesia. Philadelphia, Lea & Febiger, 1951.
4. Courville, C. B.: Untoward Effects of Nitrous Oxide Anesthesia. Mountain View, Calif., Pacific Press Publishing Association, 1939.
5. Eastwood, D. W. (ed.): Clinical Anesthesia—Nitrous Oxide. Philadelphia, F. A. Davis Co., 1964.
6. Faulconer, A., Pender, J. W., and Bickford, R. G.: Influence of partial pressure of nitrous oxide on depth of anesthesia and the electroencephalogram in man. Anesthesiology, 10:601, 1949.
7. Gellhorn, E.: Automatic Regulation. New York, Interscience Publishers, 1943.
8. McKesson, E. I.: Nitrous Oxide and Oxygen Anesthesia. Toledo, Ohio, Conjure House Printing, Business News Publishing Co., 1953.
9. Zelinigher, J.: Behavior of N_2O in Anesthesia and Analgesia, p. 111, Sept.–Oct., 1949.
10. Menken, N.: Nitrous oxide–oxygen analgesia, clinical safety matched by technical safety. J. Am. Anal. Soc., 12:7–10, 1974.

CASE REPORTS AND A QUESTION AND ANSWER REVIEW

11

CASE REPORTS

The following case reports are taken from the author's personal experience. For other case reports, see Chapter 9, *Relative Analgesia for the Handicapped Child.*

Gagging

EPILEPSY AND GAGGING

A 14 year old boy, normal in height and weight, had a medical history that was negative except for epilepsy. His last dental visit took place two years previously, at which time he had two restorations placed. The boy's mother had tried unsuccessfully several times to have her family dentist treat him. The dentist had earnestly attempted treatment, but the patient was an extreme gagger.

An attempt to make a clinical examination met with an extreme gag response as soon as the mirror went past the lips. The same result was obtained in an effort to take an anterior roentgenogram. At the next visit, analgesia was introduced, the reaction was optimal, permitting a thorough clinical examination. At the succeeding visit a full series of intra-oral roentgenograms was taken without difficulty.

The diagnosis disclosed 45 carious surfaces with possible pulpal involvement of five molars. Treatment proceeded uneventfully. About one-half of the work was accomplished with analgesia alone, the remainder with a combination of analgesia and local anesthesia. In four visits, the 45 surfaces were restored and three pulpotomies completed.

Dosage. Fifteen to 25 per cent nitrous oxide at 2 mm. pressure was delivered from an intermittent flow machine with the air valve closed.

GAGGING AS A DEFENSE MECHANISM IN A CHILD-PATIENT

The patient was 4 years old, a thin, pale, shy little girl. Her mother described her as a very poor eater, one who would readily regurgitate. Aside from this, her medical history was negative. An attempt to insert a mouth mirror produced a violent gag response; however, the introduction to analgesia proved to be no problem.

At the second visit, analgesia was accepted readily, and a complete clinical examination was made. Roentgenograms were taken under analgesia. Two large boli of food were noticed in the mucobuccal folds of the right and left molar areas. It seems that the child had been punished for regurgitating her food. She now pretended to swallow it, but actually kept it in her mouth for hours. With the gagging response controlled by analgesia, treatment was carried out uneventfully.

Dosage.   Three liters of oxygen and 4 to 5 liters of nitrous oxide were delivered from a continuous flow machine with the air valve open.

EXTREME GAGGER

A 60 year old man enjoyed good health except for diabetes, which was controlled. He declared himself an excellent dental patient who did not need any anesthesia for tooth preparation. He was a heavy cigarette smoker, with excessive amounts of calculus and stain. His last dental visit had taken place seven years ago.

All his upper teeth were present; however, the lower jaw had only a cuspid remaining on the right side and two bicuspids and two molars on the left side. Having arrived at this rather precarious situation, he had decided to have the missing teeth replaced. The indicated treatment consisted of the splinting of the four teeth on the left side, the fabrication of a crown for the lone right cuspid, and the fabrication of a partial denture.

The patient refused local anesthesia, insisting that it was not necessary for him, and analgesia because he was afraid of it. Under these conditions, work was begun. The first spray of water from the handpiece elicited an extreme gag response. Three or four more attempts were made with the same result. The patient had been right as far as not needing anesthesia for tooth preparation or band impression taking, but it proved to be impossible to do any dental work because of his extreme gagging. The use of analgesia was a perfect solution to this problem.

Dosage.   Three liters of oxygen and 3 to 4 liters of nitrous oxide were delivered from a continuous flow machine with the air valve open.

The Cardiac Patient

THE NERVOUS CARDIAC PATIENT

A 59 year old male cardiac patient was very nervous, but tried to hide it. He had suffered two coronary attacks within the last two years and had not applied for a dental checkup since the last attack. The patient's physician forbade the use of epinephrine with the local anesthetic solutions. He did not object to the use of nitrous oxide–oxygen analgesia.

Four 4-unit fixed bridges with full coverage were made, one in each quadrant of the mouth. Under analgesia, preparations for full coverage on three teeth were done at each sitting without disturbing the complete comfort of the patient. The impressions, fittings, and cementation were all done under analgesia. The treatment was uneventful.

Dosage.   Three liters of oxygen and 3 liters of nitrous oxide were delivered from a continuous flow machine with the air valve open.

THE CARDIAC PATIENT AND EXISTING MEDICATION

The patient was a 57 year old woman who had had two coronary attacks and now suffered continuous anginal pain. She required prophylactic antibiotic therapy before oral surgery or oral prophylaxis. Her current medication included Coumadin, Peritrate, and Esidrix. She had had surgery for a gallbladder condition, a hysterectomy, an appendectomy, and surgery for varicosities.

After consultation with her physician, analgesia was introduced with excellent results. The patient was completely relaxed and free from fear, tension, and apprehension.

Dosage.   Fiver liters of oxygen and 3 liters of nitrous oxide were delivered from a continuous flow machine with the air valve open.

The Psychiatric Patient

SCHIZOPHRENIA

An 18 year old girl had been under psychiatric care for five years, with intermittent periods of hospitalization. She had a completely negative personality, and her facial expression was vapid. Part of the necessary extensive dental work had been done under general anesthesia, but both the patient and her mother objected to further use of this approach.

At the first and second visits, she was very uncooperative because of fear. Nevertheless, analgesia was introduced at the second visit, and work was begun at the third visit. This patient turned out to be an ideal analgesia subject. An average dose created complete relaxation and near-perfect cooperation. Fifty surfaces were restored in eight sittings. Because of a tendency toward mouth-breathing, an intermittent flow machine was used.

Dosage.   Ten to 15 per cent nitrous oxide was delivered from an intermittent flow machine with the air valve closed.

Extreme Apprehension

EXTREME APPREHENSION: THE FEAR OF PAIN

A 43 year old man with essentially negative medical history insisted that he could not stand any pain and wanted local anesthesia for every procedure, even though he was afraid of the injection. After two administrations of analgesia, this patient was so relaxed during treatment that he often fell asleep and snored. Fortunately he slept with his mouth open. This was not general anesthesia, for the dosage was very small indeed.

Dosage. Three liters of oxygen and 2 liters of nitrous oxide were delivered from a continuous flow machine with the air valve open.

EXTREME APPREHENSION: PREMEDICATION

A 41 year old woman was just about the most apprehensive patient in the author's experience. She did not sleep for two nights preceding every dental appointment. She hesitated to sit in the dental chair and cried profusely. She could not bear the thought of a needle being used in her mouth.

Three visits were used to condition her to the effects of analgesia. She was so hysterical that normal flows of nitrous oxide had no effect whatsoever. In addition, she kept up a running conversation, which further diluted the effects of the analgesia. Premedication was used (Miltown) at the next two visits, with greatly improved results, permitting the initiation of treatment periods lasting 2 to 3 hours. She accepted local anesthetic injections for part of the work, and the remainder was carried out with analgesia alone.

Dosage. Three liters of oxygen and 8 liters of nitrous oxide were delivered from a continuous flow machine with the air valve open.

EXTREME APPREHENSION: THE FEARFUL AND SUSPICIOUS PATIENT

A 26 year old woman, who had had her last dental examination 5 years previously, was terribly afraid of the needle. She winced and contracted her lips during a gentle clinical examination. She could not bear the pain of the roentgenographic film pressing against the floor of the mouth and was suspicious of every move made by the dentist. To complete the picture, she could not bear the sight of blood.

Gaining the complete confidence of this patient was the essential prerequisite and occupied the entire first visit. At the second sitting the patient hesitantly agreed to try analgesia. No nitrous oxide (only oxygen) was used, because of her extreme fear of the nasal inhaler and the entire procedure. She did, however, signify that she wanted very much to lose her fear of dentists and dental treatment.

On the third visit, nitrous oxide and oxygen was administered successfully. Her confidence in the operator permitted her to accept the sensations of analgesia (which had been described to her in advance). The ultimate result was a patient who gave herself up to the symptoms and procedure so completely that small volume flows of nitrous oxide produced a deep analgesic level from which it was difficult to rouse her with the usual 1 to 2 minutes of oxygenation. The patient now needs 4 minutes of oxygenation, but she is completely removed from her surroundings during treatment, yet fully cooperative.

Dosage. Three liters of oxygen and 3 liters of nitrous oxide were delivered from a continuous flow machine with the air valve open.

EXTREME APPREHENSION: THE NASAL INHALER AS PLACEBO (AUTOSUGGESTION)

A quiet, kindly woman of 50 years suffered a rise in heart rate and blood pressure at every visit. It was explained that the use of analgesia would help her immeasurably. She agreed to try it. The initial symptoms were described very carefully but when she felt anything different from the normal, even when she knew that it was to be expected, fear gained the upper hand. The second trial produced the same reaction, but what was unusual and interesting was that she agreed to take analgesia a second time.

At the third visit, only oxygen was used. This pleased her (although she was not told anything about this). Since then this patient has been treated in this way. She insists on having the "analgesia" and relaxes very well, indeed.

Tolerance to Nitrous Oxide as Analgesia

AN INSTANCE OF INCREASING TOLERANCE

The patient was 25 years old, a normally "happy-go-lucky" young woman, but extremely fearful of dental treatment. Analgesia proved to be a boon to her, for a very small dose was sufficient to completely eliminate her fears and permit her to accept treatment. After several years she seemed to need a much higher flow of nitrous oxide to provide complete comfort. This individual has now been a patient in the author's office for 30 years. This is the *only instance* in the author's experience in which the nitrous oxide flows required for analgesia have risen from an extreme minimum to a maximum.

Dosage.   The *original* dose was 3 liters of oxygen and 2 liters of nitrous oxide delivered with the air valve open. The *later* dose was 3 liters of oxygen and 6 to 8 liters of nitrous oxide delivered with the air valve closed. A continuous flow machine was used throughout.

Mental Retardation

DOWN'S SYNDROME (MONGOLISM)

A short time previously, this 12 year old girl had had 12 teeth extracted under general anesthesia. When first seen by the author, she was frightened but tractable. After analgesia was introduced gently and with kindness, the dentition was seen to be in dire need of care. Twenty surfaces were restored in four sittings. Because of excessive mouth-breathing and the almost constant presence of mucoid secretions in the nose, an intermittent flow machine was used to push the gases and minimize oral inhalation.

Dosage.   Twenty to 25 per cent nitrous oxide at 3 to 4 mm. pressure was delivered from an intermittent flow machine with the air valve closed.

UNCOMPLICATED MENTAL RETARDATION

A 15 year old girl with a mental age level of about seven was completely cooperative from the outset. She was treated as one would treat a 7 year old child and, with a kindly approach, her confidence was won. She proved to be a good patient (even to the time of this writing) who looks forward to visiting the dentist.

Dosage.   Three liters of oxygen and 4 liters of nitrous oxide were delivered from a continuous flow machine with the air valve open.

MENTAL RETARDATION WITH ANKYLOSIS OF THE TEMPOROMANDIBULAR JOINT

The patient was 45 years old, a mentally retarded woman with a partial ankylosis of the temporomandibular joint. She was also very nervous and fearful and, although she tried very hard, could not seem to open her jaw more than 2 mm. anteriorly. She accepted analgesia readily. The resulting relaxation seemed to permit a much wider movement of the mandible, so that treatment was possible. Obviously only part of this problem was due to the ankylosis.

Dosage.   Three liters of oxygen and 3 to 4 liters of nitrous oxide were delivered from a continuous flow machine with the air valve open.

Mental Retardation and Epilepsy

CASE I

This patient is a 27 year old woman who has been epileptic for 19 years following a blow to the head on falling down a flight of stairs. Her parents relate that she has two to three seizures per week, and that her intelligence quotient is that of a 10 year old child. The use of Dilantin resulted in a severe case of hyperplastic gingivitis with rampant caries.

The patient responded extremely well to relative analgesia from the very first administration, and all her restorative work was completed with no local anesthesia and with no adverse effects. She has no anxiety pertaining to her dental visits, and freely admits enjoying the experience.

The wonderful, but as yet unanswered, question was posed by the patient's mother: might analgesia have a beneficial effect on seizures? Since the initiation of dental treatment with nitrous oxide and oxygen, her daughter's seizures have been reduced from two to three a week to two seizures in four months!

Dosage.   Three liters of oxygen and 3½ liters of nitrous oxide from a continuous flow machine with the air valve open.

Nitrous Oxide Analgesia for the Brain Damaged

CASE II

At the age of 22, this patient, who was in an auto accident, suffered brain damage and became totally blind. She has had a fear of men ever since the accident. Her first medical examination had to be performed under sedation because she screamed, scratched others, and would not cooperate. Her first dental examination, which was conducted at the hospital, elicited the same responses as the medical examination. Her next dental examination was performed in the dental office with analgesia (4½ liters of nitrous oxide and 6½ liters of oxygen). Bite-wing x-rays were taken and four restorations completed. Even at this level there was very little cooperation. The second dental visit went a little better and the analgesia dosage was then 3 liters of nitrous oxide and 3 liters of oxygen. A prophylaxis and restorations were completed at this time. Every visit since has been pleasant, and the patient's cooperation has improved. Her fear of men is also diminishing. She is now 29 years of age and a very cooperative dental patient.

CASE III

When this girl was 16 years of age she was involved in an auto accident and suffered brain damage and neurological impairment. She was semicomatose for about a year and she still blames herself for the death of her companion. She has since been hospitalized with severe depression and suicidal urges. She had a prophylaxis and fluoride treatment, and bite-wing x-rays were taken for her first dental experience since the accident. No analgesia was used for this work. The second visit was for restorative work and she was slightly uncooperative when 2½ liters of nitrous oxide and 3 liters of oxygen were given for analgesia. After this appointment she complained we had not finished the work. At the third visit more restorations were done, and this time the patient cooperated well, with no complaints. The cooperation of this patient had improved so much that by the fourth visit she had a third molar extracted.

Nitrous Oxide Analgesia for the Severely Mentally Retarded Child[1]

The dental treatment of the severely mentally retarded child presents a multifaceted problem from the point of view of management, prevention of disease, and restoration of oral breakdown. The approach to the management of restorative procedures for this special patient has been covered in numerous articles and texts. One author feels that attempts at using nitrous oxide analgesia with this type of patient will probably fail and that more effective types of treatment would be deep sedation or general anesthesia. Another relates that severe mental retardation is a contraindication to the use of relative analgesia. Elsewhere it is stated that if combinations of kindness and firmness do not allow the practitioner to achieve his objective, then general anesthesia may be necessary for successful treatment. This section will be concerned with ascertaining the proper management modality for the severely retarded child based on the author's experience in treating these special patients at the Dental Clinic of the Rose F. Kennedy Center for Mental Retardation and Human Development, Bronx, New York.

As with many normal children, the severely retarded individual, when faced with a new situation, has an initial fear of the unknown and of separation from his usual environment and trusted guardian. Added to this dilemma is the inability of this retarded individual to truly comprehend and respond to the oral or visual suggestions of the dentist. How then is one able to accomplish his duty—that of examining, restoring, and preventing dental disease when the patient is unable to consciously cooperate in this endeavor? The choices open to the dentist in accomplishing this task include establishing a productive rapport, tell-show-do, firmness, physical coercion, relative analgesia with or without the concurrent use of premedicants, premedicants alone, or general anesthesia.

Physical coercion or the use of restraints is outdated procedure for the severely retarded patient. Not only does it add to the already multiple problems of the patient, but it also results in a physical and mental strain upon the dentist and staff, as well as adversely affecting the quality of the dentistry performed.

General anesthesia is at the other extreme of management modalities. But, by and large, the severely retarded child can be treated by more conservative means. The use of general anesthesia in this context implies the admission of a patient to a hospital, at least overnight, during which time the patient is given an agent that causes loss of consciousness so that treatment may be accomplished. This technique has numerous disadvantages. First, the child will be separated from his usual environment for an inordinate amount of time in relation to the amount of work being accomplished. Additional strain will be placed upon the child owing to separation from his parents and protectors. An added burden will devolve on the staff, since the child will need attention above and beyond that usually given to the "normal" youngster. Finally, general anesthesia is not without its inherent complications. The general situation is not innocuous.

The use of premedicants alone leaves much to be desired. One is never sure of the effect a particular drug or dosage will have on the child. Relative analgesia added to the premedicant will overcome this problem.

The technique of tell-show-do is generally inadequate for this child; however, rapport can be established, not through verbal or visual communication, but through physical contact and voice tone. Touching the patient's cheeks or putting one's arm gently across his chest and using a soothing tone of voice can take the place of words in many situations.

Finally, there is the technique of relative analgesia. In the severely retarded patient, it can diminish fear and anxiety, produce slight euphoria, result in some degree of amnesia, and raise the pain threshold. The combination of this technique with the above-mentioned physical and voice rapport will enable the practitioner to accomplish good dental treatment. The only contraindication to the use of nitrous oxide analgesia is the situation in which the patient has an upper respiratory tract infection or some form of pulmonic dysfunction. Of course, prior to the introduction of this agent a thorough medical history, as well as an evaluation of the current physical status of the patient, should be obtained.

The technique for the administration of the nitrous oxide–oxygen combination will vary somewhat from that described here, depending upon the child and his initial reaction to the dentist and the dental environment. Each child will react differently to your technique, so you must be versatile. Analyze your patient. The child is brought to the dental operatory by his parent or other companion and is seated in the dental chair (which is either upright or already in a reclining position). The dentist and dental assistant establish rapport with the patient, as mentioned previously, and the nose-piece of the analgesia apparatus is introduced by holding it near, but not in physical contact, with the patient's nose while allowing only oxygen to flow. This will enable the patient to become used to the feeling of cool air passing over his nose. After this is accomplished, reasonably high concentrations of nitrous oxide are introduced (approximately 6 liters of nitrous oxide to 3 liters of oxygen). It must be remembered that the nose-piece is not in contact with the patient's nose and that we have an open system; thus, the patient is not breathing the actual concentration of gas emanating from the nitrous oxide equipment. As soon as the child shows signs of relaxing and appears to accept the feeling of the gases flowing past his nose, the nose-piece is gently placed on his nose and the concentration of nitrous oxide is decreased to what the dentist feels will be necessary for the situation. Again it must be stated that you must carefully watch your patient and monitor his plane of analgesia. Evaluate his respirations, pulse, pupils (are they fixed in a stare, do they react to light?), eyelids (are they closing?). Know at what level your patient is at each moment. Once the patient is in a stable plane of analgesia, dental procedures may be initiated.

In certain situations, premedication may be called for. These situations may include those in which the patient is extremely agitated and fights off the introduction of the nose-piece either because of a previous bad experience or because of apprehension. Relative analgesia may also be employed to help correct any deficits which the premedicant may have—i.e., to "top off" the premedicant.

Case histories of two patients will be presented to illustrate the successful use of relative analgesia for the severely retarded patient. The first describes results with use of premedicants and nitrous oxide as well as the effects of establishing rapport. This patient, T. G., is an 8 year old male with the diagnosis of congenital rubella syndrome, presenting with bilateral cataracts, severe mental retardation, patent ductus arteriosus, deafness, and growth retardation. He had previously been hospitalized for tonsillectomy, for three cataract operations, and for dehydration. He arrived at our dental clinic with the chief complaint from his mother that "he does not eat and pulls at his mouth." A full medical history was taken, after which the child was helped into the dental chair by his mother. Nitrous oxide–oxygen was introduced by holding the nose-piece near the patient's nose and blowing the gas past his nose. The child initially would attempt to remove the nose-piece from this position with his hand, but gradually he accepted the introduction. An oral examination, as well as a partial radiographic examination, was accomplished. The patient's oral hygiene was poor, and oral hygiene instruction was demonstrated to the parent. A thorough prophylaxis was accomplished. Although the child was relatively cooperative, he seemed tense during the initial visit, possibly as a result of his previous history of operations. The decision was made to use premedicants at subsequent visits. Vistaril was given intramuscularly 35 minutes prior to the introduction of nitrous oxide analgesia, which was easily accomplished. The child's eyes were open throughout the procedure and there was continued movement of the eyeballs, indicating his concern with the procedures. Additional radiographs were taken and one quadrant of his mouth was restored with amalgam and stainless steel crown restorations. Oral physiotherapy was again illustrated to the child's mother. At subsequent visits it was evident that the patient was more amenable to dental treatment. At the third operative visit, premedicants were not given and relative analgesia alone was used as a management aid although local anesthesia aided in pain control. The patient seemed much more relaxed in the dental chair than at his initial visit. He seemed to react positively when I touched his cheek prior to the introduction of nitrous oxide. At the final operative appointment the nitrous oxide–oxygen proportions were 1 liter of nitrous oxide to 4½ liters of oxygen with an excellent response from this severely retarded patient. It can be argued that dental treatment could have been accomplished quickly with general anesthesia, but is this our sole purpose? We now have a severely retarded patient who will accept regular dental care; in short, a good dental patient.

The second patient is a 5 year old girl who presents with the following diagnosis: severe mental retardation, hyperkinetic behavior, questionable mild ataxia, and a seizure disorder, all secondary to anoxia during uncontrolled seizures at age 7 months. Current medication consists of a multivitamins once a day, phenobarbital (15 mg. b.i.d.) and Dilantin (50 mg. b.i.d.) with no other medical complications reported. Initial oral examination was accomplished using the previously mentioned technique and relative analgesia introduced as described above (6 liters of nitrous oxide to 3 liters of oxygen initially, with 3 liters of nitrous oxide to 3 liters of oxygen for maintenance). Full mouth radiographs were taken and an oral examination was accomplished which indicated generalized Dilantin hyperplasia. It was decided to give the patient a combination oral premedication for surgery (chloral hydrate and Vistaril) in addition to relative analgesia. Her reaction to the gingivectomies was excellent and at the last visit the nitrous oxide–oxygen ratio for maintenance was (1 liter: 4 liters). It should be pointed out that the nose-piece did not interfere with the surgical procedures in the maxillary anterior section of the patient's mouth.

CONCLUSION

There are many management modalities for treatment of the severely retarded child, ranging from physical restraint to general anesthesia. Our treatment objectives should be to perform good dental treatment without adding to the already multiple difficulties of the patient and the parents. We do not want the dental experience to be a one-time affair, but to be one of continued observation and education amenable to routine office visits. Nitrous oxide analgesia in combination with premedicants can be the most judicious modality in the dental treatment of the severely mentally retarded child.

Dentistry in the Treatment of Handicapped Children[2]

Handicapped children do not receive adequate dental services because:

1. The family has not been educated fully regarding the care for the handicapped member. The expense of providing rehabilitation services can very well deplete the financial resources of a family. Also, the care for these children is such that both the patience and energy of the family frequently are exhausted. Transportation problems might also discourage the family from seeking out a dentist. Some families may need assistance at home, so that parents can accompany the child to the treatment facility.

2. It is not uncommon for parents to be unable to find a dentist to provide services for their handicapped child either because

a. The dentist feels that he is unable to manage the child.

b. The child may have medical problems, making the dentist feel insecure about treating such a child.

c. Having a busy practice, the dentist may not have sufficient time to undertake the type of treatment these children require.

d. Hospital facilities may not be available.

e. The home-bound or bedridden child presents additional problems.

3. Most communities do not provide dental services for handicapped children. This results from a fear that the cost of such services would be prohibitive.

How costly is dental care for the handicapped? Can care be given in a private office, or must the child be hospitalized and general anesthesia used? Must the dentist have special training? Answers to these questions and others were sought from a three year project that the United States Public Health Service and the Idaho Department of Health sponsored jointly.

The conclusions drawn as a result of this study were:

1. The handicapped child has greater initial dental treatment needs than the average child. This drives the cost up. However, upon periodic recall, the maintenance needs appear to be minimal. This places him on the same plane as the average child, and the costs are greatly reduced.

2. *Most handicapped children can be treated successfully in private dental offices.*

3. Hospitalization costs for providing dental treatment to handicapped children are not prohibitive.

4. The cost of treatment over a three year period will be approximately the same as the cost of diagnostic and preventive services in a population without an unusually high caries attack rate.

Many years ago, Dr. Laurence Taft, a pediatric neurologist, pioneered the establishment of a Developmental Evaluation Clinic and a separate Pediatric Rehabilitation Center at the Albert Einstein College of Medicine in New York. He was a firm believer in the principle of management which involves the treatment of all the patient's dimensions, i.e., somatic, intellectual, emotional, and social. Dr. Taft realized that dental treatment was as important as occupational or physical therapy for the handicapped. Eventually, both clinics were amalgamated into the Children's Evaluation and Rehabilitation Clinic, which is now housed in the Rose Kennedy Center for Research in Mental Retardation and Human Development at the Bronx Municipal Hospital Center.

We must emphasize the multidisciplinary appraoch, the complex knowledge, and the variety of services required to meet the needs of the handicapped. It is obvious that this segment of our society will grow with the expansion of our total population and with the increasingly higher rate of survival among the handicapped. We must find ways to utilize our present knowledge more concisely, increase the efficiency of existing services, and discover new and better methods and techniques, if we are to become effective instruments in helping to overcome the myriad problems of handicapped individuals.

Over a period of many years it definitely has been established that the utilization of relative analgesia has provided us with a multifaceted approach to the successful treatment of many, many handicapped patients in private dental offices, involving minimal office visits, and minimal trauma to patient, parent, and dentist.

Analgesia and Local Anesthesia

ANAPHYLACTIC SHOCK REACTION TO LOCAL ANESTHETICS

The patient was a 55 year old highly tensed woman with a blood pressure of 190/100. She had had a partial denture made six months previously and a bruxing habit began soon after. Her fear of the dental experience was pronounced. She gave a history of anaphylactic shock reaction to local anesthetic injection. This had occurred twice and, as a result, her physician had forbidden the use of any local anesthetic injections. As the patient described it, she was "allergic to Novocain."

The patient required extensive oral rehabilitation involving all the upper teeth and the lower posteriors. Twenty-one teeth were prepared and restored with splinted cast veneer crowns. Periodontal treatment was also instituted. A partial upper denture and a partial lower denture were fabricated. All of this dentistry was done with only analgesia at average doses. After some initial nervousness, the patient proved to be a good analgesia subject who augmented the favorable effects of the analgesia by autosuggestion.

Dosage.   Three liters of oxygen and 3 to 4 liters of nitrous oxide were delivered from a continuous flow machine with the air valve open.

SYNERGISTIC USE OF ANALGESIA AND LOCAL ANESTHESIA

The patient was 35 years old, a very obese, very distraught individual. She was recently divorced and had the responsibility of raising three children. Her history disclosed tachycardia due to "nerves," lack of sleep, and so forth; an underactive thyroid; and low blood pressure. Clinical examination showed a marked peridontitis simplex, an infected lower right first molar, and

15 surfaces to be restored. The patient stated that local anesthetic injections "never took effect" and that therefore she always had pain during cavity preparation. She "dreaded" going to the dentist.

Analgesia was introduced at the second visit, with no dental work being attempted. At the next sitting, three class 5 cavity preparations were done under analgesia, without local anesthesia. Although the patient submitted, she complained of considerable pain during the preparations. Since the first three dental visits had taken place in the evening, after her day's work, it was decided to try morning appointments. These proved to be highly successful, since she was not tired and was more relaxed. All 15 tooth surfaces were restored without the use of local anesthesia. For the extraction of the lower right first molar and the fabrication of a 4-unit fixed bridge to replace it, local anesthesia was added to the analgesia. Complete anesthesia was obtained with total comfort and freedom from pain.

Dosage.   Three liters of oxygen and 8 liters of nitrous oxide were delivered from a continuous flow machine with the air valve open.

Psychological and Emotional Problems

THE EMOTIONALLY DISTURBED PATIENT

This patient of 42 years was a large, heavy-set man with a florid complexion who had spent the previous year in a mental hospital. He was completely blind in his left eye owing to a detached retina. Several years previously two teeth had been removed under intravenous sodium Pentothal anesthesia, for he could not bear the sight of a needle.

On his first visit, he fidgeted in the chair and was loath to open his mouth. The introduction of a mouth mirror caused a gag response accompanied by a peculiar harsh and raucous yell. Since the mirror had barely gone past his lips, this was obviously psychological gagging owing to fear and apprehension. Once his confidence was gained, this reaction disappeared. However, high flows of nitrous oxide were required. This individual wanted to cooperate and was very grateful for the patience and consideration shown him.

Dosage.   Three liters of oxygen and 7 liters of nitrous oxide were delivered from a continuous flow machine with the air valve closed.

"NERVOUS BREAKDOWN"

This 56 year old man was a fearful individual, a pessimist, a worrier. His physical condition was good, but he had had two periods of hospitalization and was unable to cope with his daily problems. Analgesia was introduced after consultation with the patient's psychiatrist. Good results were obtained immediately. The patient felt more at ease and less tense after each analgesia administration.

Dosage.   Three liters of oxygen and 3 to 4 liters of nitrous oxide were delivered from a continuous flow machine with the air valve open.

A PSYCHOLOGICAL PROBLEM NECESSITATING THE WITHDRAWAL OF ANALGESIA

This 7 year old patient was a very shy, thin, quiet little girl who obeyed every direction and who submitted to analgesia without protest. She was completely cooperative during treatment, but would not talk or answer any questions put to her.

About one year later, the mother revealed that she had taken her daughter to a psychologist. It seemed that the child was content just to exist; she did not want to get involved in living and feeling. In an attempt to break through this barrier, the psychologist suggested the withdrawal of analgesia for dental treatment. He wanted the child to feel and react emotionally to life situations. The child was not as good a patient without analgesia, since gagging became a problem. But after two years, with great improvement in the patient's emotional development, the psychologist allowed the child to choose whether or not she wanted analgesia for her dentistry. She chose dentistry with analgesia.

Dosage.   Three liters of oxygen and 3 liters of nitrous oxide were delivered from a continuous flow machine with the air valve open.

The Child-Patient

EMERGENCY TREATMENT OF A CHILD-PATIENT

A 14 year old boy had fallen and fractured both upper central incisors. He was in pain and extremely frightened. Radiographic examination showed the roots of both teeth to be shattered. With a gentle but firm approach, analgesia administration was begun. Because of the patient's highly nervous state, a high volume flow of nitrous oxide was used at the outset. When it had taken effect (2 minutes), injections of a local anesthetic solution were made. The right root was removed in five fragments, the left root in two fragments. Sutures were placed and recovery was uneventful.

This patient has continued to be a good analgesia patient for the past 26 years. His wife and two children are also good analgesia patients.

Dosage.   Three liters of oxygen and 8 liters of nitrous oxide were delivered from a continuous flow machine with the air valve open.

THE RECALCITRANT CHILD-PATIENT

When first seen, this 7 year old boy was an adversely conditioned dental patient who had refused to visit a dentist until one year previously. At that time, he would not sit in the chair and would not open his mouth.

He complained of a toothache in several quadrants of the mouth. When analgesia was suggested, he refused the idea immediately. However, he seemed to like the dental assistant, who talked with him and was very patient. Although reticent at the outset, he became very voluble with the assistant. She donned the nasal inhaler and interested him sufficiently that he promised to try it at the succeeding visit. This promise was kept, and introduction of analgesia was so successful that he couldn't wait to take a ride on the "Magic Carpet" on the next visit, at which time treatment was initiated.

This youngster proved to be an ideal subject for analgesia. An average dose sufficed, because he was a good nose breather and learned to relax completely. Fifteen surfaces were restored and four pulp-cappings executed with no need for local anesthesia. Four sittings were required to complete the work.

Dosage. Three liters of oxygen and 4 liters of nitrous oxide were delivered from a continuous flow machine with the air valve open.

THE ASTHMATIC CHILD-PATIENT

A 5 year old boy had developed an asthmatic condition one year previously. One attack had been quite serious. He was a highly sensitive, but docile child who enjoyed taking analgesia from the very first time. He found it easier to breathe when he was on the "Magic Carpet" and was completely cooperative during treatment. He seemed to come out of the analgesic state feeling more refreshed and relaxed.

Dosage. Ninety per cent oxygen and 10 per cent nitrous oxide at 3 mm. pressure was delivered from an intermittent flow machine with the air valve closed.

DOSAGE AND THE CHILD-PATIENT

A 10 year old girl had adamantly refused treatment in three dental offices. On her first visit to us, she refused to accept the nasal inhaler. At the second visit, however, a combination of cajolery, bribery, and threats (this from the mother) resulted in her accepting an introductory administration of analgesia. Although the patient cried, she submitted. No work was attempted.

The next administration was more successful, and a good analgesic level was obtained with a high flow of nitrous oxide. One surface was restored at this sitting. This was a case of rampant caries with 30 surfaces to be restored. At every subsequent visit, four to six surfaces were restored, each treatment necessitating a higher than average flow of nitrous oxide.

Dosage. Three liters of oxygen and 6 to 8 liters of nitrous oxide were delivered from a continuous flow machine with the air valve open.

THE CHILD-PATIENT AND ASSOCIATION OF IDEAS

A completely deaf girl of 12 years was highly sensitive and had a lovable disposition. With a little patience, kindness, and tact, she was quickly won over to the idea of taking analgesia, which was introduced successfully.

Two years later she developed epilepsy, the first attack occurring on the street. For about one year she refused to take analgesia, because the symptoms reminded her of the vertigo suffered during the first epileptic seizure. It was difficult to treat her without analgesia. Fortunately, she accepted analgesia again after a one year lapse.

Dosage.   Three liters of oxygen and 2 to 3 liters of nitrous oxide were delivered from a continuous flow machine with the air valve open.

THE NEEDS OF THE CHILD-PATIENT: AN UNUSUAL APPROACH

A boy of 14 was frightened of all dentists and all dental treatment. His parents disclosed that he was a brilliant scholar and read a great deal. Yet he was a highly suspicious patient, watching the dentist's every move. He opened his mouth, but pursed his lips so that it was very difficult to make a clinical examination. He refused to accept the placing of the nasal inhaler, even though this had been preceded by a lengthy explanation and description of the procedure and the reasons for employing this approach. All to no avail. A reprint of one of the author's articles on analgesia was then given to this boy with instructions to read it.

At the next visit he was so greatly interested in the machine, the procedure, the volumes of gases flowing from the machine, and so on, that he lost all his fears in his anxiety to try it. He had read the article from cover to cover and seemed to understand most of it. From that day to the present (18 years later) he has been an ideal patient. (A footnote to this story: this individual is now a brilliant and successful physicist.)

Dosage.   Three liters of oxygen and 3 to 4 liters of nitrous oxide were delivered from a continuous flow machine with the air valve open.

Geriatric Dentistry

ACCEPTANCE OF ANALGESIA BY THE AGED PATIENT

A slight, debilitated little lady 78 years of age had never heard of analgesia and was highly suspicious of its use. On the other hand, she detested and feared injections. On the promise that the use of analgesia would eliminate many injections, she agreed to try it. A low minute flow of nitrous oxide seemed to suffice. Ultimately, four teeth were prepared for full coverage under analgesia without the addition of local anesthesia. The patient was perfectly comfortable and happy.

Dosage.   Five liters of oxygen and 3 liters of nitrous oxide were delivered from a continuous flow machine with the air valve open.

Nitrous Oxide Analgesia in Podiatric Medicine[3]

CASE REPORTS

Bilateral Tendo Achillis Lengthening (T.A.L.) Surgery of a Three Year Old Boy (Office Procedure).   Because of the length of the surgical procedure (3 hours) and the postsurgical foot and lower leg casts that must be placed following surgery, this child was given Vistaril (25 mg.) (oral suspension) the day before surgery.

After suggesting that the nasal inhaler was an astronaut's nose-piece, the assistant placed it in position and began administration of 8 liters of oxygen. The oxygen flow was reduced to 3 liters and nitrous oxide was introduced gradually until the proper level was attained. Because of the prone position necessary for this type of surgery, the patient's face was turned to one side. The assistant then began suggesting a pleasant excursion to the playground. Within a few minutes the patient was completely relaxed, receptive to all directions and drifted in and out of natural sleep during the entire 3 hour period. He opened his eyes from time to time, but at the suggestion of the assistant he would close them and again be "back at the park having a picnic or swinging on the swings."

This bilateral T.A.L. surgery had been in the planning stage for several months, but not having hospital staff privileges, the thought of performing this lengthy surgery on a 3 year old child conjured up many doubts in the mind of the doctor. Additionally, difficulties were envisioned in keeping this very active child lying quietly on his abdomen for three hours. Despite all, the results were ideal. During the 3 months of postoperative care, surgery, and casting, the only pain experienced by this child was at the time of suture removal 1 month postoperatively, when unfortunately no analgesia was administered. This should have been done. The little boy loves coming to the office and has no fear and no thoughts of pain connected with the office.

Dosage. Three liters of oxygen and 2½ liters of nitrous oxide from a continuous flow machine with the air valve closed.

Complete Amnesia — Neuroma Surgery. This patient is a 38 year old woman. Neuroma surgery was performed, the procedure lasting 1 hour. During the infiltration block she jerked, said "Ouch," made facial signs of pain, and seemed to stiffen from the pain of injection. Upon questioning her after completion of the procedure, she remembered nothing at all of pain or discomfort.

Dosage. Three liters of oxygen and 3 liters of nitrous oxide from a continuous flow machine with the air valve open.

Complete Amnesia — Fifth Toe (Hammer Toe) Bilateral Surgery. A 46 year old secretary, who had extreme fear of pain, made it quite clear that she did not want to "feel anything." Her secondary fear was of being tickled on the soles of her feet. Although under analgesia, she jerked excitedly throughout the entire prescrub procedure. During the second scrub, after the local anesthetic injection, she still wiggled around and made comments about the "ticklish sensations." However, after surgery she remarked that she did not remember a second scrub or the injections. The procedure took 70 minutes.

Dosage. Three liters of oxygen and 3 liters of nitrous oxide from a continuous flow machine with the air valve closed.

Complete Relaxation — Third Metatarsal Resection. This 62 year old maintenance man was completely and beautifully relaxed from the very outset of administration. The procedure lasted 1½ hours. During the last half hour only pure oxygen was administered. After surgery he said that a friend had asked him to make mental notes about the procedure because he needed a similar operation. However, he could not help his friend because he was so comfortable and completely relaxed during the procedure that he remembered nothing.

Dosage. Three liters of oxygen and 4 liters of nitrous oxide from a continuous flow machine with the air valve closed.

A Desire to be in "Complete Control" — Neuroma and Second Metatarsal Head Resection.

The patient was a 39 year old secretary who wanted always to be in "complete command of every situation" because of her managerial conditioning over the years. She jumped and made facial expressions of pain during the injection procedure. As soon as infiltration was completed she began to "fight" her sensations and became quite angry that she was being overpowered. The nitrous oxide was then turned off and only oxygen was administered. Within a minute or two she felt completely in control. The remainder of the surgery was performed without nitrous oxide but with the patient completely relaxed. Upon returning to the office two days later for postoperative care she was asked how she liked the "tranquilizing air." Her answer was "Just great!" She had no memory of becoming angry or of her feeling of losing control. She became an enthusiastic patient subsequently. It is important to add here that this patient had feared having this surgery performed for 4 years. Palliative treatment had been utilized until she could muster up enough courage.

Dosage. Three liters of oxygen and 2½ liters of nitrous oxide from a continuous flow machine with the air valve closed.

Creating Fear (Excessive Dosage) — Bunion and Metatarsal Surgery.

A 52 year old arthritic woman was given too much analgesia (for her), and became hysterical immediately after the injection of local anesthetic. Oxygenation was initiated immediately. The patient was ashamed of her reaction, but needlessly so. The remainder of the preoperative preparation and surgery were performed without analgesia. It is evident that the patient felt she was about to lose consciousness or to die. This points out the value of giving enough nitrous oxide to control the situation (but no more) as long as that depth does not create fear in the patient.

Dosage. Three liters of oxygen and 5 liters of nitrous oxide from a continuous flow machine with the air valve closed. *Proper dosage* would have been 3 liters of oxygen and 3 liters of nitrous oxide with the air valve open.

The Child-Patient — Syndactyly Surgery for Overlapping Fifth Toes.

A 9 year old girl who was a "wiggle worm" came to the office fearful of being hurt and did not want to be "stuck with needles." This was to be a 1½ hour procedure, and no preoperative medication was given. The assistant asked the child if she would like to take a ride on a "Magic Carpet." The child was encouraged to hold and fondle the nasal inhaler, and she was shown a storybook page by page. The assistant then suggested that the child close her eyes and "see" all the characters in the storybook. Soon the little girl was asleep with a low flow of nitrous oxide (2 liters) and moved only rarely throughout surgery, and then with very "sleepy" movements. Oxygenation was begun during the application of the surgical dressings and continued for 15 minutes. The patient was so completely relaxed that no one could get her to say a single word. She had a drink of water, looked at the comic books, but refused to talk. Her mother later remarked that she wouldn't talk for the rest of the day. Two days later, the child was brought to the office chattering like a parrot as usual. The only discomfort this little girl ever experienced in the office was at suture removal, when analgesia should have been, but was not, employed.

Dosage.   Three liters of oxygen and 2 liters of nitrous oxide from a continuos flow machine with air valve closed.

Note: An open air valve would have resulted in quicker return to normalcy.

Two Patients' Evaluations of Procedures Done With and Without Analgesia.   In both of these cases the first surgical procedure was done without nitrous oxide analgesia, and the second procedure performed under nitrous oxide analgesia.

Patient 1.   Dosage was 3 liters of oxygen and 2½ liters of nitrous oxide from a continuous flow machine with the air valve closed.

Upon being asked whether the second procedure was less traumatic she answered: "It was so nice not to hear all these noises; things dropping into pans, hammering noises on the bones." It should be noted that this patient experienced all of the above sensations, but could not remember them.

Patient 2.   Three liters of oxygen and 1½ liters of nitrous oxide from a continuous flow machine with air valve closed were given.

This patient did not describe as dramatic a difference, but she was highly cooperative, and commented that it had been "much easier the second time."

Note: Perhaps a slightly higher flow of nitrous oxide should have been used.

Evaluating the Reactions of the Extremely Nervous Patient.   This was a 50 year old woman who had memories of childbirth experiences. She had "pain" sensations from pressure, pulling, or suggestion. She also had a fear of losing consciousness or "saying foolish things." Although she made audible signs of being in excruciating pain, she had no memory of having experienced pain at her postoperative examinations. The procedure lasted for 70 minutes.

Dosage.   Three liters of oxygen and 1½ liters of nitrous oxide from a continuous flow machine with air valve closed.

Note: This patient could have been assured that no one speaks inappropriately while under analgesia. It is also possible that a higher flow of nitrous oxide should have been utilized (3 liters), but only after proper psychological conditioning, and after stressing that the patient can always dilute the effect simply by taking a few breaths through the mouth.

Fear of Losing Consciousness—Calcaneal Heel Spur Surgery.   Analgesia was administered for one hour to this 43 year old farmer throughout the preoperative preparation and posterior tibial block injection. He was a relaxed patient, but was also concerned about losing consciousness.

Dosage.   Three liters of oxygen and 2½ liters of nitrous oxide with air valve closed.

Note: It is very important to teach the patient how to control depth of analgesia by oral dilution. It is also important to know the patient's history, especially in relation to past experience with general anesthesia.

QUESTIONS AND ANSWERS

Q—*Why do some dental practitioners have greater success with children than with adults?*

A—First, it must be recognized that certain adults simply get along well with children. But beyond this, there are qualities in children that the successful practitioner turns to the advantage of both the child-patient and the dentist. He or she knows that a child is more open to suggestion, so that properly constructed word pictures are readily accepted. In addition, a child has little past experience, so that there is less rationalization as to possible dangers involved in the procedure, as would be the case with an average adult patient who has had opportunity to construct psychic barriers to ready acceptance. Thus, since all the equipment in a dental office is new to a child, the gas machine has no particular significance to set it aside as a special feature. The successful dentist approaches the child-patient accordingly. The relative ages of the dentist and patient may also be a factor.

Q — *How many different ways are there to modify analgesic depth?*

A — To increase the depth of analgesia:
1. Increase the proportionate flow of nitrous oxide (the most rapid method).
2. Decrease the proportionate flow of oxygen (however, never below 20 per cent).
3. Close the air valve.
4. Increase the pressure of the gases (on an intermittent flow machine).
5. Increase the minute volumes of the gases (on a continuous flow machine).

To decrease the depth of analgesia:
1. Decrease the proportionate flow of nitrous oxide.
2. Increase the proportionate flow of oxygen.
3. Open the air valve to its widest point.
4. Decrease the pressure of the gases (on an intermittent flow machine).
5. Decrease the minute volumes of the gases (on a continuous flow machine).

Q — *Does the use of relative analgesia tend to reduce the number of patients who can be treated in one day, especially with the use of more than one treatment room?*

A — The use of relative analgesia permits the dentist to accomplish more work per hour. He or she can thus treat *more* patients, not fewer, if the dentist so desires. While a filling is setting, or a local anesthetic is taking effect, the nasal inhaler is removed (without oxygenation), and the patient in the second treatment room can be treated.

Q — *Does the use of relative analgesia involve any change in the malpractice insurance policy?*

A — The introduction of relative analgesia to a practice should cause no alteration in the malpractice insurance policy. Malpractice policies do differentiate between treating a patient who is conscious, with all protective reflexes intact, and treating an unconscious patient. Relative analgesia (conscious sedation) falls into the former class and does not call for an increased premium rate.

One of the largest professional insurance carriers in this country recently pointed out to the author that one of the most frequent causes of legal actions brought against a dental practitioner is the failure to build good rapport with the patient. The utilization of relative analgesia *most certainly creates a good dentist-patient relationship.*

Q— *Is posthypnotic suggestion effective under analgesia?*

A— While it is true that analgesia, by inducing a state of well-being, euphoria, and amnesia, does produce a semihypnotic state, the author has not had any success with posthypnotic suggestion unless hypnotic induction has been utilized in conjunction with relative analgesia.

Q— *Is is true that the dentist should never carry on a conversation with a third person while the patient is under analgesia?*

A— This restriction is of the utmost importance at the introductory administration, since the patient must feel that he has the complete attention of the operator. After that, conversation with a third party will not affect the patient unless carried to excess. Excessive conversation will prevent the patient from reaching a good analgesic level.

Q— *What is the proper answer to the patient who is concerned about talking inappropriately while under analgesia?*

A— Assure the patient that this is not possible. Patients under analgesia do a great deal of thinking, but do not speak. When the plane of analgesia is light enough that the patient is able to converse, he will be fully aware and have complete control of his thoughts and words.

Q— *How does the operator know when the addition of a local anesthetic injection is necessary for the analgesia patient?*

A— This is determined by the needs and desires of the patient. If complete comfort is obtained only at an analgesic depth that is accompanied either by repeated closure of the mouth or by generation of fear, a local anesthetic injection will be necessary. If the patient asks for it initially, his wishes should be acceded to.

Q— *Can a patient under analgesia and in a reclining position tolerate water and other foreign material in the posterior area of the mouth?*

A — Since the cough reflex is completely active and the gagging reflex is slightly depressed, excessive amounts of fluids and the manipulation of instruments and materials are of no concern to the patient.

Q — *Can a rubber dam be used with the nasal inhaler in position?*

A — The rubber dam can be used. It need not be cut out to accommodate the nasal inhaler, for it will fold right over it. The use of a rubber dam limits oral inhalation.

Q — *Does the use of analgesia necessitate the introduction of additional instruments?*

A — The introduction of analgesia to a dental practice does not necessitate the introduction of additional instruments. An ordinary saliva ejector is quite compatible with analgesia; evacuators or aspirators do not have to be used because of the addition of analgesia. Mouth props are not only unnecessary but contraindicated in analgesia (except in certain handicaps), since the closing of the mouth with failure to open on direction is used as a sign of the patient's entrance into the plane of total analgesia.

Q — *Does rebreathing play any role in analgesia administration?*

A — Not as important a role as that which obtains in anesthesia administration, for the operator must modify the respiration of an unconscious patient. In contrast, the conscious analgesia patient can voluntarily, or upon direction, alter both the rate and depth of his respiration. However, in analgesia administration, some rebreathing does obviate the chilliness experienced at the end of a lengthy administration and assists a subject in obtaining smooth, deep breathing.

Q — *What are the most untoward effects that may occur in the administration of analgesia?*

A — 1. Generating fear in the patient.
    2. An occasional case of nausea or vomiting. This occurs in fewer than 1 per cent of the total number of administrations.

Q — *Can an analgesia machine be used for resuscitation in emergencies?*

A — Yes. (See Chapter 7.)

Q — *How much of the effect obtained under relative analgesia is a result of autosuggestion?*

A—A very small but significant segment of the analgesic effect is due to autosuggestion. Once the patient has accepted the symptoms and sensations of analgesia, he enhances the effects by autosuggestion.

Q—*Does a patient usually feel more relaxed after dental treatment under analgesia?*

A—Yes. Additionally, most pretreatment headaches have been dissipated at the end of treatment. This happens because many headaches are caused by tension, and analgesia eliminates tension.

Q—*Does the high, wide-backed dental chair pose a problem in positioning of the nasal inhaler?*

A—Yes, but not an insurmountable one. Possible solutions include (a) double lengths of tubings leading to the nasal inhaler, (b) a nasal inhaler with one central overhead tubing, and (c) a slit in back of dental chair. (See Chapter 7.)

Q—*Do children take the same dose of nitrous oxide as adults?*

A—No sharp differentiation can be made between the dose for a child and that for an adult. The tonsillar or adenoidal tissue of a child may be such that he is forced to inhale through the mouth a great deal. In that event, the gas machine may have to produce a dose that would be high even for the average adult in order to obtain the proper effect. The operator works from the patient to the machine; that is, the gas machine is not preset, but rather it is adjusted for the dosage that will give the desired analgesic level, whether the subject is an adult or a child.

Q—*Is the odor of the nasal inhaler objectionable?*

A—Rarely. To overcome any possible objection and to enhance the psychological effect, a pleasant smelling volatile oil is added to the alcohol solution with which the nasal inhaler is cleaned.

Q—*Do patients complain of having their hairdos disturbed?*

A—Sometimes. However, if the complainant is one whose fear of the dental experience has been eliminated by the use of analgesia, he or she will realize that this is indeed a small price to pay.

Q—*What precautions should be taken for the occasional nauseated patient?*

A—1. Instruct the patient to abstain from food for two to three hours before treatment.

2. Prescribe a drug to control the nausea.
3. Change the time of treatment from the morning to the afternoon, or vice versa.
4. Close the air valve to eliminate atmospheric air from the gas delivered.
5. Oxygenate longer than usual.
6. Use a high proportion of oxygen during administration.
7. Check to see whether the nitrous oxide cylinder is almost empty.

Note: A single occurrence of nausea in a patient does not call for any alteration in procedure. However, when there is a second occurrence in the same individual or a history of propensity to nausea, then one or more of the above modifications of treatment should be followed.

Q — *May patients experience erotic dreams under analgesia?*

A — This is possible, but rare. For this reason, a third party should always be present during the administration.

Q — *Are there any medications which would contraindicate the use of nitrous oxide analgesia?*

A — No.

Q — *Should dental treatment be undertaken during the first administration of analgesia?*

A — As a general rule, no work should be performed during the introductory administration of analgesia. The patient has his fears of the procedure and the resultant sensations to contend with. Superimposing dental treatment might result in an unsuccessful introduction. For most subjects, attaining the lightest plane of analgesia is more than enough for the first administration. Moreover, in this plane, very little pain would be obtunded. At the succeeding sitting, more nitrous oxide will be acceptable because fear is absent. As the operator gains experience in analgesia administration and in evaluating patient reactions in the chair, he or she may perform dentistry during the initial exposure when conditions are deemed favorable.

Q — *When is the exhaling valve closed?*

A — When rebreathing is desired. (See Chapter 7.)

Q — *What is the purpose of history taking prior to the introduction of analgesia?*

A — From the history the dentist learns all the important facts relative to the patient's physical and emotional status, past relationship with dentists, likes and dislikes, anxieties and fears. On the basis of this information, he or she can suggest the use of analgesia to the patient, explaining how it will solve his particular problems.

Q — *How is analgesia introduced to a patient of long standing?*

A — The fears, phobias, medical history, and reactions to dental treatment of a patient of long standing are an open book. One has only to explain how analgesia will solve his particular problems. To the question "Why was this not used on me before?" the answer could be: "I have learned how to use this instrument and, having seen how valuable and effective it is, I decided to offer the benefits of its use to my patients."

Q — *Can analgesia be safely administered during pregnancy?*

A — Yes. (See the discussion of indications for the use of relative analgesia in Chapter 7.)

Q — *What is the role of the dental assistant or secretary in analgesia administration?*

A — The secretary or assistant is very often the first individual to come into contact with the patient. It is therefore highly important that he or she experience the effects of analgesia, for the assistant can then in his or her own words effectively act as a missionary, giving the patient initial encouragement and an authentic explanation of the symptoms and benefits of analgesia. Auxiliary personnel can also be of great assistance with the recalcitrant child or fearful adult.

Q — *When a patient under analgesia winces, how can you ascertain whether he is experiencing pain?*

A — Ask him directly, or give him a direction to open wider or turn his head. If there is a ready response to your question or direction, the analgesic level is too shallow and the patient is experiencing pain. Lack of response signifies the opposite effect (the patient is approaching or is in plane 3).

Q — *When treating handicapped children under analgesia a mouth prop must sometimes be used. What signs other than mouth closure can be used as guidelines to the depth of analgesia?*

A — 1. The expression in the eyes. Excessive analgesic depth will change the relaxed, dreamy look to a vacant stare or a hard, angry look.
2. The response to a verbal direction. If the depth is too great, the patient

will not respond to directions such as "Give me your hand," "Hold this cup," "Turn your head toward me," or "Sit up straight."

3. The rapidity of winking. In the analgesic state the rate of winking slows.

Q—*What proportion of the population is amenable to treatment with relative analgesia?*

A—With proper initial conditioning, 98 per cent of those applying for dental treatment can become good analgesia patients.

Q—*How much time does it take to introduce analgesia to a patient?*

A—Between 5 and 10 minutes.

Q—*How long does it take to integrate analgesia into a dental practice?*

A—This varies with the dentist's approach to the use of this modality. The practitioner who starts using analgesia by attempting to introduce it to every patient in his (or her) practice will find himself applying it maximally within one year. Some dentists start with the thought that they will use analgesia only for those patients that they feel really need it. As a result they will not use it for more than 25 to 50 per cent of their patients. But it is almost impossible to decide who does and who does not need analgesia, for the outwardly stoical type of individual may be in need of relative analgesia more than the obviously fearful type. The fact that a patient does not cry out, wince, or cringe does not necessarily imply that he is indifferent to the experience.

Q—*Why is the introductory administration of analgesia so critical?*

A—The successful use of relative analgesia is predicated on the fact that the most important reason for using it is the elimination of fear of the dental experience. The patient who is afraid of undergoing dental treatment may be no less afraid of analgesia. Additionally, the individual who is most afraid of analgesia needs the services of such an instrument more than anyone else. If the fear of the instrument is not eliminated at the first administration, the dentist will rarely be given a second opportunity to attempt its use.

Q—*What is the importance of the word "may" when describing and predicting symptoms to a new analgesia patient?*

A—No individual ever experiences all the possible symptoms of the analgesic stage. If the operator, when enumerating these symptoms, says, "You *will* feel them," the patient infers that he should experience every one of them. When this fails to materialize, he may become fearful and begin to think that he is not reacting properly. It must be explained that these are sensations which he *may* experience, but that he will not feel all of them.

Q— *Should the patient always be reassured that he will not go to sleep?*

A— No. The patient does not always fear going to sleep. Indeed, fear may be aroused by this information, since the emphasis placed on it creates fear where none existed. The question of falling asleep should be raised by the dentist only when he feels that his patient is concerned about it or when the patient himself raises the question.

Q— *Should the safety of the procedure be stressed?*

A— The safety of the administration of relative analgesia should never be mentioned by the dentist unless the question is first raised by the patient. Then, and only then, should reassurance as to its safety be forthcoming.

Q— *What is the differential between the alveolar concentration of nitrous oxide necessary to induce analgesia and that necessary to induce anesthesia?*

A— Analgesia is induced at 10 to 50 per cent nitrous oxide by volume in the lung alveoli, whereas anesthesia is induced at 80 per cent nitrous oxide by volume in the lung alveoli.

Q— *Aside from tooth reduction, what are some of the causes of pain and discomfort to the patient in the dental chair?*

A— 1. Injections.
    2. Gagging because of the manipulation of instruments, the spray of water, impression taking, and the taking of roentgenograms.
    3. The noises of instruments, drill, etc.
    4. The sight of instruments, blood, etc.
    5. Long appointments.
    6. The fitting of restorations.

Q— *Should the nasal inhaler be pressed tightly against the face to exclude air?*

A— The nasal inhaler should *never* be pressed tightly against the face by the operator. Since the analgesia patient is conscious, it is not good procedure from a psychological viewpoint. It creates fear as well as discomfort. The nasal inhaler should be secured snugly without creating any discomfort. If a choice has to be made between some air leakage and the patient's comfort, then comfort should be paramount in importance. The diluent effects of the air leak can be compensated for by increasing the nitrous oxide flow from the machine.

Q — During the introductory administration, what is the significance of asking the patient "What do you feel?" as opposed to "How do you feel?"

A — During the introductory administration, the patient should never be asked *how* he feels. This question may initiate a form of self-analysis that could be destructive. He does feel different from normal when he is beginning to experience the sensations induced by analgesia, and this difference may be somewhat upsetting and frightening initially. The question "How do you feel?" is therefore usually answered by "Not so well," "Funny," and so forth. On the other hand, asking him *what* he feels calls for nothing but an enumeration of symptoms without adverse or unpleasant connotations.

Q — Should the flow of nitrous oxide be increased slowly at each administration?

A — The flow of nitrous oxide should and must be increased very slowly at the introductory administration to ensure success. Thereafter this slow approach is unnecessary. The dosage is estimated and the flow of nitrous oxide is set immediately to that point.

Q — How can the operator judge the depth of analgesia?

A — With a little experience the operator can judge the signs of analgesia. He will also "sense" how deep in analgesia his patient is by the way the muscles of the lips and cheeks react to his manipulations. These are some of the criteria:
   1. Maintenance of an open mouth by the patient (proper depth).
   2. Frequent closing of the mouth (proper depth, but decrease nitrous oxide).
   3. Calm, dreamy look in the eyes (proper depth).
   4. Hard, angry stare (too deep).
   5. Rapidity and lucidity of response to a question (too light).
   6. Response to a direction (proper depth).
   7. Failure to respond to a direction (too deep or proper depth if mouth is open).
   8. Strong reaction to tooth reduction (too light or approaching stage 2).
   9. Contraction of the orbicularis oris and masseter muscles (too light).
   10. Position of the patient's hands: clenched fist (too light); natural position (proper depth); hands falling off lap (proper depth if mouth is open).

11. Moderate activation of the gag reflex: (if the patient is a gagger: too light; if he is an extreme gagger: proper depth).
12. Frequent wincing signs: (if the patient responds to a query: too light; if he does not respond: too deep).

Q—*Is the dosage constant for each patient?*

A—No. Since analgesia has both a psychological and a physiological effect, the dosage for an individual patient will vary from visit to visit not only because of the strength of painful stimulus, but also because of the patient's emotional state at a given time (and the degree of nasal, as opposed to oral, inhalation).

Q—*Do large or obese patients need more nitrous oxide than others?*

A—Not necessarily. An obese person who breathes only through his nose requires a smaller volume of nitrous oxide than a slimmer individual who frequently inhales through the mouth. In like manner, a child who inspires orally needs a greater flow of nitrous oxide than the average adult.

Q—*Should less than 20 per cent oxygen ever be administered?*

A—Never should less than the metabolic requirement for oxygen (20 per cent) be used. To increase the depth of analgesia, more nitrous oxide may be administered but not beyond this proportional limitation.

Q—*Why is an open air valve unnecessary with an intermittent flow machine?*

A—The flowmeters on an intermittent flow machine are so constructed that a change in nitrous oxide flow automatically changes the oxygen flow. For relative analgesia, less than 50 per cent nitrous oxide is almost always administered with these machines. This automatically means that the concentration of oxygen is always more than 50 per cent. An open air valve may be employed for dilution effects, but it is not a necessity, since so much oxygen is being delivered. In addition, one does not have to admix air for greater volumetric flow, for this type of machine is a demand gas machine; that is, it provides any volume of gas required by the patient.

Q—*Does relative analgesia completely eliminate the gag reflex?*

A—Relative analgesia does not always completely eliminate the gag reflex. If an extreme gagger is being treated, he will gag moderately but he will not forcibly remove the impression tray or roentgenographic film. All degrees of gagging less than extreme are completely controlled under relative analgesia.

Q — *Why is the frequent use of premedication disadvantageous in the administration of relative analgesia?*

A — It is not necessary, and it creates a situation that makes the use of this modality more cumbersome and less practical. The special preparation required by premedication interferes with appointment making, and it often necessitates the patient's being accompanied by someone.

Q — *Is the recording of dosage for each administration necessary?*

A — When initiating the use of relative analgesia, it is helpful to keep a record of dosage for each patient. Even though the requirements of any one individual will vary from visit to visit, the keeping of records will afford a knowledge of the range within which most patients respond with a given machine. This procedure may be discarded after three months of experience.

Q — *Does perspiring under relative analgesia have any clinical significance?*

A — No. Nitrous oxide has a vasomotor effect that induces this reaction in some individuals. Unless it is excessive and makes the patient uncomfortable afterwards, it may be disregarded.

Q — *Why do some patients cry under relative analgesia?*

A — Their thoughts stray to some sad event in their lives. One would prefer happy thoughts, and these can be suggested as the patient goes into the analgesic state. The act of crying does point up one of the most valuable potentials of this modality: that of making the patient's thoughts wander beyond the dental treatment room and away from the dentist's manipulations.

Q — *How deep in analgesia is the patient who repeatedly closes his mouth?*

A — Repeated closure of the mouth calls for a decrease in nitrous oxide only because it becomes difficult for the operator to work properly and with dispatch. However, the patient is still in plane 2 of the maintained analgesic state.

Q — *What is the significance of a rigid mandible?*

A — In the planes of relative analgesia, the mandible is relaxed. A rigid mandible signifies the passing into plane 3 (total analgesia) of the maintained analgesic stage. It calls for a decrease in the flow of nitrous oxide.

Q—*What is the significance of a hard, angry look in the eyes?*

A—In the planes of relative analgesia the eyes assume a faraway, dreamy look. A hard, angry look means that the patient is in the stage of total analgesia, approaching the excitement stage. Decrease the flow of nitrous oxide.

Q—*How can unpleasant dreams and nightmares be forestalled?*

A—Unpleasant dreams and nightmares occur rarely, and then only when the patient is new to analgesia. They can be obviated by suggesting to the patient that he think of something pleasant as he goes into the analgesic state.

Q—*What effect does analgesia have on salivary output?*

A—Relative analgesia has no direct effect on salivary output; however, it does minimize the sudden increased secretion of saliva sometimes occasioned by pain. Additionally, the lessened activity of the tongue minimizes flooding of areas that the dentist wishes to keep dry.

Q—*Can nitrous oxide cylinders be inadvertently interchanged with oxygen cylinders?*

A—The Pin-Index Safety System and the Diameter-Index Safety System make it impossible to interchange a nitrous oxide cylinder with an oxygen cylinder. Each will fit only into its proper receptacle.

Q—*Why should grease or oil never be used on valves, gauges, machines, and so forth?*

A—Under pressure, both oxygen and nitrous oxide can form an explosive mixture in the presence of grease or oil. At high pressures their oxidizing properties are enhanced, and grease, oil, and other organic materials may oxidize with explosive speed and melt contacting metal.

Q—*What is the function of the regulator?*

A—The regulator maintains a constant gas pressure to the machine. This allows a constant flowmeter reading for any fixed setting of the flow control valve of the machine, regardless of the gas pressure in the cylinder. It also permits a more accurate adjustment of the flow control valve of the machine, since at a consistent, relatively low pressure (as compared with cylinder pressure) the valve can be turned through a relatively large turn to achieve a small change in flowmeter reading. The use of constant, relatively low pressure throughout the system precludes the possibility of a dangerous pressure build-up that could cause damage to the machine.

Q—What is the function of the pressure gauge?

A—The pressure gauge shows the pressure of the gas in the cylinder. The pressure gauge on an oxygen cylinder shows an even decrease in pressure proportionate to the volume of oxygen that has flowed from the cylinder. In contrast, since nitrous oxide is liquefied, the pressure gauge on a nitrous oxide cylinder shows an uneven decrease in pressure, for so long as sufficient liquid is present to exert pressure the gauge remains constant. Then when the liquid contents have been largely consumed, the indicator drops suddenly from its maximum reading.

Q—Is nitrous oxide eliminated solely through the lungs?

A—Nearly all of the nitrous oxide inhaled is eliminated unchanged through the lungs. A tiny fraction remains in the body for a longer period of time and is later excreted through the skin and sweat glands, in the urine, and as bowel gas.

Q—Is blood pressure or cardiac rate or output altered in the maintained analgesic stage?

A—No.

Q—How is it possible to have a conscious patient who does not feel pain?

A—Anesthetic drugs have a selectivity for the neural mechanisms subserving pain perception at dosages that may leave other perceptions relatively unaffected.

Q—How is general anesthesia produced?

A—The mechanism by which general anesthesia is produced is still unknown. Within the general theory of narcosis there are about 25 sub-theories that attempt to explain the cellular mechanisms involved.

Q—Why is the stage of relative analgesia much more effective than general anesthesia in eliminating fear of the dental experience?

A — Clinical experience has amply demonstrated that the use of general anesthesia for dental treatment, although a necessary approach in some cases, does not have a long-term effect on the patient's fear of future treatment. To be free of fear, the patient must be sufficiently aware (during and after treatment) that he has been subjected to dental treatment but that he was *not fearful at the time.* This seems to be a necessary prerequisite for favorable future conditioning. In the stage of relative analgesia, the subject is sufficiently aware and has no fear.

Q — *Why do local anesthetic injections result in complete local anesthesia more often when administered under relative analgesia?*

A — Because of the proper cooperation of the patient in the control of his musculature, the injection can be made more accurately. A patient without fear does not translate sound, pressure, or vibratory sensations into pain sensations. The relaxation and freedom from fear induced by analgesia prevent an overstimulated circulation from dissipating the effects of the local anesthetic solution too rapidly.

Q — *Why is the use of relative analgesia such an effective practice builder?*

A — The use of relative analgesia is a highly effective practice builder (and modifier) because it eliminates fear of the dental experience. This effectiveness emphasizes the fact that a great proportion of the population still fears dental treatment and consequently avoids it.

Q — *How can one prevent the formation of the facial pressure marks sometimes caused by the nasal inhaler?*

A — 1. By using small pieces of tissue paper or gauze under the lateral flanges of the nasal inhaler.
2. By using a nasal inhaler of a different size.
3. By using a nasal inhaler of lighter weight and softer rubber.

Q — *Why is a knowledge of psychology of practical importance to the dentist who administers relative analgesia?*

A — A knowledge of human behavior enables the operator (a) to accurately judge the type of individual with whom he or she is dealing, (b) to interest the patient more successfully in the idea of becoming an analgesia patient, (c) to properly condition him during the introductory administration, and (d) to evaluate more correctly the patient's reactions to the administration of relative analgesia.

Q — *Do the mood and attitude of the dentist affect the success of an analgesia administration?*

A — Yes. Even an experienced analgesia patient will sense that the dentist is curt, short, impatient, or angry, and hence will fail to relax in his usual and customary manner.

Q — *Should the parent of a child-patient under analgesia be invited into the dental treatment room?*

A — If neither the child nor the parent requests it, the dentist should not ask for the parent's presence in the dental treatment room. This is permitted only upon the request of the child or the parent and only with the express understanding that the parent refrain from all conversation with the child or doctor during the treatment period.

Q — *How does relative analgesia differ from total analgesia?*

A — In dental practice the term "analgesia" has been used with different connotations for over half a century. In one sense, this term has been used to indicate a patient in or near the state of total analgesia, a level that is near the excitement stage. An inexperienced operator would find it extremely difficult to maintain the patient at this level. Although not completely in general anesthesia, the subject is not conscious enough to follow directions, and the line of demarcation between analgesia and excitement or light anesthesia is very thin and unpredictable. In attempting to maintain this level of analgesia, most dental practitioners would find themselves confronted with a semiconscious patient constantly teetering between consciousness and unconsciousness and rarely able to cooperate with the operator.

In contrast, with the administration of relative analgesia, the operator is in control of an entirely different situation. The patient is conscious and cooperative, and there is no fine, critical line which can be crossed over easily and inadvertently to produce the symptoms of the excitement stage or general anesthesia.

Q — *How may the dentist determine when the patient is ready for treatment?*

A — This presents no problem when treating a patient who has had long exposure to analgesia. The patient himself can tell the operator when he is ready, or the operator can judge by the relaxed appearance of the patient's body, hands, or eyes. A patient new to analgesia may be asked simply, "Are you ready?" or "Do you feel it?"

A dentist relatively inexperienced in the administration of analgesia tends to wait for distinct symptoms to appear, such as tingling in the extremities or lips. This is not a good criterion, for it must be remembered that the patient is aware of these symptoms as discrete entities only in the lightest plane of analgesia. As he goes deeper into the analgesic state, all the sensations fuse so that he is no longer aware of individual symptoms—they have all merged into one overall state. It could be said, therefore, that the patient's awareness of distinct, individual symptoms denotes a light plane of analgesia. When he enters into a deeper plane he is usually ready for treatment.

Q—Can the trace gases of nitrous oxide in the dental operatory have any effect on the dentist and ancillary personnel?

A—The question of *possible* effects on the health of dental office personnel who have repeated exposure to trace quantities of anesthetic gases has been raised because there have been a succession of reports in the medical literature over the past few years *circumstantially* implicating a variety of inhalation agents (including nitrous oxide) as a possible cause of occupational disorders in operating room personnel.[4] These difficulties range from headache, fatigue, depression, and irritability at one end of the scale to a series of problems including teratogenicity and fetal mortality at the other end. Although *no direct cause and effect relationship* has been demonstrated in any of these reports, documentary evidence abounds which is fortified conceptually and by implication from positive results in some animal studies.

The results of many medical studies in anesthesiology are not usually readily transmissible to the dental situation. However, in this case, since nitrous oxide is discharged in the atmosphere during inhalation sedation at the same rate as in the open and semi-open techniques employed in medicine, all the results of the medical reports are applicable to dentistry.

According to the 20 or 30 reports and references in the medical literature, the nitrous oxide escapes into the atmosphere in varying amounts around the room. Thus, it may enter the tissues of the treatment room personnel in direct proportion to the concentration at their locale. It should again be stressed that this is a *potential* problem. A continued awareness that it is possible is necessary. The problem should neither be magnified nor minimized where *potential* harm is concerned, until further investigation either proves or disproves the present speculative findings.

Even though there is *no direct and clear evidence* in humans of teratogenicity or of the relationship to spontaneous abortion, dental personnel who are in the first trimester of pregnancy should be forewarned of the potential problem so that they can act, if they so desire, to avoid unnecessary exposure. It must be fully understood that the risk may be real or unreal, remaining to be proved by later studies.

Attention should be given to the ventilation of the operatory so that maximum circulation and venting to the outside may be achieved, together with a minimum of recirculation.

Of one thing we can be certain: The utilization of nitrous oxide will not cease, because the inventive genius of dentists and of others working with the dental profession will create technically feasible instruments designed to remove the nitrous oxide at or near its source, or at least to prevent its being inhaled and absorbed into the systemic circulation of the operating room personnel. As a matter of fact, manufacturers associated with the health professions, as well as government agencies, have begun to design equipment for scavenging trace gases in the operatory. We can be certain that there will be many such instruments offered to us for this purpose. With subsequent refinements, the problem of eliminating trace gases will be solved.

Several methods of waste gas scavenging in the dental treatment room are currently under investigation.[5] These include the use of individual fresh air breathing masks, the use of a controlled air flow pattern that rapidly evacuates the air in the immediate vicinity of the patient and dental personnel, and the use of an exhaust line attached to the exhalation part of the breathing circuit. Another possibility is breaking down the nitrous oxide into nitrogen and oxygen. Several of these methods are illustrated in Figures 10–66 to 10–71 (pages 363 to 373).

REFERENCES

1. Schmetz, S. L.: Nitrous oxide analgesia for the severely mentally retarded child. J. Am. Anal. Soc., 12:10–14, 1974.
2. Sesken, L. A.: Dentistry in the treatment of handicapped children. Bull. Dental Guidance Council for Cerebral Palsy, 11:2–10, 1971.
3. Harris, M. D.: Nitrous oxide analgesia in podiatric medicine. J. Nat. Anal. Soc., 2:15–18, 1973.
4. Driscoll, E. J.: Inhalation of anesthetic gases. J.A.D.A., 90:1260, 1975.
5. Cohen, E. N., et al: A survey of anesthetic health hazards among dentists. J.A.D.A., 90:1295, 1975.

Index